Saunders'

Q&A for the

REVIEW

PHYSICAL THERAPIST ASSISTANT BOARD EXAMINATION

Saunders'

Q&A for the

REVIEW

PHYSICAL THERAPIST ASSISTANT BOARD EXAMINATION

BRAD FORTINBERRY, PT, DPT
President
Fortinberry Physical Therapy
Director of Rehabilitation Services
St. Luke Home Health
McComb, Mississippi

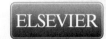

ELSEVIER
SAUNDERS

3251 Riverport Lane
St. Louis, Missouri 63043

Notices

Knowledge and best practice in this field are constantly changing. As new research and experience broaden our understanding, changes in research methods, professional practices, or medical treatment may become necessary.

Practitioners and researchers must always rely on their own experience and knowledge in evaluating and using any information, methods, compounds, or experiments described herein. In using such information or methods they should be mindful of their own safety and the safety of others, including parties for whom they have a professional responsibility.

With respect to any drug or pharmaceutical products identified, readers are advised to check the most current information provided (i) on procedures featured or (ii) by the manufacturer of each product to be administered, to verify the recommended dose or formula, the method and duration of administration, and contraindications. It is the responsibility of practitioners, relying on their own experience and knowledge of their patients, to make diagnoses, to determine dosages and the best treatment for each individual patient, and to take all appropriate safety precautions.

To the fullest extent of the law, neither the Publisher nor the authors, contributors, or editors, assume any liability for any injury and/or damage to persons or property as a matter of products liability, negligence or otherwise, or from any use or operation of any methods, products, instructions, or ideas contained in the material herein.

Vice President and Publisher: Linda Duncan
Content Strategist: Jolynn Gower
Senior Content Development Specialist: Christie M. Hart
Publishing Services Manager: Julie Eddy
Senior Project Manager: Celeste Clingan
Design Direction: Teresa McBryan

Working together
to grow libraries in
developing countries

www.elsevier.com • www.bookaid.org

Printed in the United States of America

Last digit is the print number: 9 8 7 6 5 4 3 2 1

Without the love and support of my wife, Melissa,
and the sacrifices of my children, Austin and Hayden,
this project would have never been possible.

Also, thanks to my parents, Bebo and Brenda,
who set me on the correct path many years ago.

Preface

The purpose of any exam preparation study guide is to help you find the area of weakness in your knowledge base. You should already have a vague idea of which topic in physical therapy has challenged you in the past. It is not important that you memorize answers to the questions included in this book, only that you understand how to prepare and pass the exam. Careful study of this book and its associated companion website (EVOLVE) will allow you to tackle these different areas.

This book does not attempt to take the place of the vast array of knowledge gained in course work and clinical rotations, nor should this preparation tool be used to cram for hours before taking the exam. Instead this text and accompanying online material should be used to simulate actual exam scenarios and find faults in your knowledge base. For this reason, we have divided this book into 4 sections:

CHAPTER 1 Data Collection
CHAPTER 2: Diseases and Conditions
CHAPTER 3: Interventions
CHAPTER 4: Non-System Topics

Each section has a wide variety of scenarios, diagnoses, patient populations, practice settings, and types of questions designed to help you prepare for the national examination. References were selected primarily from sources and textbooks familiar to physical therapist assistant programs across the country.

Examination Preparation

Remember, it is not as important that you get questions right or wrong when practicing, but that you understand how to prepare yourself for the exam and your career as a physical therapist assistant. You should consider several factors in preparing for the exam. First and foremost, you should consider the actual material on the test. Your knowledge in the varied subject areas of physical therapy will be tested. Although cramming for this sort of comprehensive exam is usually futile, you may prefer to study in that fashion. Previous coursework, clinical studies, peer-group study sessions, and observing experienced PTAs over the years is what prepares you for this type of national exam.

The practice exams should be administered in the same environment as the actual national exam. Rooms should be quiet and at a comfortable temperature. Limit interruptions for the duration of your simulated examination. The online material included in this book is an excellent source for practice exams. It will randomly select questions to create a practice test. Each practice test will have roughly the same percentage of questions in each of the sections as the actual exam. If you are using the actual text for your practice, block off enough time and treat the text as if it were an actual computerized test.

In the final weeks prior to the exam, concentrate study on those areas in which you have found yourself to be weak. Cramming huge amounts of facts only increases your level of anxiety. Establish a routine of sleeping, eating, and exercise before the exam. If your routine is the same day in and day out, your anxiety level will be decreased at exam time.

Familiarize yourself with the testing center. It may be a good idea to map your route to the testing center in the days before the exam. This would give you time to find alternate routes for road construction or poor weather. Make sure you have complied with your state's testing requirements. Do you have the proper identification? Do you have all the correct paperwork from your state PT association or school? Have you paid all appropriate fees? Also check with the testing center for specific rules such as: Will there be a lunch break? Can I bring lunch into the testing center? Will lockers be provided? Will scratch paper be provided?

Taking the Exam

RELAX!!! The exam allows ample time for completion, so do not get nervous about time in the first portions. The exam is computerized, so read all directions and familiarize yourself with all controls before beginning. Read each question carefully and slowly. Each question or stem will be followed by four choices. There will be one correct answer and three distracters or incorrect answers to each question. Remember that you are required to choose the correct or best answer for each question. There may seem to be more than one correct answer, but look for the most correct one for the question provided.

Bring appropriate supplies to the exam, such as pencils and erasers. Consider ear plugs if you are distracted by noise. Ask the exam center if they will provide such items in advance.

Most computerized exams offer a tutorial of the computerized controls used in the exam. Even if you feel you are very computer literate, it is still advisable to take this opportunity to familiarize yourself with the specific controls for the test. The tutorials do not usually count into your actual exam time.

Be cognizant of what exactly the question is asking. Some of the distracters are designed to lead you into an incorrect answer. Reread the stem along with each choice, if necessary, before deciding upon an answer. Determine what part of the therapy process the question is referring. For example, is the question asking you about examination, intervention, plan, or goals? Also pay attention to words related to timing of a particular action, like initial, first, next, or last step.

Answer all questions even if you have no idea of the correct answer. Unmarked and incorrect questions equally count against the tested student. Narrow the distracters to the best of your ability and guess at the answer if necessary. If applicable, skip the question and come back if you have time. Sometimes questions early in the exam can seem unfamiliar to you, but a question later can jog your memory and help you answer earlier questions.

It is certainly normal to feel a little nervous before taking on the exam. Control your emotions and breathing rate before you begin the actual test. If allowable, take a break during the exam just to clear your head and refocus your thoughts.

After the Exam

Allow some time to decompress after you leave the testing area. Most people are mentally exhausted after such an expansive test. Consider a good meal and some relaxation time for the evening after the exam. Also, plan something fun for the next day to take your mind off of the test.

It is imperative that you do not discuss the specifics after completing the exam. The organization that manages the national exam, the Federation of State Boards of Physical Therapy (FSBPT), is very explicit in their desire to stop students from discussing questions after the test. If you are found to have circulated actual test items, you could face disciplinary action from the FSBPT, such as voiding of your test score and an inability to retake the exam.

We wish you the best of luck as you prepare for the exam. This is an important step to launch a long and successful career as a physical therapist assistant.

Brad Fortinberry, PT, DPT

Contents

CHAPTER 1

Data Collection

Questions

1. What type of cartilage is normally found on joint surfaces?
   a. Hyaline cartilage
   b. Fibrocartilage
   c. Elastic
   d. Fibroelastic

2. Which of the following is a grade II muscle strain?
   a. Moderate tearing of muscle fibers, with some strength loss but without complete tearing of the muscle
   b. Tearing of a few muscle fibers without strength loss
   c. Complete tearing of the muscle with complete strength loss
   d. Complete tearing of the muscle but with preserved strength

3. A hard callus is formed in what phase of bone healing?
   a. Hemostasis
   b. Inflammatory phase
   c. Reparative phase
   d. Remodeling phase

4. At what age is the knee meniscus the most vascular?
   a. Birth
   b. 10 years old
   c. 20 years old
   d. 40 years old

5. Articular cartilage can be described as:
   a. Containing few cells
   b. Having a large neural network
   c. Having a large vascular network
   d. Being a high-friction surface

6. Which of the following is a normal response by articular cartilage to the aging process?
   a. Proteoglycan aggregation is increased.
   b. Chondroitin sulfate content is reduced.

    c. Hydrophilic proteoglycans increase their ability to hold water.

    d. Larger proteoglycans are synthesized with an increase in keratin sulfate content.

7. Which of the following is NOT a primary influence for bone remodeling?
    a. Mechanical stresses
    b. Neurologic stresses
    c. Calcium and phosphate levels
    d. Hormonal levels

8. Which of the following types of bone fractures is unique to children?
    a. Greenstick fracture
    b. Compression fracture
    c. Avulsion fracture
    d. Physeal plate fracture

9. Fatigue-resistant type I muscle fibers demonstrate which of the following attributes?
    a. They have a high capillary content.
    b. They are referred to as fast oxidative fibers.
    c. They are white in color.
    d. They fatigue rapidly.

10. Which of the following is NOT a common gait deviation seen with children who have Down syndrome?
    a. Long step length
    b. Decreased knee flexion at heel contact
    c. Hyperextension in stance
    d. Increased hip extension at push off

11. The PTA is using a scoliometer to screen for scoliosis in adolescent patients. What is the minimal degree of deviation from 0 that warrants further medical evaluation?
    a. 3 degrees
    b. 5 degrees
    c. 10 degrees
    d. 12 degrees

12. An infant has a myelomeningocele at level L4 to L5. Which of the following muscles would most likely have normal function in this individual?
    a. Tibialis anterior
    b. Gluteus medius
    c. Peroneus brevis
    d. Iliopsoas

13. An individual with a right torticollis will present with which of the following?
    a. Left side bending and left rotation
    b. Right side bending and right rotation
    c. Left side bending and right rotation
    d. Right side bending and left rotation

14. Which of the following groups of individuals are most likely to have the highest bone mass?
    a. Males 15 to 20 years old
    b. Females 15 to 20 years old
    c. Males 30 to 35 years old
    d. Females 35 to 40 years old

15. A patient reports to physical therapy and states that her bone mineral density testing T-score is −0.8. What is the correct interpretation of this datum?
    a. This is a normal score with low risk for fracture.
    b. This patient has a high risk for fracture.
    c. This patient should be classified with osteopenia.
    d. The patient should be classified with osteoporosis.

16. Which of the following is NOT a part of the axial skeleton?
    a. Cranium
    b. Femur
    c. Ribs
    d. Pelvis

17. You begin manual muscle testing on a client with osteoporosis. Which of the following muscles would you expect to be the weakest?
    a. Biceps brachii
    b. Pectoralis major
    c. Semitendinosus
    d. Quadriceps femoris

18. Which of the following statements best describes a person's base of support?
    a. The type of surface one is standing on
    b. The area, projected on the ground, of the broadest/widest part of the body
    c. The area of the body in contact with the supporting surface
    d. The feet

19. Static posture may be assessed during which activity?
    a. Sitting
    b. Walking
    c. Pushing
    d. Moving from sit to stand

20. The zero position for measuring joint range of motion for most joints is based on which of the following?
    a. Ideal alignment
    b. Anatomic position
    c. American Academy of Orthopedics standards
    d. The sagittal plane

21. Which of the following characterizes swayback posture?
    a. Anterior pelvic tilt and increased lumbar lordosis
    b. Posterior pelvic tilt and increased lumbar lordosis
    c. Anterior pelvic tilt and decreased lumbar lordosis
    d. Posterior pelvic tilt and decreased lumbar lordosis

22. During postural assessment, all of the following should be in vertical alignment EXCEPT which?
    a. External auditory meatus and greater trochanter of the hip
    b. External auditory meatus and acromion
    c. Occiput and sacrum
    d. Anterior-superior iliac spine and greater trochanter of the hip

23. Rotation is described by which of the following statements?
    a. Turning about a longitudinal axis
    b. Sliding motion usually of a flat or slightly curved surface relative to another surface
    c. Upward and downward gliding of the scapulae
    d. Anterior and posterior movements at the sternoclavicular joint

24. What is an accurate description of flexion at the lumbar spine?
    a. Increasing lordosis
    b. Decreasing lordosis
    c. Decreasing kyphosis
    d. Right rotation

25. Which of the following describes a posterior pelvic tilt?
    a. Upward movement of the anterior-superior iliac spine (ASIS), downward movement of the posterior-superior iliac spine (PSIS), and lumbar extension
    b. Downward movement of the ASIS, upward movement of the PSIS, and lumbar extension
    c. Upward movement of the ASIS, downward movement of the PSIS, and lumbar flexion
    d. Downward movement of the ASIS, upward movement of the PSIS, and lumbar flexion

26. Where is a muscle strain on the biceps brachii most likely to occur?
    a. Midpoint of the muscle belly
    b. Musculotendinous junction

c. Coracoid process of the scapula

d. Radial tuberosity

27. In the outpatient setting, you are asked by the supervising physical therapist to assess a patient with complete active range of motion against gravity of the knee. He can also tolerate minimal resistance and has full passive range of motion. What is his appropriate manual muscle testing grade?

a. 2/5

b. 4/5

c. 2+/5

d. 3+/5

28. What is the fastest, most efficient way to assess muscle strength in the clinical setting?

a. Hand-held dynamometer

b. Isokinetic testing

c. Functional testing

d. Manual muscle testing

29. In patients with spondyloarthropathies, Schober's test measures which of the following?

a. Intrinsic tightness

b. Spinal mobility

c. Ulnar drift

d. Hip mobility

30. The unique purpose of combining sequences of movement during a range-of-motion (ROM) assessment is to do which of the following?

a. Determine the presence of hypomobility

b. Determine the presence of hypermobility

c. More closely approximate functional movements that are problematic to the patient

d. Avoid nerve root irritation during the examination

31. A mechanical provocation test in which symptom relief indicates the presence of foraminal encroachment is called which of the following?

a. Cervical compression

b. Cervical distraction

c. Spurling's test

d. Quadrant test

32. The C5 nerve root can be tested with what upper extremity reflex?

a. Biceps

b. Brachioradialis

c. Triceps

d. Radial

33. Which of the following are bones that develop in tendons and areas where tendons cross the ends of long bones?
    a. Irregularly shaped bones
    b. Sesamoid bones
    c. Accessory bones
    d. Heterotopic bones

34. Which of the following defines an avulsion fracture?
    a. A fracture that runs parallel to the bone
    b. A fracture in which one fragment of the bone is driven into another
    c. A fracture caused by repeated low-force trauma
    d. A fracture caused by sudden muscular contraction wherein the ligament pulls away from the bone

35. The PTA intends to use a circumferential measurement of the involved knee to assess the edema at the suprapatellar pouch. Where should this measurement be obtained on the involved lower extremity?
    a. 20 cm proximal to the joint line
    b. 10 cm proximal to the joint line
    c. At the joint line
    d. 15 cm distal to the joint line

36. What is the phase of the gait cycle encompassing initial double support and involving approximation of the foot to the supporting surface?
    a. Initial contact
    b. Loading response
    c. Midstance
    d. Preswing

37. During normal gait, the period of double support encompasses what percentage of the gait cycle?
    a. 10%
    b. 20%
    c. 40%
    d. 60%

38. What period in the gait cycle is likely to increase when there is bilateral lower extremity weakness?
    a. Double support
    b. Acceleration
    c. Midswing
    d. Deceleration

39. Which of the following is NOT a critical functional task for successful walking?
    a. Acceptance of weight by the supporting limb
    b. Forward flexion of the trunk at initial contact

    c. A period of single limb support

    d. Advancement of the limb

40. The hamstrings do NOT perform which of the following functions during gait?
    a. Stabilize the trunk at the initial contact phase of gait
    b. Decelerate the tibia during the terminal swing phase of gait
    c. Stabilize the knee during the stance phase of gait
    d. Stabilize the hip during midstance

41. The typical times spent in swing phase and stance phase in a gait cycle are which of the following?
    a. Swing phase 60% and stance phase 40%
    b. Swing phase 40% and stance phase 60%
    c. Swing phase 50% and stance phase 50%
    d. Swing phase 70% and stance phase 30%

42. Using Rancho Los Amigos gait terminology, what period of gait is defined as the period when the body's center of gravity moves anterior to the supporting limb until the opposite limb makes contact with the support surface?
    a. Initial contact
    b. Loading response
    c. Midstance
    d. Terminal stance

43. Which of the following would be the correct definition of step length?
    a. The distance between the point of initial contact of one extremity and the point of initial contact of the opposite extremity
    b. The distance between the point of initial contact of one extremity and the next point of initial contact of the same extremity
    c. The point of initial contact of one extremity and the point of terminal stance at the opposite extremity
    d. The point of initial contact of one extremity and the next point of terminal stance of the same extremity

44. At what point during the gait cycle is the knee in maximum flexion?
    a. Preswing
    b. Initial swing
    c. Terminal stance
    d. Initial contact

45. When are the ankle dorsiflexors the least active during the gait cycle?
    a. Initial swing
    b. Midswing
    c. Terminal swing
    d. Terminal stance

46. Which of the following conditions is an irritation of the fluid-filled sacs designed to decrease friction between structures in the body?
    a. Tendinopathy
    b. Nerve entrapment
    c. Fracture
    d. Bursitis

47. A sprain occurs when what structure is stressed?
    a. Tendon
    b. Ligaments
    c. Muscle
    d. Bone

48. Which of the following is the ability of the patient to voluntarily move a limb through an arc movement?
    a. Passive range of motion
    b. Manual muscle testing
    c. Active range of motion
    d. Gait

49. What type of tool is used to measure range of motion at a joint?
    a. Isokinetic dynamometer
    b. Goniometer
    c. Spirometer
    d. Barometer

50. Using the 0 to 5 manual muscle testing grade scale, what level of strength would a muscle receive if it were able to move the body segment to the complete range of motion with gravity eliminated?
    a. 0/5
    b. 2/5
    c. 3/5
    d. 4/5

51. What is the term for the property of joints that allows the joint surfaces to glide, roll, and spin on each other allowing increased range of motion?
    a. Accessory motion
    b. Primary motion
    c. Secondary motion
    d. Available motion

52. Which of the following tests objectively measures the flexibility of the hamstring muscles?
    a. Hamstring stretch
    b. 90/90 test
    c. 100/100 test
    d. Bending over to touch the toes from a standing position

53. Which of the following are standardized instruments that measure an individual's actual or perceived activity limitations?
    a. Goals
    b. Activities of daily living
    c. Interventions
    d. Outcome measures

54. Getting out of the bed, drinking from a cup, and putting on shoes are all examples of what?
    a. Outcome measures
    b. Activities of daily living
    c. Interventions
    c. Special tests

55. If a therapist uses palpation to assess the patient, what is the therapist doing?
    a. Assessing activities of daily living
    b. Touching the patient
    c. Taking an accurate history
    d. Consulting another health care professional

56. Which of the following is a test for shoulder impingement?
    a. Phalen's test
    b. Lachman's test
    c. Thomas' test
    d. Hawkins' test

57. During the opening of a patient's mouth, a palpable and audible click is discovered in the left temporomandibular joint. The physician informs the therapist that the patient has an anteriorly dislocated disk. What does this click most likely signify?
    a. The condyle is sliding anterior to obtain normal relationship with the disk.
    b. The condyle is sliding posterior to obtain normal relationship with the disk.
    c. The condyle is sliding anterior and losing normal relationship with the disk.
    d. The condyle is sliding posterior and losing normal relationship with the disk.

58. In what position should the PTA place the upper extremity to palpate the supraspinatus tendon?
    a. Full abduction, full flexion, and full external rotation
    b. Full abduction, full flexion, and full internal rotation
    c. Full adduction, full external rotation, and full extension
    d. Full adduction, full internal rotation, and full extension

59. A 17-year-old athlete has just received a posterior cruciate ligament reconstruction. The PTA is attempting to explain some of the characteristics of the posterior cruciate ligament. Which of the following is incorrect information?
   a. The posterior cruciate ligament prevents posterior translation of the tibia on the femur.
   b. Posterior bands of the posterior cruciate ligament are tightest in full knee extension.
   c. The posterior cruciate ligament is attached to the lateral meniscus and not to the medial meniscus.
   d. The posterior cruciate ligament helps with medial rotation of the tibia during full knee extension with open chain activities.

60. Components of lower extremity alignment that contribute to toe in include which of the following?
   a. Femoral retroversion
   b. Femoral anteversion
   c. Calcaneovalgus feet
   d. External tibial torsion

61. Which of the following patients is most likely to have osteophyte formation that leads to rotator cuff damage?
   a. 16-year-old baseball player
   b. 34-year-old factory worker
   c. 45-year-old tennis player
   d. 75-year-old sedentary individual

62. The cuboid bone is located just posterior to what structure?
   a. Base of the first metatarsal
   b. Head of the first metatarsal
   c. Medial cuneiform bone
   d. Tuberosity of the fifth metatarsal

63. The metacarpophalangeal joints are classified as what type of joint?
   a. Plane
   b. Hinge
   c. Condyloid
   d. Saddle

64. Which muscle would move the abducted (90-degree) arm anteriorly?
   a. Sternocostal head of the pectoralis major
   b. Clavicular head of the pectoralis major
   c. Inferior fibers of the serratus anterior
   d. Pectoralis minor

65. Which of the following structures does NOT pass through the foramen magnum of the occipital bone?
    a. Spinal cord
    b. Meninges
    c. Cranial nerve XII
    d. Vertebral artery

66. Contraction of which muscle produces extension of the head?
    a. Spinalis cervicis
    b. Longus capitis
    c. Longus colli
    d. Sternocleidomastoid

67. The nucleus pulposus is thickest in which region of the spine?
    a. Lumbar spine
    b. Inferior half of the thoracic spine
    c. Superior half of the thoracic spine
    d. Cervical spine

68. The speed of muscle contraction is a function of which of the following factors?
    a. Resting length of the muscle fiber
    b. Cross-sectional diameter of the muscle
    c. Creatine phosphate of the muscle
    d. Glycolytic capacity of the muscle

69. Which of the following describes the proper normal anatomy of the proximal carpal row, from lateral to medial?
    a. Capitate, lunate, triquetrum, pisiform
    b. Lunate, trapezium, capitate, hamate
    c. Scaphoid, lunate, triquetrum, pisiform
    d. Scaphoid, hamate, lunate, capitate

70. A physician notes a vertebral fracture on the radiograph of a patient involved in a car crash. The fractured vertebra has a bifid spinous process. Which of the following vertebrae is the most likely to be involved?
    a. 4th lumbar vertebra
    b. 5th cervical vertebra
    c. 12th thoracic vertebra
    d. 1st sacral vertebra

71. If the line of gravity is posterior to the hip joint in standing, on what does the body first rely to keep the trunk from moving into excessive lumbar extension?
    a. Iliopsoas muscle activity
    b. Abdominal muscle activity

   c. Anterior pelvic ligaments and the hip joint capsule
   d. Posterior pelvic ligaments and the hip joint capsule

72. What is the closed-packed position of the shoulder?
   a. Internal rotation and abduction
   b. External rotation and abduction
   c. Internal rotation and adduction
   d. External rotation and adduction

73. A patient with a diagnosis of a rotator cuff tear has just begun active range of motion. The PTA is strengthening the rotator cuff muscles to increase joint stability and oppose the superior shear of the deltoid. Which of the following rotator cuff muscles participates least in an opposing the superior shear force of the deltoid?
   a. Infraspinatus
   b. Subscapularis
   c. Teres minor
   d. Supraspinatus

74. What portion of the adult knee meniscus is vascularized?
   a. Outer edges
   b. Inner edges
   c. The entire meniscus is vascular
   d. The entire meniscus is avascular

75. At what age does a human have the greatest amount of fluid in the intervertebral disk?
   a. 1 year
   b. 4 years
   c. 7 years
   d. 10 years

76. Which of the following is NOT an example of a synarthrodial joint in the body?
   a. Coronal suture
   b. The fibrous joint between the shaft of the tibia and fibula
   c. Symphysis pubis
   d. Metacarpophalangeal

77. Observing a patient in a standing position, the PTA notes that an angulation deformity of the left knee causes it to be located medially in relation to the left hip and left foot. This condition is commonly referred to as which of the following?
   a. Genu varum
   b. Genu valgum
   c. Pes cavus
   d. None of the above

78. Which of the following is the most vulnerable position for dislocation of the hip?
    a. 30 degrees of hip extension, 30 degrees of hip adduction, and minimal internal rotation
    b. 30 degrees of hip flexion, 30 degrees of hip adduction, and minimal external rotation
    c. 30 degrees of hip flexion, 30 degrees of hip abduction, and minimal external rotation
    d. 30 degrees of hip extension, 30 degrees hip abduction, and minimal external rotation

79. A physician ordered a splint for a patient who should keep the thumb of the involved hand in abduction. A new graduate PTA is treating the patient and is confused about the difference between thumb flexion, extension, abduction, and adduction. Which of the following lists is correct?
    a. Extension is performed in a plane parallel to the palm of the hand, and abduction is performed in a plane perpendicular to the palm of the hand.
    b. Flexion is performed in a plane perpendicular to the palm of the hand, and adduction is performed in a plane parallel to the palm of the hand.
    c. Extension is performed in a plane perpendicular to the palm of the hand, and adduction is performed in a plane parallel to the palm of the hand.
    d. In referring to positions of the thumb, flexion and adduction are used synonymously, and extension and abduction are used synonymously.

80. Which of the following is NOT part of the triangular fibrocartilage complex of the wrist?
    a. Dorsal radioulnar ligament
    b. Ulnar collateral ligament
    c. Radial collateral ligament
    d. Ulnar articular cartilage

81. What is the normal low-end range for interincisal opening with a temporomandibular joint dysfunction patient?
    a. 50 mm
    b. 30 mm
    c. 40 mm
    d. 60 mm

82. The PTA is analyzing a patient's gait with descending stairs. During left single-limb stance, the patient demonstrates a right pelvic drop with left trunk lean. What is the physical therapy hypothesis in this case?
    a. Weak right gluteus medius with left trunk lean to move center of mass toward stronger side
    b. Weak left gluteus medius with left trunk lean to move center of mass toward weaker side

    c. Weak left quadratus lumborum producing left trunk lean

    d. Weak right gluteus medius with left trunk lean to move center of mass toward stronger side

83. Which is true about the hip joint?

    a. Its closed pack position is extension with full external rotation.

    b. Its loose pack position is 30 degrees of abduction, 70 degrees of flexion with lateral rotation.

    c. With its capsular pattern of restriction, medial rotation is most restricted.

    d. With its capsular pattern of restriction, flexion is most restricted.

84. Whiplash injury from a rear-end collision would tear which of the following ligaments?

    a. Posterior longitudinal ligament

    b. Anterior longitudinal ligament

    c. Ligamentum nuchae

    d. Ligamentum flavum

85. A PTA should place the knee in which of the following positions to palpate the lateral collateral ligament?

    a. Knee at 60 degrees of flexion and the hip externally rotated

    b. Knee at 20 degrees of flexion and the hip at neutral

    c. Knee at 90 degrees of flexion and the hip externally rotated

    d. Knee at 0 degrees and the hip at neutral

86. A patient is in prone position with her head rotated to the left side. The left upper extremity is placed at her side and fully internally rotated. The left shoulder is then shrugged toward the chin. The PTA then grasps the midshaft of the patient's left forearm. The patient is then instructed to "try to reach your feet using just your left arm." This movement is resisted by the PTA. This test is assessing the strength of what muscle?

    a. Upper trapezius

    b. Posterior deltoid

    c. Latissimus dorsi

    d. Triceps brachii

87. Which of the following is the normal end-feel perceived by a PTA assessing wrist flexion?

    a. Bone to bone

    b. Soft tissue approximation

    c. Tissue stretch

    d. Empty

88. A PTA is assessing radial deviation range of motion at the wrist. The correct position of the goniometer should be as follows: the proximal

arm aligned with the forearm and the distal arm aligned with the third metacarpal. What should be used as the axis point?
a. Lunate
b. Scaphoid
c. Capitate
d. Triquetrum

89. The PTA is assessing a patient's strength in the right shoulder. The patient has 0 degrees of active shoulder abduction in the standing position. In the supine position, the patient has 42 degrees of active shoulder abduction and 175 degrees of pain-free passive shoulder abduction. What is the correct manual muscle testing grade for the patient's shoulder abduction?
a. 3−/5 (fair−)
b. 2+/5 (poor+)
c. 2−/5 (poor−)
d. 1/5 (trace)

90. Which of the following statements best describes lower extremity positioning in standing during the first 2 years of life of a child with no dysfunction?
a. Femoral anteversion, femoral external rotation, foot pronation
b. Femoral anteversion, femoral internal rotation, foot supination
c. Femoral retroversion, femoral external rotation, foot pronation
d. Femoral retroversion, femoral internal rotation, foot supination

91. What are signs and symptoms of an acute temporomandibular joint (TMJ) anterior displaced disk without reduction?
a. Clicking and pain in the TMJ joint
b. Absence of clicking and opening limited to 26 to 30 mm, lateral movements limited to contralateral side, deflection to same side with protrusion
c. Crepitation and limitation to 26 mm
d. Absence of clicking and opening limited to 26 to 30 mm, lateral movements limited to ipsilateral side, deflection to same side with protrusion

92. A PTA is performing manual muscle testing (MMT) of a patient with right lateral hip pain. The standing alignment reveals anterior pelvic tilt and associated hip flexion. During the MMT of the right posterior gluteus medius, which substitution is likely to occur?
a. Increase in hip flexion angle to substitute with the tensor fascia latae
b. Increase in lateral rotation to substitute with the tensor fascia latae
c. Forward rotation of the pelvis to substitute with the gluteus minimus
d. Knee flexion to substitute with the lateral hamstrings

93. A cause of a noncapsular pattern might be which of the following?
    a. Arthrosis in the knee
    b. Hemarthrosis of the shoulder
    c. Septic arthritis in the knee
    d. Loose body in the shoulder

94. A PTA is assessing passive range of motion in a patient reporting hip pain. When measuring with a goniometer, the patient had 0 to 60 degrees of passive hip internal rotation. This finding is considered which of the following?
    a. Normal
    b. Indicative of hypomobility
    c. Indicative of hypermobility
    d. Indicative of a capsular pattern

95. The skin and its mucosal barriers are an example of what type of immunity?
    a. Innate
    b. Active acquired
    c. Passive acquired
    d. Acquired

96. Inflamed lymph nodes as a result of infection are LEAST likely to be palpated in which of the following areas?
    a. Popliteal area
    b. Cervical area
    c. Axillary area
    d. Inguinal area

97. Which of the following is NOT a risk factor for pressure ulcer formation?
    a. Friction
    b. Shear
    c. Pressure
    d. Dry skin

98. Tissue anoxia and resulting cell death can occur if the external pressure is greater than the capillary closing pressure. Which of the following statements is TRUE about capillary closing pressure?
    a. Capillary closing pressure is defined as the pressure that occludes the smallest blood vessels.
    b. The average capillary closing pressure in a healthy adult is greater than 40 mm Hg.
    c. The closing capillary pressure adjusts and increases with the amount of pressure exerted on the tissue.
    d. Capillary closing pressure is the same for all patients.

99. Which of the following is NOT a mechanism by which moisture contributes to the formation of pressure ulcers?
   a. Changing the pH of the skin
   b. Increasing bacterial load of an existing skin lesion
   c. Increasing tissue destruction from shear and friction
   d. Occlusion of capillaries

100. Thick necrotic drainage often accompanied by a foul odor is termed which of the following?
   a. Serous
   b. Sanguineous
   c. Exudate
   d. Purulence

101. The fan-shaped subcutaneous wound extension that is the result of destruction of the connective tissue between the dermis and subcutaneous tissue is termed which of the following?
   a. Undermining
   b. Sinus
   c. Tunneling
   d. Fistula

102. In which stage of healing does the body produce new capillaries?
   a. Hemostasis
   b. Inflammation
   c. Proliferation
   d. Remodeling

103. What structure in the cranium has the closest contact with the brain?
   a. Dura mater
   b. Arachnoid
   c. Subarachnoid space
   d. Pia matter

104. What cranial nerve is involved with tic douloureux?
   a. Trigeminal
   b. Optic
   c. Olfactory
   d. Spinal accessory

105. After a severe concussion, a football player has difficulty with visual-spatial processing. Where did this lesion most likely occur?
   a. Left-side cortical area
   b. Right-side cortical area
   c. Amygdala area
   d. Brainstem

106. What is the lowest possible score for a patient on the Glasgow Coma Scale?
   a. 0
   b. 1
   c. 2
   d. 3

107. Damage to what structure in the brain would most likely lead to ataxic breathing?
   a. Diencephalon
   b. Pontine
   c. Medulla
   d. Pons

108. What excessive position is responsible for most spinal cord injuries?
   a. Excessive flexion
   b. Excessive extension
   c. Excessive rotation
   d. Excessive lateral flexion

109. Lower motor neuron involvement occurs with trauma to several sites. Damage to which of the following sites will NOT produce lower motor neuron symptoms?
   a. Cerebellum
   b. Cell body of alpha motor neuron located in the spinal cord or brainstem
   c. Motor endplate of the axon
   d. Muscle fibers innervated by the motor nerve axon

110. Which test is considered the gold standard for carpal tunnel syndrome?
   a. Phalen's test
   b. Tinel's test
   c. Nerve conduction velocity testing
   d. Carpal compression test

111. Disruption of which cranial nerve will result in Bell's palsy?
   a. Trochlear
   b. Trigeminal
   c. Facial
   d. Vagus

112. Which of the following body systems is NOT directly involved in balance?
   a. Visual system
   b. Somatosensory system
   c. Vestibular system
   d. Olfactory system

113. Which of the following is NOT a primary role of the vestibular system?
    a. Sensing self-motion
    b. Controlling center of mass
    c. Anticipating possible responsive postural control
    d. Stabilizing the head

114. Which body system is directly involved when a patient has a diagnosis of vertigo?
    a. Olfactory
    b. Vestibular
    c. Somatosensory
    d. Visual

115. Which of the following tests assesses a patient's anticipatory postural control?
    a. Timed up-and-go test
    b. Berg's balance scale
    c. Functional reach test
    d. Dynamic gait index

116. What motor level would be given to a patient with myelomeningocele that has 4/5 strength in the abdominals, hip flexion 3+/5, hip adduction 3+/5, and 1/5 knee extension?
    a. T10
    b. T12
    c. L3
    d. L4

117. Typical examination findings for a patient with peripheral neuropathy include all of the following EXCEPT which?
    a. Muscle weakness
    b. Muscle atrophy
    c. Diminished sensation
    d. Increased reflexes

118. Which of the following tests would NOT be expected to reproduce the patient's symptoms in a patient with a peripheral nerve injury?
    a. Upper limb neural tension test
    b. Deep tendon reflex
    c. Tinel's test
    d. Phalen's test

119. The autonomic nervous system does NOT innervate which of the following types of muscle?
    a. Skeletal muscle
    b. Smooth muscles

c. Cardiac muscle
d. Glandular activity

120. Motor neurons of which of the following nerves extend from the brainstem?
a. Sympathetic nerves
b. Parasympathetic nerves
c. Cranial nerves
d. Spinal nerves

121. Which of the following is TRUE when a nerve is elongated by movement over one or more joints?
a. The nerve becomes narrower.
b. Pressure inside the nerve decreases.
c. Blood flow increases.
d. Strain decreases.

122. A high school football player has just received anterior shoulder dislocation following a tackle. Which of the following nerves is most likely damaged in this scenario?
a. Ulnar nerve
b. Median nerve
c. Radial nerve
d. Axillary nerve

123. A patient presents to physical therapy with damage to the radial nerve. What would be the most likely clinical signs of this injury?
a. Weakened shoulder abduction
b. Weakened pronation
c. Diminished elbow flexion
d. Diminished supination and loss of extension

124. A peripheral nervous system dysfunction of the spinal roots is which of the following?
a. Polyradiculoneuropathy
b. Polyradiculopathy
c. Mononeuropathy multiplex
d. Multiple mononeuropathy

125. Where on the body would you find sebaceous glands?
a. Shoulders
b. Soles of the feet
c. Palms of the hands
d. Lower lip

126. Apocrine glands are found in what two locations on the body?
a. Soles of the feet and axillary areas
b. Anogenital and axillary areas

c. Soles of the feet and anogenital areas

d. Elbows and knees

127. Which of the following layers of the epidermis is responsible for the constant renewal of epidermal cells?
    a. Stratum germinativum
    b. Stratum granulosum
    c. Stratum lucidum
    d. Stratum corneum

128. An 80-year-old woman has been diagnosed with a stage IV pressure sore on the sacrum. She was transferred to the hospital from a subacute facility and is being followed by the wound care team. After 2 weeks of wound care treatment, the physical therapist assistant is reassessing the wound and determines that the bone is no longer visible. How would the physical therapist document the stage of the wound at this time?
    a. Stage IV
    b. Stage III
    c. Stage II
    d. Stage I

129. A 21-year-old woman has sustained a traumatic brain injury and is demonstrating significant neurologic impairments. The PTA notices a blister with surrounding erythema on the patient's sacrum. Which of the following stages would best describe the wound?
    a. Stage I pressure ulcer
    b. Stage II pressure ulcer
    c. Stage III pressure ulcer
    d. Stage IV pressure ulcer

130. It is noted on the patient's chart that the current platelet level is 50,000. Which of the following exercise routines would be most appropriate for this patient?
    a. Exercise is contraindicated at this time.
    b. Low-intensity exercise with no weights or resistance would be appropriate.
    c. Exercise at intense levels would be appropriate.
    d. Low-load resistance exercise with 1- to 2-pound weights would be appropriate.

131. Upon review of a medical chart, a physical therapist assistant (PTA) finds a patient has a PaO_2 of 90 mm Hg. From this information alone, the PTA should expect which of the following?
    a. The patient will complain of lightheadedness.
    b. The patient will have marked confusion.
    c. The patient is possibly experiencing cardiac arrest.
    d. This is a normal finding.

132. The primary cause of atelectasis is obstruction of the which of the following serving the area?
    a. Trachea
    b. Bronchus
    c. Bronchioles
    d. Alveolar ducts

133. What medication is most effective to decrease the risk for stroke in patients with atrial fibrillation?
    a. Warfarin sodium (Coumadin)
    b. Aspirin
    c. Clopidogrel
    d. Ticlopidine

134. All of the following are accepted peripheral sites for pulse assessment EXCEPT which?
    a. Carotid artery
    b. Radial artery
    c. Axillary artery
    d. Femoral artery

135. Which of the following is defined as velocity-dependent hypertonia?
    a. Flaccidity
    b. Rigidity
    c. Spasticity
    d. Akinesia

136. What is the purpose of a screening examination in pediatric physical therapy?
    a. To gain a comprehensive profile of the child's needs
    b. To act as a guide for initial frequency and duration of service
    c. To distinguish children with behavior different from that of other children of the same age
    d. To determine the need for disability-related adaptive equipment

137. Which of the following is least likely to be used as a documentation method for pediatric patients?
    a. Individualized Family Service Plan (IFSP)
    b. Individualized Education Program (IEP)
    c. SOAP (subjective, objective, assessment, and plan) note
    d. Gross Motor Function Measure

138. A PTA is working with a client who has visual field deficit. The PTA asks the client to look straight ahead and presents a stimulus at the outer margins of the person's visual fields. The technique checks which cranial nerve (CN) function?
    a. CN II
    b. CN III, CN IV, and CN VI

c. CN V

d. CN VIII

139. Your patient had a laceration anterior to the medial malleolus, which required stitches. He is now complaining of pain along the medial border of the foot. Which nerve is most likely involved?
    a. Sural nerve
    b. Deep fibular nerve
    c. Tibial nerve
    d. Saphenous nerve

140. Which named peripheral nerve is responsible for pain sensation from the pericardium, mediastinal pleura, diaphragmatic pleura, and diaphragmatic peritoneum?
    a. Vagus nerve
    b. Phrenic nerve
    c. Greater thoracic splanchnic nerve
    d. 10th intercostal nerve

141. The neural canal is smallest and circular in shape in what region of the vertebral canal?
    a. Cervical
    b. Thoracic
    c. Lumbar
    d. Sacral

142. Ascending tracts in the white matter of the spinal cord carry what kind of information?
    a. Sensory
    b. Motor
    c. Both sensory and motor
    d. Autonomic

143. Which of the following cranial nerves does NOT contain parasympathetic fibers?
    a. Oculomotor
    b. Facial
    c. Trigeminal
    d. Vagus

144. Which of the following neural fibers are the largest and fastest?
    a. C fibers
    b. A fibers
    c. A and C fibers are equal
    d. None of the above

145. A posterior lateral herniation of the lumbar disk between vertebrae L4 and L5 most likely results in damage to which nerve root?
    a. L4
    b. L5
    c. L4 and L5
    d. L5 and S1

146. A patient has traumatically dislocated the tibia directly posteriorly during an automobile accident. Which of the following structures is the least likely to be injured?
    a. Tibial nerve
    b. Popliteal artery
    c. Common peroneal nerve
    d. Anterior cruciate ligament

147. Nerve regeneration occurs at which pace per month?
    a. 5 mm
    b. 1 inch
    c. 1 cm
    d. 2.5 inches

148. Which of the following muscles of the pharynx is supplied by the glossopharyngeal nerve (cranial nerve IX)?
    a. Palatopharyngeus
    b. Stylopharyngeus
    c. Superior constrictor
    d. Middle constrictor

149. Nerve conduction velocity/electromyography studies of motor nerves are NOT able to differentiate which of the following?
    a. Peripheral nerve disease from anterior horn cell disease
    b. The specific location of the cord, nerve, root, plexus, or peripheral nerve
    c. Neuromuscular junction disease from peripheral nerve disease
    d. The specific cause or nature of the neural lesion

150. Which statement below best describes the difference in motor function for a nerve root deficit versus a peripheral nerve deficit?
    a. In peripheral nerve deficit, the motor weakness is evident more rapidly when applying resistance compared with nerve root deficit.
    b. In nerve root deficit, the motor weakness is evident more rapidly when applying resistance compared with peripheral nerve deficit.
    c. In peripheral nerve deficit, the motor weakness is only evident when applying resistance without gravity.
    d. In nerve root deficit, the motor weakness is only evident when applying resistance without gravity.

151. The L4 deep tendon reflex is elicited at which of the following?
    a. Achilles tendon
    b. Femoral tendon
    c. Medial hamstring tendon
    d. Patella tendon

152. This descending tract originates in the superior colliculus and is involved with the orientation toward a stimulus in the environment by reflex turning of the head.
    a. Rubrospinal
    b. Reticulospinal
    c. Tectospinal
    d. Vestibulospinal

153. Decerebrate posturing is indicative of what stage of hepatic encephalopathy?
    a. Stage I
    b. Stage II
    c. Stage III
    d. Stage IV

154. What happens when an action potential reaches the neurons terminal?
    a. Sodium channel blockers bind the outer axonal surface of the channel and prevent the flux of sodium.
    b. The cell membrane is depolarized.
    c. There is an increase in sodium permeability.
    d. There is a release of chemical neurotransmitter through the presynaptic terminals.

155. Almost all communication between neurons occurs through what process?
    a. Electrical
    b. Mechanical
    c. Chemical
    d. Gravity dependent

156. Which of the following structures in the brain is most involved in extremity movement?
    a. The pons
    b. Reticular formation
    c. Substantia nigra
    d. Medulla

157. Which of the following cranial nerves innervates the superior oblique muscle of the eye?
    a. Optic
    b. Oculomotor

    c. Trochlear

    d. Trigeminal

158. Which of the following cranial nerves does NOT have a sensory function?
    a. Olfactory
    b. Optic
    c. Vagus
    d. Spinal accessory

159. What part of the cerebellum controls gait and dynamic standing balance?
    a. Anterior lobe
    b. Spinocerebellum
    c. Vestibulocerebellum
    d. Cerebrocerebellum

160. What part of the brain is responsible for behavior and personality?
    a. Parietal lobe
    b. Broca's area
    c. Temporal lobe
    d. Frontal lobe

161. Which characteristic of an acute wound would predispose it to become a chronic wound?
    a. Ischemia
    b. Rolled wound edges
    c. Minimal necrotic tissue
    d. Overgrowth of epithelium

162. A patient presents to inpatient physical therapy with a pressure ulcer. The supervising physical therapist has noted that the wound has a sinus tract associated with it. What is the most likely mechanism of injury for this pressure wound?
    a. Shear
    b. Friction
    c. Pressure
    d. Moisture

163. Which mechanism of pressure ulcer is characterized by changes in skin surface pH?
    a. Shear
    b. Friction
    c. Pressure
    d. Moisture

164. A patient with a stage II pressure ulcer presents with blanched white skin around the wound. What is the most likely cause of this skin color?
    a. Friction
    b. Pressure
    c. Moisture
    d. Shear

165. A pressure ulcer is described according to what?
    a. The layer of tissue involved at the time of examination
    b. The healing phase at the time of examination
    c. The stage of wound changes as it heals
    d. The deepest layer of tissue involvement at the initial examination and the healing phase at the time of assessment

166. A noninvasive test therapists may use to screen for lower extremity arterial compromise is which of the following?
    a. Magnetic resonance imaging
    b. Manual muscle testing
    c. Ankle-brachial index (ABI)
    d. Radiograph

167. Inspection of the neuropathic foot EXCLUDES which of the following?
    a. Skin
    b. Nails
    c. Shoes and socks
    d. Areas above the malleoli

168. What size of monofilament should be used on the plantar surface of the foot in a patient with diabetic neuropathy to determine protective sensation?
    a. 2.83
    b. 3.61
    c. 4.31
    d. 5.07

169. A patient has a burn over the anterior thigh. In which of the following situations would it be appropriate to use manual muscle testing to determine the strength of the quadriceps?
    a. The burn is in the remodeling phase.
    b. The patient's resting pain level is 8/10 on the Visual Analogue Scale.
    c. It is 1 day after surgical skin grafting.
    d. It is the same day as surgical skin grafting is scheduled.

170. When using the rule-of-nines chart for estimating surface area of a burn, what score would be given to a burn covering the entire left upper extremity only?
    a. 4.5%
    b. 9%
    c. 18%
    d. 27%

171. Which structure is located in the epidermis only?
    a. Stratum corneum
    b. Hair follicle
    c. Sebaceous glands
    d. Apocrine glands

172. Which of the following is a typical examination finding in a patient with polyneuropathy?
    a. Unilateral decrease or loss of reflexes
    b. Distal decrease or loss of reflexes
    c. Change in proximal but not distal reflexes
    d. No change in reflexes

173. Which of the following is FALSE regarding the Glasgow Coma Scale (GCS)?
    a. The GCS is the most widely used coma scale.
    b. The GCS consists of three categories: eye opening, best motor response, best verbal response.
    c. The lowest possible total score on the GCS is 0, indicating coma.
    d. A total score of 12 or more indicates minor injury.

174. A stroke in which of the following structures of the brain could lead to a locked-in syndrome?
    a. Thalamus
    b. Hypothalamus
    c. Cerebral cortex
    d. Brainstem

175. Most complex partial seizures arise from what area of the brain?
    a. Frontal lobe
    b. Parietal lobe
    c. Temporal lobe
    d. Occipital lobe

176. In the semicircular canals, the ampulla moves in which direction in relation to head movement?
    a. The ampulla moves in the same direction as head movement.
    b. The ampulla moves in the opposite direction of head movement.

    c. The ampulla remains constant without movement regardless of the movement of the head.

    d. The ampulla moves with rotational movement only.

177. Which pathway between the vestibular system and the motor system receives the majority of its input from the otoliths in the cerebellum?
    a. Medial vestibulospinal tract
    b. Lateral vestibulospinal tract
    c. Dorsal horn of the spinal cord
    d. Reticulospinal

178. Which pathway that receives its signals from the vestibular system is responsible for postural changes in response to angular head motion?
    a. Medial vestibulospinal tract
    b. Lateral vestibulospinal tract
    c. Dorsal horn of the spinal cord
    d. Reticulospinal tract

179. What is the primary blood supply to the components of the vestibular system?
    a. Posterior cerebellar artery
    b. Inferior cerebellar artery
    c. Circle of Willis
    d. Vertebral basilar artery

180. Which of the following tests is specific to dysfunction of the otolith?
    a. Vestibular-evoked myogenic potentials
    b. Electrocochleography
    c. Posturography
    d. Rotational chair testing

181. Which of the following is NOT a function of the vestibular system?
    a. Maintaining our orientation in space
    b. Allowing us to hear
    c. Controlling our posture
    d. Maintaining our balance

182. A resting pulse of more than 100 beats/minute is considered:
    a. Tachycardia
    b. Bradycardia
    c. Tachypnea
    d. Hypertension

183. Respirations less than 10 breaths/minute in a resting adult are considered which of the following?
    a. Apnea
    b. Bradypnea

     c. Hypoventilation

     d. Tachypnea

184. Which is the most common site for taking blood pressure?
     a. Upper arm
     b. Thigh
     c. Wrist
     d. Foot/ankle

185. A transient decrease in blood pressure that occurs when changing to a more upright position is known as what?
     a. Hypertension
     b. Autonomic dysreflexia
     c. Orthostatic hypotension
     d. Prehypertension

186. Which of the following correctly matches the normal value range with the parameter it is measuring?
     a. Adolescent respiratory rate: 20 to 40 breaths/minute
     b. Adult resting heart rate: 80 to 140 beats/minute
     c. O_2 saturation: 95% to 100%
     d. Adult blood pressure: 140/90 mm Hg

187. Which of the following is NOT considered a traditional vital sign?
     a. Temperature
     b. Pulse
     c. Respiration rate
     d. Urinary voiding

188. Where should the thermometer be placed in the mouth to obtain the most accurate body temperature measurement?
     a. Inside the cheek and gum
     b. In the sublingual pocket
     c. At the roof of the mouth
     d. Behind the first molar

189. The PTA is attempting to obtain the blood pressure of a patient. After the PTA has heard the systolic blood pressure, there is a loud noise in the room, and the diastolic pressure cannot be heard. What should the PTA do next?
     a. Reinflate the blood pressure cuff and try again immediately.
     b. Record the systolic blood pressure only.
     c. Wait at least 2 minutes before repeating the test.
     d. Attempt to take the blood pressure at the calf.

190. In which of the following scenarios is it considered satisfactory to take a patient's blood pressure in the right upper extremity?
    a. The patient underwent right mastectomy 2 years ago.
    b. The patient has an intravenous line on the right upper extremity.
    c. The patient has an arteriovenous fistula in the right upper extremity.
    d. The patient had right rotator cuff repair 1 week ago.

191. What is considered the best indicator of cardiopulmonary fitness?
    a. Respiration rate at rest
    b. Heart rate at rest
    c. Maximum oxygen uptake (VO_{2max})
    d. Blood glucose level at rest

192. What is the best way to estimate a maximum heart rate for a 70-year-old man?
    a. 220 minus 70
    b. 180 minus 70
    c. 220 plus 70
    d. 180 plus 70

193. The normal inspiratory-to-expiratory ratio is approximately which of the following?
    a. 1:1
    b. 1:2
    c. 1:4
    d. 2:1

194. Fluid retention can be used to assess the severity of heart disease. Which of the following should NOT be used to assess fluid levels in a patient?
    a. Subjective complaints by the patient
    b. Body weight
    c. Jugular venous distention
    d. Palpating for peripheral edema

195. Which of the following is TRUE regarding the diaphragm?
    a. It is innervated by roots of C4, C5, and C6.
    b. It is innervated by the vagus nerve.
    c. It originates from the lower three lumbar vertebrae.
    d. It has a boney origin but not a boney insertion.

196. What is the volume of air in the lungs at the end of a maximum inspiration?
    a. Forced vital capacity
    b. Residual volume
    c. Inspiratory capacity
    d. Total lung capacity

197. What pulmonary test would most likely be decreased in a patient with an obstructive lung disease?
    a. Tidal volume
    b. Total lung capacity
    c. Forced vital capacity
    d. Forced expiratory volume in 1 second

198. Lymphedema caused by malformations of the lymphatic system is known as which of the following?
    a. Primary lymphedema
    b. Lipolymphedema
    c. Secondary lymphedema
    d. Phlebolymphedema

199. When examining a patient with lymphedema, it is important to measure the unaffected as well as the affected extremity because of which of the following?
    a. The patient needs to know these measurements to receive insurance reimbursement.
    b. It will help monitor weight gain and joint mobility measurements.
    c. Measurements of the unaffected extremity can provide a goal for the affected extremity.
    d. Measurements will determine the number of bandages needed to reduce the swelling in a limb.

200. Lymphedema resulting from breast cancer surgery is classified as which of the following?
    a. Dynamic lymphedema
    b. Primary lymphedema
    c. Secondary lymphedema
    d. Idiopathic lymphedema

201. What is the correct procedure to take girth measurements of an affected extremity with lymphedema with a tape measure?
    a. The tape measure should barely touch the skin in two to three places.
    b. The tape measure should not indent the tissue.
    c. The tape measure should slightly indent the tissue.
    d. The tape measure should firmly indent the tissue.

202. The PTA is determining intervention for a patient in the hospital. A review of the chart finds that the patient has a positive Doppler signal. What information does this convey to the PTA?
    a. The pulses of the lower extremity are normal.
    b. The pulses are absent in the lower extremity and nonaudible with a Doppler.

   c. Pulses in the lower extremity are absent to palpation with an audible Doppler signal.

   d. The patient should immediately be referred to the physician for further medical evaluation.

203. Which metabolic equivalent is associated with the slowest walking speed?

   a. 3

   b. 4

   c. 5

   d. 6

204. A client is scheduled to begin physical therapy at an outpatient clinic. The PTA performs a chart review and finds that the patient has a body mass index of 21.3. What should the PTA expect from this information only?

   a. A patient who is underweight

   b. A patient who is of normal weight

   c. A patient who is overweight

   d. A patient who is morbidly obese

205. Which of the following is not included in a basic metabolic panel?

   a. Acid-base balance

   b. Blood sugar

   c. Cerebral-spinal fluid level

   d. Kidney status

206. Which of the following values is most likely to be increased with infection?

   a. Magnesium

   b. Red blood cells

   c. Platelets

   d. White blood cells

207. Which of the following patient populations will have the highest hematocrit percentage?

   a. Newborns

   b. Children

   c. Adult men

   d. Adult women

208. Which of the following is the maximum volume of air that can be expired after a normal inspiration?

   a. Vital capacity

   b. Inspiratory capacity

   c. Expiratory reserve volume

   d. Inspiratory reserve volume

209. What quadrant of the heart receives venous blood first?
    a. Left atrium
    b. Right atrium
    c. Left ventricle
    d. Right ventricle

210. Which is the correct action of the pulmonary veins?
    a. Take oxygenated blood to the lungs
    b. Take oxygenated blood to the heart
    c. Take deoxygenated blood to the lungs
    d. Take deoxygenated blood to the heart

211. Which chamber of the heart has the highest muscle mass?
    a. Left atrium
    b. Right atrium
    c. Right ventricle
    d. Left ventricle

212. What structure is referred to as the pacemaker of the heart?
    a. Atrioventricular node
    b. Sinoatrial node
    c. Purkinje fibers
    d. Right ventricle

213. Damage to which of the following structures will cause a heart attack or myocardial infarction?
    a. Sinoatrial node
    b. Coronary arteries
    c. Purkinje fibers
    d. Pulmonary veins

214. Which of the following is not part of the upper conducting airway?
    a. Nose
    b. Pharynx
    c. Larynx
    d. Trachea

215. Pulmonary function tests are accomplished by which of the following?
    a. Computed tomography
    b. Magnetic resonance imaging
    c. Spirometry
    d. Sphygmomanometry

216. When you palpate thoracic expansion of the patient with severe pulmonary emphysema and chronic obstructive pulmonary disease, you would expect which of the following physical findings?
    a. Asymmetrical chest expansion
    b. Increased lateral expansion of the thorax—"bucket handle"

    c. Pain on attempts to expand

    d. Reduced chest expansion in all planes

217. The sinoatrial node is located in what chamber of the heart?
    a. Left atrium
    b. Right atrium
    c. Left ventricle
    d. Right ventricle

218. Where in the tissues does nutrient exchange take place?
    a. Capillaries
    b. Interstitial spaces
    c. Arterioles
    d. Venules

219. During which phase of the cardiac cycle is ventricular volume the lowest?
    a. Atrial systole
    b. Isovolumetric ventricular contraction
    c. At the onset of rapid ventricular ejection
    d. Isovolumetric ventricular relaxation

220. The heart contains a variety of different types of muscle fibers, each with a different frequency of spontaneous contraction. Which of the following has the shortest period (highest frequency) of spontaneous contraction?
    a. Purkinje fibers
    b. Sinoatrial node
    c. Atrioventricular node
    d. Myocardium

221. The volume of air moved when going from full forced expiration to full forced inspiration is known as which of the following?
    a. Inspiratory capacity
    b. Vital capacity
    c. Total lung capacity
    d. Inspiratory reserve volume

222. A patient with cardiac arrhythmia is referred to physical therapy services for cardiac rehabilitation. The PTA is aware that the heart receives nerve impulses that begin in the sinoatrial node of the heart and then proceed to which of the following?
    a. Atrioventricular node, then to the Purkinje fibers, and then to the bundle branches
    b. Purkinje fibers, then to the bundle branches, and then to the atrioventricular node

     c. Atrioventricular node, then to the bundle branches, and then to the Purkinje fibers

     d. Bundle branches, then to the atrioventricular node, and then to the Purkinje fibers

223. Which of the following describes lymphedema?
     a. Pathologic accumulation of white blood cell–filled fluid
     b. Accumulation of lymphocytes in the blood and tissues
     c. Pathologic accumulation of protein-rich fluid in the tissue
     d. Leakage of red blood cells into the surrounding tissue

224. The PTA is working with a patient in cardiac rehabilitation under direct supervision of a physical therapist. During a rest break for the patient, the PTA attempts to assess heart sounds with a stethoscope. Which of the following is true about the first sound during auscultation of the heart?
     a. The first sound is of the closure of the aortic and pulmonic valves.
     b. The first sound is of the closure of the mitral and tricuspid valves.
     c. The first sound is of the beginning of ventricular diastole.
     d. The first sound is usually the loudest.

225. A patient presents to a clinic with decreased tidal volume. What is the most likely cause of this change in normal pulmonary function?
     a. Chronic obstructive pulmonary disease
     b. Restrictive lung dysfunction
     c. Emphysema
     d. Asthma

226. Besides the anterolateral abdominal muscles, which muscle assists in forced expiration, coughing, sneezing, vomiting, urinating, defecating, and fixation of the trunk during strong movements of the upper limb?
     a. Piriformis
     b. Pelvic diaphragm
     c. Trapezius
     d. Gluteus maximus

Answers

1. a. Fibrocartilage is normally found on tendon and ligament insertions. Elastic cartilage is found either in the trachea or earlobe, and fibro-elastic cartilage is found in the meniscus of the knee.

2. a. Choice b refers to a grade I strain, and choice c is a grade III strain. Choice d is incorrect because if there is a complete tear, then there will be significant strength loss.

3. c. The reparative phase begins during the first few weeks and includes the formation of a soft callous about 2 weeks after injury. This is eventually replaced by a hard callus. The remodeling phase begins once the fracture has united solidly with woven bone.

4. a. At birth the entire meniscus is vascular, and by age 9 months the inner one third has become avascular. By adulthood, only the outer 10% to 30% of the meniscus is vascular.

5. a. Articular cartilage cushions the subchondral bone and provides a low friction surface necessary for free movement. It contains few cells, is aneural, and avascular, and often starts to break down with increasing age.

6. b. With age, proteoglycan aggregation is reduced, and small proteogly-cans are synthesized with an increase in keratin sulfate and reduced chondroitin sulfate content. The hydrophilic proteoglycans have been shown to become shorter with age and therefore lose their ability to hold water in the matrix.

7. b. The three primary influences that affect bone remodeling are mechanical stresses; calcium and phosphate levels in the extracel-lular fluid; and hormonal levels of parathyroid hormone, calcitonin, vitamin D, cortisol, growth hormone, thyroid hormone, and sex hormones.

8. d. The physeal or growth plates provide axial and circumferential growth of bones. After the bone has completed the growth process, these plates fuse together. These plates are only present in children.

9. a. Type I muscle fibers, also known as slow oxidative/slow twitch fibers, are the fatigue-resistant red fibers. The red color is the result of high amounts of myoglobin and a high capillary content. The other choices refer to type II, or fast twitch fibers.

10. a. Because of hypotonia and decreased strength, children with Down syndrome have several common gait deviations. Smaller step lengths and increased hip flexion are normally seen in this population in addition to choices b, c, and d.

11. b. A scoliometer is used by asking the patient to bend forward so that the shoulders are level with the hips. The scoliometer is then placed over the level of possible scoliosis. A measurement of 5 degrees or more in this screening test is considered positive and requires medical follow-up.

12. d. Any muscle innervated by the L4-L5 segment (and any segment below that) would be affected by an L4-L5 myelomeningocele. The iliopsoas is innervated by levels L1 to L3. It would not be affected in this scenario.

13. d. Torticollis is a contracted state of the sternocleidomastoid muscle, producing head tilt to the affected side with rotation of the chin to the opposite side.

14. c. Bone mass is known to reach its peak maximum size and density by the time an adult reaches age 30 years. Women have a tendency to lose bone mass sooner than men, often beginning in their late 30s.

15. a. A T-score of −1.0 or higher represents a normal score. Patients with scores of −1.5 to −2.5 have osteopenia, whereas patients with scores of −2.5 or lower have osteoporosis.

16. b. The appendicular skeleton consists of the upper and lower extremities. The axial skeleton consists of the trunk, including the cranium, ribs, vertebral column, and pelvis.

17. c. The anterior musculature in patients with osteoporosis is typically short and tight, whereas the extensors are long and weak because of constant stretch.

18. c. The base of support in normal static standing is the outer portion of the feet.

19. a. Static means "not moving." Static posture could also be assessed while the patient is standing, but that is not a choice. All other choices are dynamic "moving" postures.

20. b. In anatomic position, the body is erect with the head and torso upright. The arms are at the sides of the torso with the shoulders in neutral rotation, the elbows are extended, the cubital fossae of the elbow and the palms face forward, the fingers are extended, and the

thumbs are adducted with the pad of each thumb facing forward. The lower extremities are straight and parallel, with the second toe facing straight forward.

21. d. Choice a defines a kyphosis-lordosis posture. Although choice d could define flat back as well, there is usually increased thoracic kyphosis in swayback with decreased kyphosis in flat back.

22. d. The anterior-superior iliac spine should be anterior to the greater trochanter in normal vertical alignment.

23. a. Choice b refers to gliding, choice c refers to elevation and depression, and choice d refers to protraction and retraction.

24. b. In flexion of the lumbar spine, the back flattens, leading to a decrease in lordosis. Extension increases lordosis.

25. c. Choice b describes an anterior pelvic tilt. The other choices are not natural movement.

26. b. The most common area for strain or tear of any muscle is the musculotendinous junction. Damage at the origin or insertion is possible, but choice b is the most common.

27. d. A 4/5 grade requires moderate resistance by the particular muscle group. Choice g requires full range-of-motion gravity eliminated, and in choice c the muscle group would initiate movement against gravity.

28. d. Choices a and b require equipment and some knowledge of the equipment. Functional testing can be used to assess muscle strength, but choice d is the fastest.

29. b. This test is performed by placing marks at the lumbosacral junction and 10 cm up along the spine, with the patient standing. The patient then bends forward as far as possible, and the increase in distance between the two marks is measured with a flexible tape measure. This distance should increase by at least 5 cm if lumbar spine mobility is normal.

30. c. During an examination, it is important to find what movements exacerbate the patient's pain. It is also important to find what movements decrease the patient's pain. The particular ROM deficits of the patient would lead the therapist to the correct diagnosis and thus the correct interventions. The presence of hypomobility and hypermobility is determined with one single ROM plane, not with the combination of ROM sequences.

31. b. In the other choices, the therapist is attempting to cause the patient's symptoms of radiculopathy into the involved upper extremity. The cervical distraction test involves unloading of the cervical foramen. A decrease in pain with unloading of the cervical foramen denotes a positive test.

32. a. The C6 nerve root is tested with the brachioradialis reflex, and the C7 nerve root is tested with the triceps reflex.

33. b. These bones protect the tendons from excessive wear and sometimes increase the mechanical advantage of the involved muscle. Irregularly shaped bones are found throughout the body, and accessory bones are formed when additional ossification centers appear and form extra bones. Heterotopic bone forms in soft tissue after injury.

34. d. Choice a describes a linear fracture, choice b an impaction fracture, and choice c describes a stress fracture.

35. b. Measurements 20 cm proximal to the joint line are attempted to assess quadriceps atrophy. General joint effusion is measured at the joint line, and gastrocnemius/soleus atrophy or lower leg edema is measured at 15 cm distal to the joint line.

36. b. Loading response is the part of the initial double support characterized by the movement of the ankle into plantar flexion. This allows for the gradual contact of the foot with the supporting surface and movement of the knee into flexion. These movements at the lower extremity transfer weight, help with energy conservation, and help with shock absorption.

37. b. Double support is defined as the time in which both feet are in contact with the supporting surface. This is 20% of the gait cycle. In dysfunctional gait the period of double support often increases.

38. a. Choices b, c, and d all involve the swing phase of gait. Bilateral lower extremity weakness would often find an increase in double support cycle of gait.

39. b. The body should not forward-flex at initial contact during the gait cycle. Choices a, c, and d all must be mastered for successful ambulation.

40. d. The gluteus maximus is responsible for stabilizing the hip during initial contact, loading response, and midstance. The hamstrings perform choices a, b, and c.

41. b. In normal gait, the stance phase encompasses 60% of the gait cycle, and the swing phase is present during 40% of the gait cycle.

42. d. Initial contact is defined as the point at which the heel makes contact with the supporting surface. Loading response is the period of initial double support characterized by movement of the ankle into plantar flexion. Midstance begins with the contralateral limb leaving the supporting surface and ends as the body's center of gravity moves directly over the reference supporting limb.

43. a. Choice a is the correct definition of step length. Choice b characterizes stride length. A single right step and single left step make up one stride.

44. b. The knee moves from 0 degrees of flexion to 60 to 65 degrees of flexion during initial swing. There is also 60 to 65 degrees of knee flexion in midswing.

45. d. During the swing phase of gait, the ankle dorsiflexors are responsible for the dorsiflexion movement of the ankle before initial contact. During terminal stance, the ankle dorsiflexors are silent.

46. d. Bursitis is inflammation of the bursae, which are the fluid-filled sacs located throughout the body that decrease friction between structures. Bursae become irritated and painful when they are repeatedly pinched between two structures.

47. b. Ligaments are supporting structures that serve to stabilize the joint and prevent excess movement. When ligaments are overstretched, their fibers can tear and cause pain and instability of the joint, resulting in a sprain.

48. c. Active range of motion refers to the ability of the patient to voluntarily move the limb through an arc of movement. Passive range of motion refers to the amount of movement that a joint obtains by the therapist moving the segment without resistance or assistance from the patient.

49. b. The goniometer may be used to document range of motion. The most common measurement technique, goniometry is performed with a goniometer and measures joint angles.

50. b. If no contraction is felt or seen in the muscle, it receives a grade of 0/5. If the patient is able to hold the test position with no added pressure, the muscle receives a grade of 3/5. If the patient is able to hold against moderate pressure, a grade of 4/5 is recorded.

51. a. The soft tissue surrounding the joint must be pliable to allow movement between the surfaces. This feature is referred to accessory motion in the joint. Accessory motion is the ability of the joint surfaces to glide, roll, and spin on each other.

52. b. The PTA may perform a number of tests to determine flexibility. One common test for lower extremities is the 90/90 straight leg raise test. This test objectively measures flexibility of the hamstring muscles, located on the posterior aspect of the thigh.

53. d. Outcome measures are standardized instruments that measure individual's actual or perceived activity limitations and participation restrictions, quality of life, or health status.

54. b. Other examples of activities of daily living are transferring to a toilet, getting in and out of a car, dialing a telephone, and washing your hands.

55. b. A comprehensive understanding of anatomy is essential for any PTA. In the clinical situation, the therapist uses the sense of touch, known as palpation, to assess what is occurring below the skin and what musculoskeletal structures are involved in an injury.

56. d. Phalen's test is for nerve compression at the carpal tunnel, and Lachman's test is for anterior cruciate ligament instability. Thomas' test is used to determine hip flexor tightness.

57. a. In the case of a reciprocal click, the initial click is created by the condyle slipping back into the correct position under the disk with opening of the mouth. In this disorder, the condyle is resting posterior to the disk before jaw opening. With closing, the click is caused by the condyle slipping away from the disk.

58. d. The supraspinatus tendon is best palpated by placing the patient's involved upper extremity behind the back in full internal rotation.

59. d. The posterior cruciate ligament becomes tight in full knee extension. This assists the tibia in external rotation, which is needed for the screw home mechanism with open-chain activities.

60. b. Femoral anteversion is the only option that would account for the internal rotation seen in toe in.

61. d. Older adults are more likely to have osteophyte formation. All other populations can have rotator cuff damage, but it will most likely come from another source.

62. d. The tuberosity of the fifth metatarsal is at the base of the metatarsal. The base of the metatarsal is proximal, and the head is distal. The medial cuneiform is on the high medial side of the transverse arch of the foot. The cuboid bone is on the lower lateral side of the foot.

63. c. Metacarpophalangeal joints are condyloid joints. These are biaxial joints allowing flexion and extension around one axis and abduction and adduction around another axis.

64. b. These actions can be easily demonstrated and palpated. Resisting anterior movement of the arm abducted to 60 degrees tests the sternocostal head of the pectoralis major; the clavicular head is tested after the arm is abducted to 90 degrees.

65. c. The structures that pass through the foramen magnum include the spinal cord, the meninges, the spinal components of cranial nerve XI, and the vertebral arteries. Cranial nerve XII exits the skull through the hypoglossal canals.

66. a. The longus capitis, longus colli, and sternocleidomastoid muscles are all associated with the anterior aspect of the cervical vertebrae and thus produce flexion of the head.

67. a. The nucleus pulposus is thickest in the lumbar spine, followed by the cervical region; it is thinnest in the thoracic spine.

68. a. The speed of contraction is directly related to the resting length of the muscle fiber, whereas the force of contraction depends on the cross-sectional diameter. Creatine phosphate content ensures availability of adenosine triphosphate for the contraction–relaxation cycles, and glycolytic capacity is important for endurance.

69. c. This is the normal anatomy, lateral to medial of the proximal row of the carpus. The distal row, lateral to medial, is the trapezium, trapezoid, capitate, and hamate.

70. b. Bifid spinous processes (spinous processes that are split) are found only in the cervical spine.

71. c. In static standing, the line of gravity is posterior to the hip joint. The body relies on the anterior pelvic ligaments and the hip joint capsule. The iliopsoas may be recruited at times, but anterior ligaments are used first to keep the trunk from extending in static stance.

72. b. The area of contact between the humerus and the glenoid fossa is maximum in this position.

73. d. The subscapularis, teres minor, and infraspinatus muscles oppose the superior pull of the deltoid muscle. The supraspinatus does not oppose the pull of the deltoid but is important because (along with the other cuff muscles) it provides a compression force to the glenohumeral joint.

74. a. Only the edges of the adult meniscus are vascularized by the capillaries from the synovial membrane and joint capsule.

75. a. The intervertebral disk has the greatest amount of fluid at the time of birth. The fluid content decreases as a person ages.

76. d. The metacarpophalangeal joint is enclosed in a joint capsule and therefore is considered a diarthrodial joint.

77. b. Genu valgum is a term used to describe a deformity of the knee causing an inward bowing of the legs. Genu varus is an outward bowing of the legs. Coxa valgum is a deformity at the hip in which the angle between the axis of the neck of the femur and the shaft of the femur is greater than 135 degrees. In coxa varus, this angle is less than 135 degrees. Pes cavus is an increase in the arch of the foot. Pes planus is flat foot.

78. c. This is the loose-packed position of the hip.

79. a. Flexion and extension of the thumb are performed in a plane parallel to the palm of the hand. Abduction and adduction are performed in a plane perpendicular to the palm of the hand.

80. c. The triangular fibrocartilage complex is made up of the dorsal radioulnar ligament, ulnar collateral ligament, ulnar articular cartilage, volar radioulnar ligament, ulnocarpal meniscus, and sheath of the extensor carpi ulnaris.

81. c. The normal end range of opening is 40 mm.

82. b. Weak left gluteus medius with left trunk lean is to move the center of mass toward the weaker side. A pelvic drop in single limb midstance is a classic positive Trendelenburg sign of gluteus medius weakness. The compensatory trunk lateral lean is to bring the center of mass closer to the weaker side to decrease the external moment arm on the weak muscle.

83. d. According to Cyriax's classic description, flexion in the hip is limited the greatest in its capsular pattern.

84. b. Whiplash injury includes hyperextension of cervical vertebrae that may tear the anterior longitudinal ligament that limits extension of cervical spine. All the other ligaments limit flexion of the cervical spine; accordingly, they may be torn in hyperflexion injuries.

85. c. The lateral collateral ligament of the knee is best palpated with the patient in the sitting position. The patient then places the foot of

the involved lower extremity on the knee of the uninvolved lower extremity. This maneuver places the involved knee in 90 degrees of flexion and the hip in external rotation.

86. c. This test assesses the strength of the latissimus dorsi. One of the functions of the latissimus is to push up from a sitting position. This test simulates that movement.

87. c. A tissue stretch end-feel is also felt with ankle dorsiflexion. An example of a bone-to-bone end-feel is with knee or elbow extension. Knee flexion is an example of soft tissue approximation. In an empty end-feel, the patient stops the movement because pain.

88. c. The capitate is the axis.

89. c. Because the patient does not have 50% of normal range of motion in the gravity eliminated position, 2−/5 is the appropriate grade. Some therapists argue that this is an example of a 1+/5 grade. Sources used in preparation of this exam indicate that there is no grade of 1+/5 with manual muscle testing.

90. a. After the first 2 years of life, the femurs rotate to a more neutral position, and the amount of anteversion decreases.

91. b. For example: the right joint is locked. Anterior translation primarily occurs after 26 mm; therefore, opening will be restricted at 26 mm, and deflection will occur to the right (same side). Lateral movement to the opposite side (movement to the left, or contralateral side) will be restricted because the right joint cannot translate, and protrusion will deflect to the hypomobile side (right) and be restricted.

92. a. Patients tend to posteriorly rotate the pelvis to substitute with the tensor fascia latae or the gluteus minimus. These muscles are medial rotators, not lateral rotators like the posterior gluteus medius. The lateral hamstrings are not hip abductors.

93. d. Choices a, b, and c will present with the typical capsular patterns in their respective joints. A loose body in the shoulder will inhibit one plane of motion but will not limit any other motions. Hence it would not be a capsular pattern.

94. c. Based on the values provided by the American Academy of Orthopedic Surgeons, the clinical finding exceeds the expected normal range of motion for hip internal rotation, which is 0 to 45 degrees.

95. a. The innate immunity system does not distinguish between different types of invaders and is nonadaptive. Innate immunity also encompasses the nonspecific inflammatory response to all forms of cellular injury or death.

96. a. Lymph nodes can be inflamed from infection and are most often palpated in the submandibular, cervical, inguinal, and axillary areas.

97. d. Friction, shear, pressure, and moisture are all risk factors for developing pressure ulcers.

98. a. Capillary closing pressure for a healthy adult ranges from 20 to 40 mm Hg. The capillary closing pressure does not adjust in the individual, and it is different for all patients. It changes between patients because of body size and type.

99. d. Occlusion of the capillaries is caused by pressure, not moisture. The other choices may be caused by excessive moisture.

100. d. Serous exudate is usually a thin, clear, watery secretion from a wound, and sanguineous drainage is characterized by the presence of blood. Exudate is a pale yellow fluid drainage composed of blood cells, serum, and lysed debris.

101. a. A sinus tract is a long, narrow opening along a plane that may connect to a deeper abscess. Tunneling is a tract that connects two open wounds, and a fistula is tunneling that connects with a body cavity or organ.

102. c. During the proliferation phase, endothelial cells produce new capillaries, and fibroblasts produce collagen. Collagen is the connective tissue that gives granulation tissue structure.

103. d. The pia matter is the structure that has contact with brain tissue in the cranium.

104. a. Although it is an uncommon finding, tic douloureux is highly characteristic of multiple sclerosis in a young person. Tic douloureux (also called trigeminal neuralgia) is a shocklike pain in the face.

105. b. A right-sided cortical lesion could cause problems of visual-spatial processing, whereas a left-sided lesion can result in verbal processing deficits. Damage in the area of the amygdala may lead to heightened arousal, which enhances sensory information processing and is linked to emotional responses. Brainstem dysfunction could lead to decreased blood pressure, heart rate, and respiratory rate.

106. d. Scores of "no response" on eye opening, verbal, and motor sections of the Glasgow Coma Scale are each worth one point. The lowest possible score on the Glasgow Coma Scale is 3 points.

107. c. Cheyne-Stokes breathing often presents in individuals with hemispheric lesions that are bilateral or can be the result of lesions in the diencephalon. Hyperventilation is seen in individuals as pontine or midbrain lesions, and apneustic breathing is characterized by a prolonged pause at the end of inspiration and indicates lesions of the pons.

108. a. About one half of injuries come from excessive flexion of the spinal column; about one third of these injuries result in complete spinal cord lesions.

109. a. Motor involvement, termed lower motor neuron involvement, occurs when any of the following sites is affected: cell body of the alpha motor neuron located in the spinal cord or brainstem, axons that arise from the anterior horn cell form spinal and peripheral nerves and cranial nerves, motor endplate of the axon, and muscle fibers innervated by the motor nerve axon.

110. c. The criterion standard to confirm carpal tunnel syndrome is nerve conduction velocity testing. Changes in the sensory conduction across the wrists are the most sensitive indicator of carpal tunnel syndrome. Phalen's, Tinel's, and carpal compression tests are all provocation tests that are used to replicate carpal tunnel syndrome symptoms. These tests are available to the PTA.

111. c. Because the facial nerve lies in the auditory canal, any agent that causes inflammation and swelling creates a compression that initially causes demyelination

112. d. The olfactory system is the sense of smell and plays no part in balance and postural awareness. The other three choices work together to correct balance.

113. c. The visual system can detect possible changes in body control secondary to the environment. The vestibular system acts only on this information after the body has moved.

114. b. Vertigo is the sensation of the person or room spinning, resulting in reduced balance. This condition involves the vestibular system only. There is a marked increased risk for falls in patients with this diagnosis.

115. c. The functional reach test is performed by having the patient reach forward as far as possible without moving the feet or losing balance.

A reach of 6 inches or less indicates limited functional balance. The risk for falls is increased if the patient cannot anticipate the anterior displacement from this test.

116. c. The motor level grade given to a patient with myelomeningocele is named by the lowest motor level that has intact functional musculature. In this case, the patient has good L3 spinal segment function.

117. d. Neuropathy is essentially damage to the nerve. With nerve damage, one would expect to see choices a, b, and c. Reflexes would possibly be decreased in this scenario rather than increased.

118. b. Choices a, c, and d are all tests that detect possible nerve injury. Each test has a desired response to test the integrity of the nerve. Although the peripheral nerve is involved with the deep tendon reflex, it will generally not elicit a painful response from the patient as the other tests would.

119. a. Somatic motor nerves innervate skeletal muscles. The autonomic nervous system controls all the other choices. Both are considered efferent pathways.

120. c. Sympathetic nerves originate in the lateral horn of the spinal cord, and parasympathetic nerves originate in the brain and lateral gray matter of the spinal cord. Spinal nerves originate in the spinal column.

121. a. Movement in one joint may require the nerve to lengthen and can pull on the nerve where it crosses other joints. As the nerve is elongated, pressure inside the nerve will increase, blood flow will decrease, and strain will increase.

122. d. Because the axillary nerve travels near the humerus, it is most likely injured during anterior shoulder dislocation or fracture of the humeral neck.

123. d. Because the radial nerve innervates the triceps, brachioradialis, and wrist extensors, choice d is the most likely clinical scenario.

124. b. Choice a refers to involvement of peripheral nerve trunks. Choices c and d are multifocal isolated lesions of more than one peripheral nerve.

125. a. Some sebaceous glands produce a fatty secretion and are found in association with every hair follicle. Some sebaceous glands not associated with hair follicles are also found in the general distribution of the body, with the exception of the soles of the feet, the palms of the hands, and the lower lip.

126. b. The apocrine glands begin to secrete a commonly odorless and colorless oily sweat at the onset of puberty. These glands are localized in the anogenital and axillary areas.

127. a. The stratum germinativum (basale) contains stem cells characterized by intense mitotic activity indicative of cellular division because the main function of this layer is the continual renewal of epidermal cells.

128. a. The wound would be documented as a healing stage IV pressure sore. You cannot reverse staging of pressure sores. Healing of pressure ulcers should be documented by objective parameters such as size, depth, amount of necrotic tissue, amount of exudate, and presence of granulation tissue.

129. b. A stage II pressure sore results in partial-thickness skin loss involving the epidermis, dermis, or both. The ulcer is superficial and presents clinically as an abrasion, blister, or shallow crater.

130. d. Patients with platelet values between 60,000 and 40,000 can participate in low load resistance with 1- to 2-pound weights. Safe exercises also include walking, stationary bicycling with light resistance, and performing minimal activities of daily living. Patients with platelet counts of 40,000 to 20,000 require low-intensity exercise with no weights and no resistance during stationary biking. Platelet counts below 20,000 have stringent activity restrictions.

131. d. Eighty to 100 mm Hg of PaO_2 is considered normal. Patients will complain of lightheadedness and nausea at about 50 to 60 mm Hg, whereas 35 to 50 mm Hg of PaO_2 will lead to marked confusion. A PaO_2 level of 25 to 35 mm Hg is indicative of cardiac arrest.

132. b. If the bronchus is obstructed, atelectasis occurs while air in the alveoli is slowly absorbed into the bloodstream with the subsequent collapse of the alveoli.

133. a. Although aspirin has been used to decrease the risk for myocardial infarction, warfarin sodium has been proved to be significantly more effective than aspirin in the prevention of stroke in individuals with atrial fibrillation.

134. c. The axillary artery is too deep for pulse assessment. The other choices are much more superficial, which allows accurate pulse assessment.

135. c. In certain conditions, tone is disturbed, and a patient may present with hypotonia (low tone) or hypertonia (high tone). The disturbance in tone may be evident at rest, during activities, or both. Spasticity varies with the speed and direction of joint movement.

136. c. The other choices are part of a pediatric physical therapy assessment. Screening is usually indicated when a child is at risk for developmental delay or disability and is a quick way to determine whether the child is in need of further diagnostic services. Assessment measures are used to gain more in-depth information about the child's strength and needs in all developmental domains.

137. c. The SOAP note format is rarely used as a documentation method for pediatric patients. Instead, the necessary information is contained in the IFSP or an IEP developed for each child. The Gross Motor Function Measure is a tool for assessment of a pediatric patient. It can be used to assess the child's progress as therapy continues.

138. a. Of the choices listed, CN II, or the optic nerve, functions to constrict the pupil and vision. Ischemia, resulting from stroke or head injury, and pressure from tumors are two of the factors that can adversely affect the function of the nerve. Visual field loss depends on the location of the lesion. A lesion occurring before the optic chiasm results in loss of vision in the fields on the same side. After the optic chiasm, a lesion will cause loss of vision in both fields. The visual field affected will be opposite the side of the lesion and is also known as homonymous hemianopsia.

139. d. The saphenous nerve lies just anterior to the medial malleolus and runs parallel the great saphenous vein. This nerve is most likely to be injured by the sutures.

140. b. The phrenic nerve arises from ventral rami of C3, C4, and C5 spinal nerves. The sensory neurons of the dorsal root ganglia of C3, C4, and C5 supply axons for somatic pain from the named area of parietal serous membranes. C3, C4, and C5 also supply the shoulder with the cutaneous innervation by the supraclavicular nerves. This is why pericardial or diaphragmatic pain will refer to the shoulder.

141. b. The neural canal (vertebral canal) is the largest and most triangular in the cervical region and the smallest and most circular in the thoracic region.

142. a. The white matter of the spinal cord carries ascending (sensory) tracts and descending (motor) tracts.

143. c. The four cranial nerves that contain parasympathetic fibers are oculomotor, facial, glossopharyngeal, and vagus nerves.

144. b. A fibers are the largest in diameter and conduct faster than C fibers.

145. b. The fifth lumbar nerve root is impinged because it arises from the spinal column superior to the L4-L5 lumbar disk.

146. c. The common peroneal nerve travels over the lateral knee. It is the least likely to be injured. The other structures are either within the knee or directly posterior.

147. b. A nerve regenerates at an approximate rate of 1 inch per month.

148. b. All the pharyngeal muscles are supplied by the vagus nerve (CN X), except the stylopharyngeus muscle, which is supplied by the glosso-pharyngeal nerve (CN IX).

149. d. Nerve conduction/electromyographic studies are useful for identifying the possible injury site along the lower motor nerve reflex but cannot provide a definitive clinical diagnosis.

150. a. A lesion of a peripheral nerve produces a complete paralysis of the muscles innervated by this nerve. Weakness is immediately apparent when testing the motor function. A lesion of a unique nerve root produces paresis of the myotome (group of muscles innervated by a single nerve root) innervated by this nerve root. Some time is necessary for the weakness to become apparent when testing for motor function. The isometric contraction must be held for a minimum of 5 seconds.

151. d. According to Hoppenfeld, the patella deep tendon reflex muscles (the quadriceps muscle group) are innervated by the L4 nerve root through the femoral nerve.

152. c. The rubrospinal tract originates in the red nucleus; the reticulospinal tract originates in the medullary and pontine reticular formation; and the vestibulospinal tract originates in the lateral vestibular nucleus.

153. d. Stage I of hepatic encephalopathy is characterized by tension and depression disorders with minor tremor and incoordination. Hepatic encephalopathy can then proceed to stage IV, in which the patient is considered comatose with a positive Babinski's reflex and possibly decerebrate posturing.

154. d. As the action potential reaches the neuron's terminal, it stimulates the release of a chemical neurotransmitter cell through the presynaptic terminals. The intensity of the conducting signals is determined by the frequency of individual action potentials.

155. c. The chemical communication involved in this process is universally known as either neurotransmission or neuromodulation.

156. b. The reticular formation is a diffuse network of neurons extending through the brainstem to higher levels and is important in influencing movement.

157. c. The optic nerve is involved in visual acuity, and the oculomotor nerve innervates many muscles of the eye, including the inferior oblique muscle and medial, inferior, and superior rectus muscles of the eye. The trigeminal nerve is involved in sensation of the face.

158. d. The spinal accessory nerve innervates the trapezius and sterno-cleidomastoid muscles. The other nerves listed have the ability to transmit sensory signals.

159. a. The vestibulocerebellum connects to the cortex and brainstem, and the spinocerebellum connects to the somatosensory tracts of the spinal cord. It receives input from the cortex regarding ongoing motor command. The cerebrocerebellum is involved in complex motor and cognitive tasks.

160. d. The parietal lobe is responsible for body sensations and visual-spatial perception. The temporal lobe is responsible for hearing and language, and Broca's area is responsible for language expression.

161. c. Moderate to large amounts of necrotic tissue will predispose a wound to become chronic. Ischemia will not allow proper blood flow to the wound, and rolled edges of a wound include signs of unresponsive growth factors. Insufficient underlying connective tissue will often lead to an overgrowth of epithelium.

162. a. Shear forces can damage subcutaneous capillaries, resulting in tissue ischemia in the deeper tissues and subsequently in the skin. Because of this, tissue destruction occurs in deep tracts along fascial planes. This type of pressure ulcer is known as a sinus tract.

163. d. Normal skin is slightly acidic to protect it from bacterial penetration and infection. Skin exposed to urinary or fecal incontinence increases surface pH of the skin and bacterial exposure.

164. c. When moisture is inadequately managed, the periwound skin is often macerated. The therapist should check the patient's skin for further moisture, and possibly contact nursing services.

165. d. The wound stage will not change as it heals. If the wound is stage III, it does not become stage II as it granulates. The correct nomenclature would be a stage III wound in the proliferation phase or a stage III wound in the remodeling phase.

166. c. The ABI is a common noninvasive test used to determine the ratio of systolic pressure in the ankle relative to the systolic pressure in the brachial artery in the upper extremity. Normally, blood pressure at the ankle is equal to or slightly higher than brachial blood pressure.

The ABI should be 1 to 1.4. An ABI of less than 0.9 indicates the presence of lower extremity arterial disease.

167. d. Ulcers on the neuropathic foot occur either on the weight-bearing surfaces or where the shoe is in contact with the foot. This would occur in choices a and b and not in choice d. Shoes and socks should be inspected for damage that could cause an ulcer.

168. d. The test for protective sensation on the plantar surface of the foot uses the 5.07 filament that bends on 10 g of pressure. The inability to feel this monofilament on the plantar aspect of the foot has been shown to predict foot ulceration in patients with type 2 diabetes.

169. a. The patient's wound has neared completion of healing as it enters the remodeling phase. In the other choices, the injuries are too acute or the patient is in too much pain to tolerate manual muscle testing. There is no need for manual muscle testing on an open burn injury before skin grafting.

170. b. Both the anterior and posterior surfaces of the upper extremity count as 4.5% of the total body surface area. A burn covering the entire upper extremity would then be classified as 9% of total body surface area.

171. a. The stratum corneum is the most superficial layer of the epidermis. The other structures arise in the dermis and pass through the epidermis.

172. b. Because of the length-dependent phenomenon of polyneuropathies, the distal portion of the limb will be more affected than the proximal portion of the limb.

173. c. The GCS is widely used because of its simplicity. The score ranges from a low of 3 to a high of 15.

174. d. Patients with locked-in syndrome have intact normal consciousness, but all motor pathways to the face, trunk, and limbs are damaged. These patients are awake and fully aware of their condition, but cannot move.

175. c. About 70% to 80% of complex partial seizures arise from the temporal lobe. Remaining cases of complex partial seizures arise mainly from the frontal lobe, with smaller percentages originating in the parietal and occipital lobes.

176. b. The ampulla is directed away from the direction of head movement by the movement of the endolymph.

177. b. The lateral vestibulospinal tract receives the majority of its input from the otoliths in the cerebellum. It is responsible for postural activity in the lower extremities in response to head position changes that occur with respect to gravity.

178. a. The medial vestibulospinal tract gets its input from the circular canals and triggers postural responses with regard to angular head motion.

179. d. The vertebral basilar artery supplies blood to the components of the vestibular system. The posterior and inferior cerebellar arteries feed the central nervous system. Because there is redundant blood supply through the circle of Willis, ischemia in this area is rare.

180. a. Vestibular-evoked myogenic potential (VEMP) is an excellent way to test otolith function in the clinic. VEMP testing generally involves a standard sound set and looking for inhibition of the sternocleidomastoid recorded during electromyography.

181. b. The vestibular system, in conjunction with other systems, allows us to maintain our orientation in space, controls our posture, and maintains our balance. Although the vestibular system is in the ear, it does not function in the sense of hearing.

182. a. Tachycardia is defined as a pulse above 100 beats/minute, and bradycardia is defined as a heart rate of less than 60 beats/minute at rest.

183. b. Bradypnea is defined as less than 10 breaths/minute in a resting adult, and tachypnea is defined as more than 20 breaths/minute in an adult. Choice a is the absence of breathing, and choice c occurs when ventilation is inadequate to perform needed gas exchange.

184. a. The upper arm is the most common site because of ease of measuring blood pressure. Blood pressure can be taken at all the other sites mentioned, but it is more difficult, and sometimes specialized blood pressure cuffs are needed.

185. c. Orthostatic hypotension occurs when a patient has been confined to bed rest for an extended amount of time. It is primarily caused by gravity-induced blood pooling in the lower extremities, which in turn compromises venous return. There is a decrease in cardiac output and lowering of arterial pressure. The overall effect of this is insufficient blood to the upper part of the body. There is a vasoconstriction response to move blood superiorly to counteract the decreasing blood pressure.

186. c. The normal adolescent respiratory rate is 18 to 22 breaths/minute, and a normal resting heart rate for an adult is between 60 and 100 beats/minute. Normal adult blood pressure is 120/80 mm Hg.

187. d. The four traditional vital signs are temperature, pulse, respiratory rate, and blood pressure. Two additional measures—pain level and oxygen saturation—were more recently added to these.

188. b. The sublingual pocket is on both sides of the frenulum under the tongue and is closest to the sublingual arteries. This gives the most accurate oral temperature.

189. c. Reinflating the cuff and repeating the test could cause an inaccurate result. The therapist should wait at least 2 minutes before attempting to obtain a blood pressure again.

190. d. Choices a, b, and c could all give an inaccurate blood pressure reading. The recent rotator cuff surgery would not affect blood pressure in the involved extremity.

191. c. Maximal oxygen uptake or VO_{2max} is the maximum amount of oxygen in milliliters that the body can use in 1 minute per kilogram of body weight. This is considered the best indicator of cardiopulmonary fitness.

192. a. Maximum heart rate is sometimes used to prescribe exercise intensity. It can be estimated by subtracting the patient's age from 220. This patient's age adjusted maximum heart rate would be 150 beats/minute.

193. b. Normally, expiration lasts twice as long an inspiration.

194. a. Because a patient's subjective comments can sometimes mislead the examiner, they should not be used solely to determine the severity of heart failure. The other three choices are objective signs to determine fluid status.

195. d. The diaphragm is innervated by the phrenic nerve, which originates from cervical roots C3, C4, and C5. It originates on the upper three lumbar vertebrae, the lower border of the rib cage, and the xiphoid process. The fibers converge to form and insert on the common central tendon.

196. d. Forced vital capacity is a volume of air forcefully exhaled from maximum inspiration to maximum expiration. The volume of air in the lungs after maximum expiration is called residual volume. Inspiratory capacity is the volume of air from tidal expiration to maximum inhalation.

197. d. Although any of these measures could be decreased, decreases in flow rates are more often associated with obstructive lung diseases. Compromised lung volumes and capacities are often associated with restrictive lung diseases.

198. a. Secondary lymphedema occurs in the absence of an anatomic malformation. This is usually caused by a traumatic injury, tumor obstruction of lymph flow, or breast cancer treatments.

199. c. Just as testing of the noninvolved lower extremity is important in a knee evaluation, measurements of the unaffected extremity are important in patients with lymphedema. The PTA should understand what is considered normal for each patient before beginning treatment.

200. c. Primary lymphedema involves a malformation of the lymph vessels and lymph nodes. It may be congenital or develop later in life.

201. b. To provide consistent measurements over time, the tape should not indent the tissue, but rather should be in firm contact with the skin throughout the circumference of the involved extremity.

202. c. A positive Doppler signal is defined as absent pulses to palpation but an audible Doppler signal. These pulses are usually not graded on the 0 to 4+ scale.

203. a. The lower the metabolic equivalent, the lower the oxygen consumption in kilocalories expended. This would translate to lower work or, in this case, lower walking speed.

204. b. A body mass index of 18.5 to 24.9 is considered a normal weight. Morbidly obese clients have a body mass index higher than 40.

205. c. The basic metabolic panel is a group of age-specific tests for electrolyte level, acid-base balance, blood sugar, and kidney status.

206. d. White blood cell count can be provided as a total or a count of individual types or subtypes of leukocytes. In general, an increase suggests infection or other inflammatory response.

207. a. Newborns have up to 60% hematocrit level, with adult men having 30% to 39%. Children have a normal hematocrit percentage of 30% to 49%, with adult women having 36% to 46%. Hematocrit is a simple test involving a small quantity of blood that can be obtained with a simple skin prick.

208. d. Vital capacity is the volume of air that is measured in slow maximal respiration after a maximal inspiration. The largest volume of air that can be inhaled from a resting expiratory volume is inspiratory capacity. The largest volume of air that can be exhaled from resting in expiratory level is the expiratory reserve volume.

209. b. The right atrium receives venous blood from the body through the superior and inferior venae cavae.

210. b. The left atrium receives oxygenated blood through the pulmonary veins coming from the lungs.

211. d. The greater muscle mass of the left ventricle provides enough force to flow the blood through the peripheral arteries. Oxygenated blood leaves the left ventricle through the aortic valve into the aorta and is transported to the body through the systemic circulation.

212. b. The sinoatrial node initiates the impulse in the heart and is referred to as the pacemaker.

213. b. The myocardium of the heart receives its blood supply from two major vessels: the right and upper coronary arteries. A blockage that prevents oxygen supply to the heart, causing permanent damage to the heart cells, is known as a heart attack or myocardial infarction.

214. d. The upper conducting airway includes the nose, pharynx, and larynx. The lower conducting airway is made of the trachea and bronchiole system.

215. c. Generally, in a pulmonary function test, the patient blows as hard as possible with the biggest breath into a machine called a spirometer. This device measures the various volumes in airflow rates, which are compared with a normal scale. The degree of change from normal helps assess the seriousness of the lung disease.

216. b. The term "bucket handle" refers to the ribs protruding from the lateral side of the thorax. Severe chronic obstructive pulmonary disease does not produce asymmetrical chest expansion; instead, chest expansion is increased bilaterally.

217. b. The sinoatrial node is located in the right atrium of the heart. It serves as the pacemaker for the heart. Impulses generated there are passed on from right to left and inferiorly to the atrioventricular node in the lower end of the interatrial septum.

218. b. The vessels of various sizes provide transmission conduits for body fluids, but the exchange described takes place between cell surfaces and the interstitial fluid.

219. d. During this phase, all of the ventricular volume has been ejected. The semilunar and atrioventricular valves are closed, and no volume is changing in the ventricles. This phase has the lowest volume.

220. b. The sinoatrial node has a frequency of 70 to 80 depolarizations per minute; the atrioventricular node frequency is 40 to 60; the Purkinje cell frequency is 15 to 40; and the myocardium is even slower. This question refers to how often these fibers will have action potentials, not how fast they travel.

221. b. Inspiratory capacity is the volume of air moved going from normal expiration to full forced inspiration. Total lung capacity is the volume of air in the lung on full forced inspiration and cannot be measured on spirometry. Inspiratory reserve volume is the volume of air moved going from normal inspiration to full forced inspiration.

222. c. The heart receives nerve impulses that travel through the sinoatrial node to the ventricles by way of the atrioventricular node, bundle branches, and Purkinje fibers.

223. c. Lymphedema is swelling that occurs when protein-rich lymph fluid accumulates in the interstitial tissue. This lymph fluid may contain plasma proteins, extravascular blood cells, excess water, and parenchymal products.

224. b. The first sound heard corresponds to closing of the mitral and tricuspid valves. The second sound corresponds to closing of the aortic and pulmonic valves. Therefore, the first sound is indicative of the onset of ventricular systole, and the second sound is indicative of the onset of ventricular diastole. The first sound is usually lower in pitch and longer than the second.

225. b. A decreased tidal volume is caused by a restrictive lung dysfunction. An increased tidal volume is caused by an obstructive lung dysfunction. Choices c and d are in the family of obstructive pulmonary disease.

226. b. The pelvic diaphragm is composed of the levator ani and coccygeus muscles. This pelvic diaphragm assists in forced expiration, coughing, sneezing, vomiting, urinating, defecating, and fixation of the trunk during strong movements of the upper limb.

CHAPTER 2

Diseases and Conditions

Questions

1. Which of the following is an example of an organ-specific autoimmune disorder?
    a. Crohn's disease
    b. Multiple sclerosis
    c. Myasthenia gravis
    d. Rheumatoid arthritis

2. A PTA begins intervention for a patient diagnosed with liver cancer. Which of the following choices is a normal complication of liver cancer and would NOT require the PTA to contact the referring physician or the supervising physical therapist?
    a. Chest pain
    b. Unusual pain
    c. Night pain
    d. Shoulder pain

3. Which of the following is associated with strenuous exercise?
    a. Anorexia
    b. Belching
    c. Constipation
    d. Achalasia

4. Which of the following is NOT considered a major cause of upper gastrointestinal bleeding?
    a. Major trauma or systemic illness
    b. Peptic ulcers
    c. Chronic alcohol abuse
    d. Failure of the lower esophageal sphincter

5. Which of the following could cause decreased pressure of the lower esophageal sphincter, predisposing an individual to gastroesophageal reflux disease?
    a. Obesity
    b. Caffeine
    c. Antacids
    d. Histamines

6. Which of the following medications will stop acid production in the stomach?
   a. Tums
   b. Mylanta
   c. Zantac
   d. Prilosec

7. Presence of a peptic ulcer will radiate pain to what part of the body?
   a. Right upper quadrant
   b. Right lower quadrant
   c. Left upper quadrant
   d. Left lower quadrant

8. Which of the following conditions is considered a chronic inflammatory disorder of the mucosa and submucosa of the colon in a continuous manner?
   a. Crohn's disease
   b. Regional enteritis
   c. Ulcerative colitis
   d. Terminal ileitis

9. What type of hernia occurs when a sac formed from the peritoneum and intestines pushes outward through the abdominal wall?
   a. Sports hernia
   b. Inguinal hernia
   c. Femoral hernia
   d. Umbilical hernia

10. Which of the following symptoms are most likely to raise suspicion of liver disease?
    a. Fever, melena, urinary frequency
    b. Left shoulder pain, pallor, coffee-ground emesis
    c. Jaundice, ascites, asterixis
    d. Left upper quadrant pain, nausea, diaphoresis

11. Cheyne-Stokes respiration is common with which of the following?
    a. Anxiety
    b. Renal failure
    c. Strenuous exercise
    d. Chronic fatigue syndrome

12. All of the following can be described as a type of chronic obstructive pulmonary disease EXCEPT which?
    a. Asthma
    b. Acute bronchitis
    c. Obstructive bronchiolitis
    d. Emphysema

13. Which of the following is NOT a sign or symptom of pulmonary edema?
    a. Hypoventilation
    b. Engorged neck and hand veins
    c. Pitting edema of the extremities
    d. Nocturnal dyspnea

14. Hyperventilation is least likely to occur in which of the following scenarios?
    a. After severe exertion
    b. After a period of high anxiety
    c. With fever
    d. After a head injury

15. What system of the body is most affected by deconditioning?
    a. Integumentary
    b. Neurologic
    c. Musculoskeletal
    d. Cardiovascular

16. What is the primary impairment for a patient with limited functional activities related to deconditioning?
    a. Abnormal posture
    b. Muscle weakness
    c. Pain
    d. Endurance

17. Which of the following would be the first to decline after a period of bed rest for a healthy 45-year-old man?
    a. Pulmonary function
    b. Heart rate
    c. Muscle metabolism
    d. Maximum oxygen consumption rate

18. The inspiratory-to-expiratory ratio you would expect to see in the patient with chronic obstructive pulmonary disease is which of the following?
    a. 1:1
    b. 1:2
    c. 1:4
    d. 2:1

19. The thoracic index (anteroposterior-to-lateral thoracic diameter ratio) in an individual with severe pulmonary emphysema would likely be which of the following?
    a. 1:1
    b. 1:2
    c. 1:3
    d. 2:1

20. Which of the following breath sounds is always considered abnormal no matter where it is heard on the thorax using auscultation?
    a. Tracheal
    b. Bronchial
    c. Wheezing
    d. Vesicular

21. Which of the following is TRUE about systolic heart failure?
    a. It is most prevalent in males.
    b. It is difficult to diagnose.
    c. It may have ischemic or nonischemic causes.
    d. It is defined by an ejection fraction greater than 35%.

22. What is the hallmark symptom of heart failure?
    a. Cyanosis of the lips
    b. Difficulty standing
    c. Decreased exercise tolerance
    d. Chest pain with exertion

23. In which stage of lymphedema is there no measurable increase in limb volume?
    a. Stage 0
    b. Stage I
    c. Stage II
    d. Stage III

24. Which stage of lymphedema is characterized by hyperkeratosis?
    a. Stage 0
    b. Stage I
    c. Stage II
    d. Stage III

25. What are the two most common chronic obstructive pulmonary disease conditions?
    a. Respiratory failure and asthma
    b. Emphysema and chronic bronchitis
    c. Chronic bronchitis and respiratory failure
    d. Emphysema and asthma

26. If the left ventricle does NOT contract appropriately as in congestive heart failure, where will an abnormal amount of blood collect?
    a. Liver
    b. Abdominal cavity
    c. Lungs
    d. Legs

27. Which of the following is considered an invasive procedure for the cardiovascular system?
    a. Echocardiography
    b. Transesophageal echocardiography
    c. Cardiac catheterization
    d. Electrocardiogram

28. Which of the following is indicative of left heart failure?
    a. Pitting pedal edema
    b. Neck vein distention
    c. Orthopnea
    d. Ascites

29. A patient asks the PTA to explain the function of his medication verapamil (a calcium antagonist). Which of the following points should be conveyed in the explanation?
    a. Verapamil causes decreased contractility of the heart and vasodilation of the coronary arteries.
    b. Verapamil causes decreased contractility of the heart and vasoconstriction of the coronary arteries.
    c. Verapamil causes increased contractility of the heart and vasodilation of the coronary arteries.
    d. Verapamil causes increased contractility of the heart and vasoconstriction of the coronary arteries.

30. Which of the following statements is NOT a common physiologic change of aging?
    a. Blood pressure taken at rest and during exercise increases
    b. Maximal oxygen uptake decreases
    c. Residual volume decreases
    d. Bone mass decreases

31. A patient whose resting and exercise-induced heart rates are less than they were before is most likely starting therapy with which of the following?
    a. Anticholinergic drugs
    b. Alpha blockers
    c. Beta blockers
    d. Antianginal drugs

32. A patient inhales a beta agonist to relieve her asthma. You may notice which of the following after its use?
    a. An increase in heart rate
    b. A few moments of incoordination
    c. Flushing with red face
    d. A decrease in blood pressure

33. Statin drugs lower cholesterol by which of the following?
    a. Preventing cholesterol absorption
    b. Binding to cholesterol in the intestines
    c. Inhibiting HMG-CoA reductase
    d. Inhibiting lipoprotein lipase

34. A patient is being treated with an antiarrhythmic drug. The drug might cause all of the following adverse reactions EXCEPT which?
    a. Dizziness and fainting
    b. Stevens-Johnson syndrome
    c. Irregular heart beats
    d. Joint and muscle pain

35. An asthmatic patient is to be exercised in a rather cool environment. It is recommended that he should use the inhaler at what frequency?
    a. About 1 hour before the exercise
    b. About 20 minutes before exercise
    c. Just at the beginning of exercise
    d. At the first onset of breathing problems during exercise

36. A patient using a beta blocker is exercised and might experience all of the following EXCEPT which?
    a. Some breathing difficulties
    b. Muscle cramps and pain
    c. A smaller than expected increase in heart rate
    d. Some drowsiness

37. A beta blocker reduces blood pressure by all of the following actions EXCEPT which?
    a. A reduction in cardiac output
    b. A reduction in central sympathetic outflow
    c. Inhibition of renin release
    d. A reduction in peripheral resistance

38. A patient on calcium channel blocker therapy might complain during therapy sessions about all of the following EXCEPT which?
    a. Lightheadedness and dizziness
    b. Muscle pain and joint stiffness
    c. Tremors
    d. Edema

39. Your patient is a 48-year-old man who reports to physical therapy with complaints of left shoulder and neck pain. Symptoms began insidiously 3 weeks ago and have been increasing in frequency and duration since that time. He notices the symptoms with lifting heavy objects and shoveling dirt for a garden that he is building. Walking fast elicits symptoms. Symptoms abate after several minutes of rest. He is

in relatively good health with the exception of high blood pressure and shortness of breath. What system is most likely affected?

a. Cardiovascular
b. Pulmonary
c. Musculoskeletal
d. Hepatic

40. Your patient is a 38-year-old man who is a patient that you have been treating for left shoulder pain. He was in a motor vehicle crash since you last treated him 2 days ago. He was the driver and was rear-ended. He hit his left side on the door handle and has been having sharp pain in his ribs. Radiographs the day of the accident revealed fractured ribs (ribs 6 and 7 on the left). He has been having difficulty breathing and has been very short of breath. Sharp pain is noted on the left with breathing and coughing. He has also noticed some blood in his sputum. What is system is mostly likely the source of the patient's symptoms?

a. Musculoskeletal
b. Pulmonary
c. Cardiovascular
d. Hepatic

41. Aspirin and clopidogrel (Plavix) fall into which class of antithrombics?

a. Thrombolytics
b. Platelet aggregator inhibitors
c. Anticoagulants
d. Fibrinolytics

42. Which of the following drugs should patients with angina always carry in case of an anginal attack?

a. Nitroglycerin patch
b. Angiotensin-converting enzyme inhibitor
c. Digoxin
d. Sublingual nitroglycerin

43. Some of the classes of drugs used to treat angina include which of the following?

a. Nitrates
b. HMG-CoA reductase inhibitors
c. Alpha blockers
d. Diuretics

44. Beta blockers that are useful in the treatment of hypertension are characterized by which of the following?

a. Work by competitively inhibiting beta receptors, thereby decreasing heart rate
b. Are always selective for beta-1 receptors

    c. Do not cause bronchoconstriction in patients with asthma

    d. Should not be combined with any other type of antihypertensive medication

45. Which of the following medications should be used to treat an acute asthma attack?

    a. Oral steroid such as prednisone

    b. Long-acting beta agonist such as salmeterol

    c. Inhaled steroid such as fluticasone

    d. Short acting beta agonist such as albuterol

46. Primary lymphedema occurs in which of the following patients?

    a. Older, who have had surgery

    b. Younger, who have had surgery

    c. Younger, who have not had surgery

    d. Older, who have not had surgery

47. A patient using diuretics might experience during strenuous exercise all of the following EXCEPT which?

    a. Easy bruising

    b. Dehydration

    c. Muscle cramping

    d. Dyspnea

48. A PTA is working with a patient who has chronic obstructive pulmonary disease. If the patient's level of oxygen being carried by arterial blood is measured, a PaO^2 finding of what is considered normal?

    a. 35 to 45 mm Hg

    b. 60 to 80 mm Hg

    c. 80 to 100 mm Hg

    d. 100 to 120 mm Hg

49. The most serious complication of lower extremity thrombophlebitis is which of the following?

    a. Cerebral infarction

    b. Pulmonary infarction

    c. Myocardial infarction

    d. Kidney infection

50. At a team meeting, the respiratory therapist informs the rest of the team that the patient, just admitted to the subacute floor, experienced breathing difficulty in the acute care department. The respiratory therapist describes the breathing problem as a pause before exhaling after a full inspiration. Which of the following is the therapist describing?

    a. Apnea

    b. Orthopnea

c. Eupnea

d. Apneusis

51. A PTA is performing chest physiotherapy on a patient who is coughing up a significant amount of sputum. The PTA later describes the quality of the sputum in his notes as mucoid. This description tells other personnel which of the following?

a. The sputum is thick.

b. The sputum has a foul odor.

c. The sputum is clear or white in color.

d. The patient has a possible bronchopulmonary infection.

52. A PTA is sent to provide passive range of motion to a patient in the intensive care unit. The chart reveals that the patient is suffering from pulmonary edema. The charge nurse informs the PTA that the patient is coughing up thin white sputum with a pink tint. Which of the following terms best describes this sputum?

a. Purulent

b. Frothy

c. Mucopurulent

d. Rusty

53. Which of the following conditions is a generalized connective tissue disorder of unknown origin cause characterized by thickening and fibrosis of the skin?

a. Rheumatoid arthritis

b. Systemic lupus erythematosus

c. Systemic sclerosis

d. Sarcoidosis

54. Where on the body are herpes simplex virus type 1 skin lesions most likely to appear?

a. On the genitals

b. In distal sensory nerve distributions

c. On the mouth or lips

d. In the nose

55. Which of the following populations is considered at low risk for cellulitis?

a. Patients diagnosed with diabetes

b. Patients older than 80 years

c. Patients with pressure ulcers

d. Patients diagnosed with fibromyalgia

56. What is the most commonly recognized skin manifestation of systemic lupus erythematosus?

a. Discoid lesions

b. Venostasis ulcers

c. Butterfly rash over the nose

d. Rash on the posterior surface of the knee

57. A full-thickness burn has what feature?
    a. Is painful
    b. Usually requires surgical intervention
    c. Is caused by sunburn
    d. Is wet or shiny in appearance

58. Which of the following areas is the most common location for a diabetic ulcer?
    a. Plantar surface of the metatarsal head
    b. Dorsal surface of the metatarsals
    c. Lateral malleolus
    d. Medial malleolus

59. Which of the following is indicative of an arterial ulcer?
    a. Edema in the involved lower extremity, superficial wound with red wound base
    b. Wound over the lateral malleolus with minimum exudate and a dry wound bed
    c. Nonpainful wound with a craterlike center with an elevated rim
    d. Weeping wound above malleoli

60. Which of the following areas would NOT be a concern for possible skin breakdown for a patient with spina bifida?
    a. Greater trochanter
    b. Sacrum
    c. Heels
    d. Lumbar spine

61. Infection may not be obvious in patients with arterial compromise because of which of the following?
    a. Reduced perfusion
    b. Sensory loss
    c. Trophic changes
    d. Bony deformities

62. Which of the following statements about venous ulcers is TRUE?
    a. The ulcer tends to be deep and dry.
    b. The ulcer tends to be shallow and wet.
    c. The ulcer has a punched-out appearance.
    d. The wound bed is most often necrotic.

63. Kyphoscoliosis primarily affects what part of the spine?
    a. Cervical
    b. Thoracic
    c. Lumbar
    d. Sacral

64. Which of the following spinal cord disorders describes external protrusion only of the meninges?
    a. Spina bifida occulta
    b. Myelomeningocele
    c. Meningocele
    d. Spondylitis

65. Why does osteomyelitis in the adult population lead to pathologic fracture?
    a. The epiphyseal growth plate is usually involved.
    b. The periosteum is loosely attached to bone and moves away easily.
    c. Osteomyelitis is rare in adults.
    d. Infection disrupts and weakens the cortex inside the bone without pain.

66. How does back pain associated with osteomyelitis react with patient activity?
    a. Back pain would diminish with activity.
    b. Back pain would not be present in a radicular distribution.
    c. Back pain would be intermittent only.
    d. Back pain would commonly be accompanied by spinal tenderness.

67. Which of the following is indicative of mechanical loosening of a prosthetic joint?
    a. A wound over the surgical incision with drainage
    b. Constant joint pain
    c. Pain with motion or weight bearing through the joint
    d. Complaints of pain accompanied by fever

68. Which of the following is a malignant tumor of the bone marrow?
    a. Osteoma
    b. Leukemia
    c. Chondroma
    d. Fibroma

69. Which of the following bones is least likely to develop osteosarcoma?
    a. Vertebra
    b. Femur
    c. Humerus
    d. Tibia

70. What type of benign soft tissue tumor is usually seen in the popliteal area?
    a. Lipoma
    b. Baker's cyst
    c. Nerve sheath tumor
    d. Schwannoma

71. What is the most common osteoporosis-related fracture?
    a. Vertebral compression fracture
    b. Rib fracture
    c. Metacarpal fracture
    d. Hip fracture

72. What are the two primary causes of osteomalacia?
    a. Diabetes mellitus and increased renal phosphorus loss
    b. Insufficient intestinal calcium absorption and diabetes mellitus
    c. Excessive corticosteroid use and increased renal phosphorus losses
    d. Insufficient intestinal calcium absorption and increased renal phosphorus losses

73. What is the most common presenting symptom in Paget's disease?
    a. Fatigue
    b. Tendonitis
    c. Pain
    d. General stiffness

74. What type of fracture most commonly occurs in distance runners?
    a. Pathologic fracture
    b. Stress fracture
    c. Traumatic fracture
    d. Compound fracture

75. What is the most common site of osteochondritis dissecans?
    a. Lateral femoral condyle
    b. Medial femoral condyle
    c. Tibial tubercle
    d. Calcaneus

76. What age group is most likely to suffer from Osgood-Schlatter syndrome?
    a. Infants
    b. Toddlers
    c. Adolescents
    d. Elderly people

77. Definitive osteophyte formation occurs at what grade of osteoarthritis?
    a. Grade I
    b. Grade II
    c. Grade III
    d. Grade IV

78. Which of the following signs/symptoms is indicative of osteoarthritis?
    a. Its onset may be sudden over several weeks or months.
    b. Inflammation, redness, and warmth are always present.

  c. Osteoarthritis usually begins on one side of the body.

  d. Systemic presentation with fatigue, weight loss, and fever is characteristic of osteoarthritis.

79. Which of the following is indicative of swan-neck deformity?
  a. Hyperflexion of the proximal interphalangeal joint and flexion of the distal interphalangeal joint
  b. Flexion of the proximal interphalangeal joint and hyperextension of the distal interphalangeal joint
  c. Hyperextension of the proximal interphalangeal joint and extension of the distal interphalangeal joint
  d. Hyperextension of the proximal interphalangeal joint and partial flexion of the distal interphalangeal joint

80. Which of the following is FALSE regarding heterotopic ossification (HO)?
  a. HO usually appears 4 to 12 weeks after the injury.
  b. Usually the first sign of HO is loss of range of motion around a joint.
  c. HO is not associated with traumatic brain injury.
  d. There is erythema, swelling, and pain with movement of the affected joint.

81. At what age would a person be considered to have peak bone mass?
  a. 12 years
  b. 24 years
  c. 36 years
  d. 56 years

82. Which of the following clients would have the greatest risk for developing osteoporosis?
  a. An Asian man who weighs 175 pounds
  b. An African American woman who weighs 150 pounds
  c. A Caucasian woman who weighs 120 pounds
  d. A Caucasian man who weighs 285 pounds

83. What is the most common manifestation of osteoporosis?
  a. Hip fractures
  b. Rib fractures
  c. Loss of wrist range of motion into extension
  d. Vertebral compression fractures

84. Which of the following is TRUE regarding age-related muscle strength?
  a. Loss is generally uniform for most muscle groups
  b. Upper extremity strength declines faster than lower extremity strength
  c. Strength potential is at its greatest between 18 and 30 years of age
  d. Changes in strength are not generally associated with less use

85. The patient history helps in selection of interventions for patients with connective tissue dysfunctions. Which of the following is NOT true?
    a. Many of these pathologies are chronic and systemic; thus, lifestyle adaptations need to be developed.
    b. Selection of interventions should not be previous experiences and outcomes.
    c. The behavior of symptoms may vary based on activity level, medications, and compensatory mechanisms.
    d. It identifies patient education opportunities to help them become self-managers.

86. Which of the following is NOT a joint manifestation of rheumatoid arthritis?
    a. Acute synovitis
    b. Morning stiffness
    c. Swan-neck deformities
    d. Heberden's nodes

87. Which of the following diseases could be categorized as an autoimmune disease that results from the body producing antibodies directed against its own tissue?
    a. Rheumatoid arthritis
    b. Osteoarthritis
    c. Systemic lupus erythematosus
    d. Ankylosing spondylitis

88. What is the clinical presentation of a boutonniere deformity?
    a. Flexion at the proximal interphalangeal (PIP) joint and hyperextension at the distal interphalangeal (DIP) joint
    b. Extension at the PIP joint and flexion at the DIP joint
    c. Flexion at the PIP joint and flexion at the DIP joint
    d. Extension at the PIP joint and extension at the DIP joint

89. Which of the following conditions is most likely to involve weakness in the proximal musculature?
    a. Polymyositis
    b. Osteoarthritis
    c. Systemic lupus erythematosus
    d. Ankylosing spondylitis

90. Gout is caused by high blood levels of which of the following?
    a. Potassium
    b. Sodium
    c. Uric acid
    d. Lactic acid

91. What is the first effect of osteoarthritis on a healthy joint?
    a. Subchondral bone will be eroded.
    b. Fragments of cartilage fall into the joint.
    c. Inflammatory mediators damage healthy cartilage.
    d. Structure of articular cartilage is compromised.

92. Which of the following is NOT a risk factor for development of osteoarthritis?
    a. Male gender
    b. Age
    c. Obesity
    d. Developmental hip disorders

93. Sequestrated intervertebral disk herniation is characterized by which of the following?
    a. Bulging of the outer annular fibers because of migration of nuclear material through annular tears, although outer annular fibers remain intact
    b. Vertical extrusion of nuclear material through the vertebral end plate into the substance of the vertebral body
    c. Nuclear material travels from its central location posterolaterally into the annular fibers
    d. Nuclear material, extruded through a rupture of annular fibers, forms a free fragment within the spinal canal

94. A fracture that runs at approximately a 30-degree angle to the long axis of the bone is called which of the following?
    a. Transverse fracture
    b. Spiral fracture
    c. Oblique fracture
    d. Compression fracture

95. Which of the following type of fracture is typically seen only in children?
    a. Greenstick
    b. Avulsion
    c. Spiral
    d. Stress

96. All of the following are associated with delayed or nonunion of fractures EXCEPT which?
    a. Smoking
    b. Diabetes
    c. Infection
    d. Hypertension

97. Which of the following fractures is least likely to heal quickly and without complication?
    a. Hip fractures in a 6-month-old
    b. Clavicle fracture in a 17-year-old
    c. Tibial fracture in a 35-year-old
    d. Hip fracture in a 70-year-old

98. Which of the following patients is most likely to receive a lower extremity stress fracture?
    a. A military serviceman during marching
    b. A female swimmer
    c. A female basketball player
    d. A male baseball player

99. How does extended immobilization affect a healing ligament?
    a. Causes a loss of tensile strength
    b. Increases the amount of collagen in the ligament
    c. Increases collagen fiber bundle diameter
    d. Accelerates functional recovery

100. Which of the following statements is TRUE regarding aging and skeletal muscle?
    a. The size of type II fibers decreases with age.
    b. There will be a smaller percentage of type I fiber mass.
    c. There will be an increase in the number of muscle fibers.
    d. There will be a decrease in fatty tissues within the muscle.

101. Which of the following groups of people are most likely to see a damaged patellar tendon?
    a. Carpenters
    b. Dancers
    c. Football players
    d. Tennis players

102. In children with osteogenesis imperfecta, fractures heal in what time frame?
    a. Within the normal healing time
    b. More quickly than normal
    c. More slowly than normal
    d. Only with assistance of medication

103. Osteochondritis dissecans occurs most commonly in which of the following?
    a. Capitellum
    b. Humeral condyle
    c. Medial femoral condyle
    d. Lateral femoral condyle

104. Which joint is most frequently involved in pauciarticular juvenile rheumatoid arthritis?
    a. Cervical spine
    b. Lumbar spine
    c. Knee
    d. Wrist

105. What is the most common onset type of juvenile rheumatoid arthritis?
    a. Systemic
    b. Juvenile ankylosing spondylitis
    c. Polyarticular
    d. Pauciarticular

106. Considering an injury to the medial collateral ligament of the knee, when does the inflammatory phase of healing begin?
    a. First days after injury
    b. 2 to 3 weeks after injury
    c. 4 to 6 weeks after injury
    d. 6 to 8 weeks after injury

107. A patient who just had received a steroid injection into one of the joints is seen by you. What should you do?
    a. Treat this joint vigorously
    b. Treat this joint gently
    c. Not touch this joint at all
    d. Postpone the session for at least 1 week

108. A patient with osteoporosis might be treated with all of the following drugs EXCEPT which?
    a. Bisphosphonates
    b. Calcitonin
    c. Calcium with vitamin D
    d. Thyroid hormones

109. A patient has been told to use Advil for rheumatoid arthritis. You notice that the patient uses acetaminophen because a friend uses it and it is cheaper. What can you can tell the patient about acetaminophen?
    a. It can be used because it is the same as Advil.
    b. It is different from Advil but has the same therapeutic action.
    c. It is actually more effective than Advil.
    d. It does not work in rheumatoid arthritis.

110. Skeletal muscle relaxants have what characteristic?
    a. May interfere with walking in patients who use their spasticity to control balance
    b. Paralyze selectively certain muscle groups

    c. Should be stopped quickly after long-term use when problems have
       been resolved
    d. Have never been proved effective

111. A 27-year-old woman is referred to a physical therapy clinic with a
     diagnosis of torticollis. The right sternocleidomastoid is involved. What
     is the most likely position of the patient's cervical spine?
    a. Right lateral cervical flexion and left cervical rotation
    b. Right cervical rotation and right lateral cervical flexion
    c. Left cervical rotation and left lateral cervical flexion
    d. Left lateral cervical flexion and right cervical rotation

112. What is dental trismus?
    a. Capsulitis of the temporomandibular joint (TMJ)
    b. Osteoarthritis of the TMJ
    c. Muscle spasm of the TMJ
    d. Trigger point of the TMJ

113. Where does temporomandibular anterior disk displacement without
     reduction occur?
    a. Between the disk and the lower joint compartment
    b. Between the disk and the ementia articularis
    c. Between the disk and the lateral pterygoid muscle
    d. Between the disk and the upper joint compartment

114. What is the normal temporomandibular joint arthrokinematics for
     lateral movements?
    a. Bilateral translation
    b. Bilateral rotation
    c. Contralateral rotation and ipsilateral translation
    d. Ipsilateral rotation and contralateral translation

115. What is the normal temporomandibular joint arthrokinematics for
     protrusion?
    a. Bilateral anterior translation
    b. Bilateral posterior translation
    c. Ipsilateral rotation with contralateral translation
    d. Bilateral rotation

116. What is the normal temporomandibular joint arthrokinematics for wide
     opening?
    a. Bilateral translation
    b. Combination of rotations occur in the first 26 mm, then anterior
       translation
    c. Combination of anterior translations occur in the first 26 mm, then
       anterior rotation
    d. Bilateral rotation

117. A patient is suffering from chronic back pain as a result of a recent automobile accident. He is currently taking an opioid medication for relief of this pain. Which of the following medications is an opioid?
    a. Ibuprofen
    b. Aspirin
    c. Codeine
    d. Acetaminophen

118. An athlete has been complaining of muscle spasms. Her physician decided to treat her with a medication called cyclobenzaprine, which is a muscle relaxant. She is unfamiliar with this medication and asks if you can tell her anything about it. Which of the following is a correct statement?
    a. There are no such medications as muscle relaxants.
    b. Muscle relaxants are the same thing as antiinflammatory medications.
    c. Drowsiness, blurred vision, and dry mouth are some of the side effects of muscle relaxants.
    d. You cannot overdose on muscle relaxants.

119. All nonsteroidal antiinflammatory drugs inhibit which of the following in some manner or another?
    a. Bradykinin
    b. Cyclooxygenase
    c. Prostaglandins
    d. Lipoxygenase

120. Which nonsteroidal antiinflammatory drug (NSAID) has been used because of its lower incidence of gastrointestinal complications?
    a. Naproxen
    b. Aspirin
    c. Ketoprofen
    d. Celecoxib

121. A patient taking opioid pain medications might experience all of the following EXCEPT which?
    a. Seeing poorly in the dark
    b. Some respiratory depression
    c. Motor incoordination
    d. Severe diarrhea

122. Whiplash injury from a rear-end collision would tear which of the following ligaments?
    a. Posterior longitudinal ligament
    b. Anterior longitudinal ligament
    c. Ligamentum nuchae
    d. Ligamentum flavum

123. What is the most common site of fracture in osteoporosis?
    a. Metacarpals
    b. Skull
    c. Proximal radius
    d. Vertebral bodies

124. Which of the following conditions is descriptive of osteoarthritis?
    a. It provokes giant cell pigmented villonodular synovitis.
    b. It is associated with decreased type II collagen, cytokines, and chondrolysis.
    c. Ankylosis and follicular inflammation are predominant.
    d. It is associated with increased cartilage matrix synthesis and deposition.

125. Which of the following is a defining symptom of fibromyalgia?
    a. Fatigue
    b. Diffuse pain
    c. Regional pain
    d. Unexplained weight loss

126. In the geriatric population, which condition usually occurs after which defect is present?
    a. Spondylolisthesis; spondylolysis
    b. Spondylolysis; spondylolisthesis
    c. Spondyloschisis; spondylolysis
    d. Spondylolisthesis; spondyloschisis

127. A patient is referred to physical therapy with a diagnosis of arthritis. What type of arthritis would the PTA expect if the patient presented with the following signs and symptoms: (1) bilateral wrists and knees involved, (2) pain at rest and with motion, (3) prolonged morning stiffness, and (4) crepitus?
    a. Osteoarthritis
    b. Rheumatoid arthritis
    c. Degenerative joint disease
    d. Not possible to determine with the given information

128. The signs and symptoms of juvenile rheumatoid arthritis include all of the following EXCEPT which?
    a. Swollen joints
    b. Neurologic impairments
    c. Stiffness
    d. Muscle weakness

129. Osgood-Schlatter disease is primarily which of the following?
    a. An inflammatory process
    b. An injury to apophyseal cartilage

c. An injury in adolescent females

d. A disease caused by tight calf muscles

130. Which orthopedic complication is NOT probable in a child with tetraplegic spinal cord injury?
    a. Shoulder subluxation
    b. Scoliosis
    c. Heterotopic ossification
    d. Hip dislocation

131. A person with injury to the brain in the right hemisphere would most likely exhibit which of the following cognitive deficits?
    a. Decreased executive functions
    b. Poor complex problem solving
    c. Slowed information processing
    d. Memory deficits

132. The PTA begins treatment on a patient diagnosed with Parkinson's disease (PD). The patient informs the assistant that she has a thalamic stimulator to help control her PD. What symptom of PD will best be controlled with the thalamic stimulator?
    a. Festinating gait
    b. Dyskinesia
    c. Rigidity
    d. Tremor

133. The patient suffers a stroke with medial temporal lobe involvement of the posterior cerebral artery. Which of the following would the PTA NOT expect to see when providing intervention for this patient?
    a. Memory loss
    b. Foot drop
    c. Agnosia
    d. Anomia

134. What adverse drug reaction would be expected with the long-term use of neuroleptic drugs in the elderly population?
    a. Abdominal cramps
    b. Hypertension
    c. Tardive dyskinesia
    d. Pulmonary edema

135. Which of the following is a delayed complication of radiation to the brain?
    a. Debilitating fatigue
    b. Dry skin
    c. Lhermitte's sign
    d. Radionecrosis

136. Which stage of HIV infection is characterized by central nervous system (CNS) involvement?
    a. Asymptomatic stage
    b. Early symptomatic stage
    c. HIV advanced disease
    d. End-stage HIV

137. What is often the first sign of facioscapulohumeral dystrophy?
    a. Forward shoulders and scapular winging
    b. Difficulty raising the arms overhead
    c. Tibialis anterior weakness
    d. Inability to close the eyes

138. What type of spinal muscular atrophy is the most severe?
    a. Type I
    b. Type II
    c. Type III
    d. Type IV

139. Erb-Duchenne palsy affects which nerve roots?
    a. C3 to C4
    b. C5 to C6
    c. C5 to T1
    d. C8 to T1

140. Posterior dislocation of the radial head is usually a sign of what type of brachial plexus injury at birth?
    a. Erb-Duchenne palsy
    b. Klumpke's palsy
    c. Proximal plexus palsy
    d. Cerebral palsy

141. What follows a lesion on one side of the spinal cord?
    a. Decrease in sensation to touch on the same side of the lesion and decrease in pain sensation on the same side of the lesion
    b. Decrease in sensation to touch on the opposite side of the lesion and decrease in pain on the opposite side of the lesion
    c. Decrease in touch on the same side of the lesion and decrease in pain sensation on the opposite side of the lesion
    d. Decrease in touch on the opposite side of the lesion and decrease in pain sensation on the same side of the lesion

142. Which of the following is indicative of damage to the thalamus?
    a. Personality change
    b. Declarative memory deficit
    c. Myoclonus
    d. Cortical blindness

143. Which of the following is a normal response of the central nervous system to aging?
    a. Increased population of reactive glia
    b. Overall increase in brain tissue
    c. Increased size of nerve cells
    d. Increased nerve conduction velocity

144. Which of the following is the most severe form of meningitis?
    a. Viral meningitis
    b. Bacterial meningitis
    c. Fungal meningitis
    d. Infective meningitis

145. What is the cardinal sign of meningitis?
    a. Balance disturbances
    b. Tinnitus
    c. Headache
    d. Confusion

146. Brain infection can cause which of the following to occur?
    a. Increased antibodies in the cerebrospinal fluid (CSF)
    b. More white blood cells than blood in the CSF
    c. Brain infarction and decreased cerebral blood flow
    d. Increase in the level of blood glucose in the CSF

147. Which of the following is a potential complication of bacterial meningitis?
    a. Hypernatremia, increased sodium ions in blood
    b. Hypercalcemia, increased calcium ions in blood
    c. Hyponatremia, decreased sodium ions in blood
    d. Hypocalcemia, decreased calcium ions in blood

148. What type of agent typically causes encephalitis?
    a. Bacteria
    b. Fungus
    c. Trauma
    d. Virus

149. Symptoms of encephalitis can be described as which of the following?
    a. Symptoms of encephalitis always include coma.
    b. Symptoms of encephalitis vary widely depending on the individual and degree of infection.
    c. Symptoms of encephalitis always include aphasia.
    d. Symptoms of encephalitis always include hemiparesis.

150. Which of the following symptoms of amyotrophic lateral sclerosis are considered signs of lower motor neuron involvement?
    a. Lack of dexterity
    b. Spasticity
    c. Decreased movement of the tongue
    d. Positive Babinski's response

151. Which of the following functions will remain normal throughout the course of amyotrophic lateral sclerosis?
    a. Bowel and bladder function
    b. Speech
    c. Dexterity
    d. Proprioception

152. What is the most common type of dementia?
    a. Pick's disease
    b. Lewy body dementia
    c. Alzheimer's disease
    d. Frontotemporal dementia

153. Loss of which neurotransmitter activity in the brain correlates to the severity of Alzheimer's disease?
    a. Glutamate
    b. Serotonin
    c. Norepinephrine
    d. Acetylcholine

154. Which of the following is considered a sign of dementia rather than a normal sign of aging?
    a. Periodic minor memory lapses
    b. Unpredictable mood changes
    c. Increasingly cautious behavior
    d. Normal sense of smell

155. What type of multiple sclerosis (MS) describes an initial pattern of relapse and remission and changes into a steadily progressive pattern over time?
    a. Relapsing-remitting MS
    b. Secondary progressive MS
    c. Primary progressive MS
    d. Progressive relapsing MS

156. What is the single most common and disabling symptom of multiple sclerosis?
    a. Visual disturbances
    b. Fatigue
    c. Sensory changes
    d. Muscular rigidity

157. What is the most common initial manifestation of Parkinson's disease?
    a. Rigidity
    b. Bradykinesia
    c. Tremor
    d. Festinating gait

158. Which of the following is associated with an improved prognosis of multiple sclerosis?
    a. Motor and cerebellar symptoms
    b. Disability after the first attack
    c. Short time interval between attacks
    d. Sensory symptoms intact

159. What is the primary cause of stroke?
    a. Hypertension
    b. Trauma
    c. Cerebral vascular disease
    d. Hyperglycemia

160. What is the most common source of embolitic occlusion that causes ischemic stroke?
    a. The pia mater
    b. The heart as a result of atherothrombotic disease
    c. Deep vein thrombosis secondary to immobility
    d. Ventricular fibrillation

161. Which of the following is true regarding traumatic brain injury?
    a. When the injury is a result of a missile wound, the size of the missile will determine the extent of the damage.
    b. A contrecoup injury is frequently worse than the initial injury.
    c. There is always a loss of consciousness.
    d. For fatal damage to occur, there must be a contusion in the brain.

162. Contusions of the brain are most likely to occur with which type of blow?
    a. Frontal
    b. Lateral
    c. Occipital
    d. Inferior

163. Damage to which cranial nerve would lead to a failure of the eye to abduct when the head is passively turned away from the side of the lesion?
    a. Abducens nerve
    b. Trochlear nerve
    c. Oculomotor nerve
    d. Trigeminal nerve

164. What is the correct term for the expression of one thought after another in disconnected or unrelated sequences using rambling speech after traumatic brain injury?
    a. Excessive verbal output
    b. Inappropriate topic selection
    c. Inappropriate word choice
    d. Tangential verbal output

165. What type of spinal cord injury occurs when there is a loss of central gray and white matter creating a cavity surrounded by a rim of intact white matter at the periphery of the spinal cord?
    a. Concussion
    b. Contusion
    c. Laceration
    d. Maceration

166. What type of spinal cord injury is characterized by a more severe loss of upper extremity movement than lower extremity movement?
    a. Anterior cord syndrome
    b. Central cord syndrome
    c. Posterior cord syndrome
    d. Conus medullaris syndrome

167. Which of the following is true regarding heterotopic ossification and spinal cord injury?
    a. It is usually found above the level of the lesion.
    b. It begins to develop 2 to 3 years after injury.
    c. It often develops near the large joints.
    d. It is usually pain free.

168. What type of cerebral palsy is most common?
    a. Hemiplegia
    b. Ataxia
    c. Spastic
    d. Dystonia

169. What type of spastic cerebral palsy involves the trunk and lower extremities, with the upper extremities to a lesser degree?
    a. Monoplegia
    b. Diplegia
    c. Hemiplegia
    d. Quadriplegia

170. Which of the following is NOT a normal aging effect on the peripheral nervous system?
    a. The perineurium will thicken.
    b. The epineurium will thicken.

c. The size and number of fascicles will decrease.

d. The endoneurium will become fibrosed.

171. Which of the following is a TRUE statement regarding neuropathy?
    a. There is hypertonia of muscles involved.
    b. Motor symptoms tend to occur first distally.
    c. Deep tendon reflexes are increased.
    d. The most proximal deep tendon reflexes will be affected first.

172. Which of the following disorders is NOT common with Charcot-Marie-Tooth disease?
    a. Distally symmetrical muscle weakness
    b. Increased deep tendon reflexes
    c. High arch deformities
    d. Hammertoes

173. Which of the following diabetic neuropathies is considered rapidly reversible?
    a. Acute sensory neuropathy
    b. Chronic sensorimotor
    c. Autonomic
    d. Hyperglycemic neuropathy

174. Why does demyelination occur in Guillain-Barré syndrome?
    a. Schwann cells die too fast for the body to replenish them.
    b. Macrophages strip myelin from the nerves.
    c. There is a lack of acetylcholine at the presynaptic junction.
    d. There is a lack of blood flow to the outermost covering of nerves.

175. When a peripheral stretch reflex is hyporeactive, what type of motor neuron lesion is involved?
    a. Upper motor neuron
    b. Lower motor neuron
    c. Both
    d. Neither

176. Which of the following is caused by a nonprogressive lesion of the brain during development?
    a. Myasthenia gravis
    b. Cerebral palsy
    c. Carpal tunnel syndrome
    d. Muscular dystrophy

177. Which of the following has been shown to be associated with an increased risk for falls?
    a. Taking less than four medications
    b. A history of previous falls

  c. Home exercise programs

  d. A high score on the dynamic gait index

178. A patient stands quickly after sitting for several moments. The patient complains of dizziness, and you notice rapid circular eye movements. What is the term for this patient's condition, and what should the therapist do?

  a. Nystagmus; the assistant should walk slowly with the patient

  b. Saccades; the assistant should walk slowly with the patient

  c. Nystagmus; the assistant should help the patient sit down immediately

  d. Saccades; the assistant should help the patient sit down immediately

179. A child is described as having athetoid cerebral palsy. Which of the following descriptions is most likely to describe his presentation?

  a. Increased resistance to fast passive movement of his extremities

  b. Impaired volitional activity encompassing slow, irregular, and writhing movements of the extremities, face, and neck that are perceived as uncontrolled and purposeless

  c. Wide-based gait with poor foot placement

  d. Reduced resistance to fast passive movement of his extremities; generally "floppy" appearing

180. Botulinum toxin injections are used in children with cerebral palsy for which of the following?

  a. To strengthen muscles

  b. To alter bony abnormalities

  c. To lengthen muscles

  d. To reduce spasticity

181. The clinical manifestations of cerebral palsy can be described as which of the following?

  a. Often change over time

  b. Are progressive because of increasing damage to the central nervous system

  c. Are acute and generally resolve within 3 to 4 years

  d. Remain static (unchanging)

182. Clinical neurologic findings of abnormal consciousness, altered tone and reflexes, feeding and respiration difficulties, and/or seizures seen in early infancy is termed which of the following?

  a. Cerebral palsy

  b. Myelomeningocele

  c. Acute hypoxia

  d. Neonatal encephalopathy

183. A child with the diagnosis of diplegic cerebral palsy is likely to present with which of the following patterns of involvement?
    a. Involvement of one side of the body (right or left)
    b. Uncontrolled movements of all extremities
    c. Involvement of the entire body but with the lower extremities more involved than the upper extremities
    d. About equal involvement of all four extremities

184. Selective dorsal rhizotomy is used in children with cerebral palsy for the purpose of which of the following?
    a. Strengthening muscles
    b. Altering bony abnormalities
    c. Lengthening muscles
    d. Reducing spasticity

185. Congenital malformations of the spine and spinal cord, including anomalies of the skin, muscles, vertebrae, meninges, and nervous tissues, is a condition termed which of the following?
    a. Spinal dysraphism
    b. Cerebral palsy
    c. Neonatal encephalopathy
    d. Chiari II malformation

186. Impairments often associated with myelomeningocele may include all of the following EXCEPT which?
    a. Paralysis
    b. Musculoskeletal deformities
    c. Spastic hemiplegia cerebral palsy
    d. Cognitive delays

187. A patient who has intact vision in all visual fields but seems not to attend to things or people on his left would be described as having which of the following?
    a. Left homonymous hemianopsia
    b. Left-side neglect
    c. Left hemiplegia
    d. Left hemianesthesia

188. Which of the following is NOT associated with both traumatic brain injury and stroke?
    a. Clinical presentation varies in severity.
    b. Brain damage can be from hemorrhage.
    c. Area of injury is diffuse.
    d. Abnormal synergy patterns are seen.

189. After a recent stroke, a patient does not use the left upper or lower extremity for any functional tasks. When asked why, the patient reports, "That is not my arm and leg." What type of neglect does this patient present with?
    a. Sensory neglect
    b. Motor neglect
    c. Personal neglect
    d. Spatial neglect

190. Which of the following is NOT a common characteristic of Huntington's disease?
    a. Spasticity
    b. Dystonia
    c. Chorea
    d. Bradykinesia

191. What is the pathologic hallmark of Alzheimer's disease?
    a. Degeneration and loss of upper motor neurons in the brain
    b. Degeneration of neurons that produce dopamine
    c. Demyelination in the brain
    d. Development of neurofibrillary tangles within the neurons of the brain

192. What is the most common secondary condition that will develop from progressive central nervous system disorders that will lead to death of the patient?
    a. Urinary tract infections
    b. Decubitus ulcers
    c. Respiratory failure
    d. Hip fractures from falls

193. What type of multiple sclerosis is characterized by episodes of acute attacks followed by recovery and stability between disease episodes?
    a. Relapsing-remitting
    b. Primary progressive
    c. Secondary progressive
    d. Progressive relapsing

194. Which of the following diseases has as primary symptoms tremor and rigidity?
    a. Alzheimer's disease
    b. Parkinson's disease
    c. Multiple sclerosis
    d. Huntington's disease

195. Which of the following diseases would show significant cognition deficits early in its disease process?
    a. Amyotrophic lateral sclerosis
    b. Parkinson's disease
    c. Alzheimer's disease
    d. Multiple sclerosis

196. Which degree of nerve injury requires surgical repair to join proximal and distal stumps of transected nerve?
    a. Axonotmesis
    b. Neurapraxia
    c. Neurotmesis
    d. Third degree

197. With peripheral nerve injury, the deep tendon reflexes can be described as which of the following?
    a. Hyporeactive
    b. Hyperreactive
    c. Normoreactive
    d. Over-reactive

198. Which of the following is NOT a mechanism of peripheral nerve injury?
    a. Radiation
    b. Stretch
    c. Compression
    d. Disuse

199. Patients with Charcot-Marie-Tooth syndrome typically present with which of the following?
    a. Proximal muscle weakness
    b. Structural foot abnormalities
    c. Sudden onset of signs and symptoms
    d. Hyperactive deep tendon reflexes

200. Which of the following is NOT associated with slowed nerve conduction velocity?
    a. Increased age
    b. Decreased limb temperatures
    c. Increased limb temperatures
    d. Demyelination

201. Which of the following is NOT a characteristic of Guillain-Barré syndrome?
    a. Predominantly affects sensory nerves
    b. Predominantly affects motor nerves
    c. Has axonal degeneration
    d. Demyelination

202. Which of the following is TRUE regarding chronic inflammatory demyelinating polyradiculoneuropathy (CIDP)?
    a. Symptoms peak in less than 4 weeks.
    b. Symptoms can be reduced with corticosteroids.
    c. Respiratory muscles are always involved.
    d. Prognosis for recovery is good.

203. The damage to the spinal cord above the cauda equina is characterized by what condition?
    a. Hyperreflexia
    b. Flaccid paralysis
    c. Loss of reflexes
    d. Fibrillations

204. Which of the following is a reflexive movement?
    a. Eyes closing in response to bright lights.
    b. Turning toward a loud noise.
    c. Pulling away from a noxious stimulus to the fingers.
    d. Blinking in response to touching the cornea.

205. A patient with a diminished conscious state can follow simple commands, has some purposeful movement of the upper extremities, and has reliable verbal yes/no responses. What is the correct term for the patient's current level of arousal?
    a. Coma
    b. Vegetative state
    c. Minimally conscious state
    d. Locked-in syndrome

206. A patient with severe brain damage is supine with upper extremity flexion and lower extremity extension. What posture is this patient exhibiting?
    a. Decorticate posture
    b. Decerebrate posture
    c. Reflex posture
    d. Cerebellar posture

207. A Charcot foot is which of the following?
    a. Collapse of the foot arch resulting in a rocker sole
    b. Condition caused by consistently wearing shoes that are too short
    c. Condition not severe enough to be of concern to a patient with diabetes
    d. Condition caused by macrovascular disease

208. Which of the following condition has the highest risk factor for neuropathic ulcers?
    a. Peripheral neuropathy with loss of sensation
    b. Peripheral vascular disease

c. High blood glucose levels

d. Foot deformities

209. Neuropathic ulcers usually do NOT occur on which of the following?
   a. The distal digits
   b. An area above the ankle
   c. The weight-bearing surfaces of the foot
   d. The dorsal interphalangeal joints

210. Which of the following structures is NOT well developed in infants and puts them at greater risk for developing central nervous system complications from environmental contaminants?
   a. Surfactant in the lungs
   b. Blood-brain barrier
   c. Epiphyseal plates
   d. Neural tube

211. A brain tumor in Broca's area will produce what signs or symptoms?
   a. Receptive dysphasia
   b. Hydrocephalus
   c. Sixth cranial nerve involvement
   d. Motor dysphasia

212. Astrocytomas in children often present with which of the following symptoms first?
   a. Expressive dysphasia
   b. Lack of concentration
   c. Unilateral ataxia
   d. Nausea and vomiting

213. Which of the following is considered the most effective brain-imaging tool?
   a. Magnetic resonance imaging
   b. Computed tomography
   c. Plain film radiograph
   d. Positron emission tomography

214. The physician decides to use corticosteroids for emergency treatment of elevated intracranial pressure. When will the physician begin to see the results of this medication?
   a. In seconds
   b. In minutes
   c. In hours
   d. In days

215. What is the most common symptom of cancer metastasis to the spinal column?
   a. Decreased deep tendon reflexes
   b. Pain
   c. Loss of sensation below the level of the lesion
   d. Loss of motor innervation below the level of the lesion

216. Which of the following is NOT considered a cause of seizures in an infant?
   a. Hypoglycemia
   b. Breech delivery
   c. Hypoxic-ischemic brain insult
   d. Cerebral contusion

217. What phase of a seizure ends with relaxation of all body muscles?
   a. Tonic phase
   b. Clonic phase
   c. Acute phase
   d. Chronic phase

218. Which of the following will NOT increase seizure activity in people with epilepsy?
   a. Aspirin
   b. Caffeine
   c. Amphetamines
   d. Some asthma drugs

219. Which cranial nerve can be stimulated by an implantable pulse generator to decrease seizures?
   a. Abducens
   b. Spinal accessory
   c. Vagus
   d. Oculomotor

220. Which of the following is NOT a characteristic of a simple partial seizure?
   a. Jerking of muscles
   b. Paresthesias or tingling
   c. Illusions/hallucinations
   d. Loss of consciousness

221. What type of seizures is characterized by a sudden loss of muscle tone that may result in falls?
   a. Atonic seizures
   b. Myoclonic seizures
   c. Absence seizures
   d. Tonic-clonic seizures

222. Which of the following would be classified as a primary headache?
    a. Headache associated with fever
    b. Headache associated with increased blood pressure
    c. Migraine headaches
    d. Headaches associated with trauma

223. Which of the following is usually NOT reported in tension headaches?
    a. Anorexia
    b. Mild photophobia
    c. Nausea
    d. Phonophobia

224. Which of the following medications (or dosages of medications) is least likely to increase tension headache symptoms?
    a. Overuse of analgesics
    b. Overuse of nonsteroidal antiinflammatory drugs
    c. Estrogenic hormones
    d. Beta blockers

225. Which of the following cranial nerves is often associated with the distribution of pain during migraine headache?
    a. Cranial nerve V
    b. Cranial nerve VI
    c. Cranial nerve VII
    d. Cranial nerve VIII

226. Why does disk disease in the lower neck contribute to cervicogenic headaches?
    a. This leads to disk displacement.
    b. This leads to abnormal increased muscle tone.
    c. There is compensatory increase in upper cervical spine movement.
    d. There is nerve root irritation in the lower cervical spine.

227. Which of the following situations would manifest as vertigo?
    a. A vestibular nerve on one side of the head has a loss of tonic firing.
    b. A vestibular nerve on one side of the head is hyperactive.
    c. Vestibular nerves on both sides of the head have a loss of tonic firing.
    d. Vestibular nerves on both sides of the head are hyperactive.

228. Complaints of "floating" or "swimming" head could represent which of the following conditions?
    a. Orthostatic hypotension
    b. Disruption of the vestibular/somatosensory system
    c. Unilateral disorder
    d. Abnormal otolith response

229. What is NOT a common complaint of benign paroxysmal positional vertigo?
    a. Sensation stops after 2 to 3 minutes in static position.
    b. Sensation of intense vertigo with head position changes.
    c. Autonomic changes such as sweating.
    d. Sensation of movement of the environment and blurred vision.

230. Which of the following is NOT a symptom of the unilateral vestibular neuronitis?
    a. Nausea and vomiting
    b. Rotary vertigo
    c. Spontaneous horizontal nystagmus
    d. Pain

231. What is usually the initial symptom of Ménière's syndrome?
    a. Rotational vertigo
    b. Sensation of fullness of the ear
    c. Postural imbalance
    d. Nystagmus

232. Permanent damage to which cranial nerve can result from malignant external otitis?
    a. Cranial nerve V
    b. Cranial nerve VI
    c. Cranial nerve VII
    d. Cranial nerve VIII

233. Which of the following disorders is most likely to involve a client who is younger than 30 years?
    a. Multiple sclerosis
    b. Parkinson's disease
    c. Lou Gehrig's disease
    d. Spinal cord injury

234. What type of stroke results from blockage in a blood vessel from a clot?
    a. Hemorrhagic
    b. Ischemic
    c. Traumatic
    d. Mild

235. Which of the following medications given after stroke has thrombolytic properties?
    a. Glutamate antagonists
    b. Calcium channel blockers
    c. Beta blockers
    d. Tissue plasminogen activator

236. Medications used in spinal cord injury perform all of the following tasks EXCEPT which?
    a. Enhancing muscle strength
    b. Preventing depression
    c. Preventing further damage to neural tissue
    d. Enhancing neural tissue repair and recovery

237. Which of the following is NOT a common symptom of vestibular disorder?
    a. Vertigo
    b. Dizziness
    c. Unsteadiness
    d. Pain

238. Which of the following diseases is characterized by demyelination of the nervous system?
    a. Stroke
    b. Spinal cord injury
    c. Multiple sclerosis
    d. Alzheimer's disease

239. How can the disease course in multiple sclerosis in the early stage be described?
    a. Easily controlled with medication
    b. Unpredictable
    c. Able to be controlled with aggressive physical therapy
    d. Always along the same path

240. Which type of multiple sclerosis is the most aggressive and causes severe disability?
    a. Relapsing-remitting
    b. Primary progressive
    c. Relapsing progressive
    d. Secondary progressive

241. What type of multiple sclerosis usually leaves the client with no functional disabilities?
    a. Secondary progressive
    b. Relapsing progressive
    c. Primary progressive
    d. Relapsing-remitting

242. Which of the following is NOT a classic symptom of Parkinson's disease?
    a. Tremor
    b. Pain
    c. Rigidity
    d. Bradykinesia

243. Parkinson's disease occurs when a deficiency of which neurotransmitter is produced in which region of the brain?
    a. Dopamine; substantia nigra
    b. Dopamine; thalamus
    c. Serotonin; substantia nigra
    d. Serotonin; thalamus

244. Which of the following is NOT a typical presentation of a patient with Parkinson's disease?
    a. Short shuffling steps
    b. Loss of reciprocal arm movements
    c. Erect posture
    d. Tremors

245. Which of the following conditions will always result in death?
    a. Stroke
    b. Amyotrophic lateral sclerosis
    c. Traumatic brain injury
    d. Multiple sclerosis

246. Which of the following electrodiagnostic tests is essential in the diagnosis and management of patients with seizure disorders?
    a. Electromyography
    b. Magnetic resonance imaging
    c. Electroencephalography
    d. Nerve conduction velocity

247. What type of communication deficit is referred to as a diminished ability to receive or interpret written communication?
    a. Expressive aphasia
    b. Written aphasia
    c. Receptive aphasia
    d. Agnostic aphasia

248. Which of the following characterizes a child with developmental delay?
    a. Was born to an alcoholic mother
    b. Has not obtained predictable movement patterns
    c. Has cerebral palsy
    d. Was born premature

249. Which of the following conditions is generally associated with in utero constraints?
    a. Juvenile rheumatoid arthritis
    b. Clubfoot
    c. Scoliosis
    d. Congenital muscular torticollis

250. If a child has a right congenital muscular torticollis, what will be the clinical presentation?
   a. Right head tilt and left rotation
   b. Right head tilt and right rotation
   c. Left head tilt and left rotation
   d. Left head tilt and right rotation

251. What is the cause of juvenile rheumatoid arthritis?
   a. Unknown
   b. Alcoholic mother
   c. Premature birth
   d. Inappropriate nutrition of the mother

252. If an infant had clubfoot, what would be the clinical presentation?
   a. The foot would be turned inward and slanted upward.
   b. The foot would be turned outward and slanted upward
   c. The foot would be turned outward and slanted downward.
   d. The foot would be turned inward and slanted downward.

253. What type of childhood disorders lead to developmental dysplasia of the hip?
   a. Myasthenia gravis and cerebral palsy
   b. Spina bifida and cerebral palsy
   c. Spina bifida and myasthenia gravis
   d. Cerebral palsy and premature birth

254. At what age do boys usually show signs of Duchenne's muscular dystrophy?
   a. Birth to 6 months
   b. 6 months to 18 months
   c. 2 years to 4 years
   d. 3 years to 5 years

255. What is the most severe of the neural tube defects?
   a. Meningomyelocele
   b. Meningocele
   c. Spina bifida
   d. Spina bifida occulta

256. Which of the following is NOT a characteristic of a child with Down syndrome?
   a. High muscle tone
   b. Flat facial profile
   c. Upwardly slanted eyes
   d. Short stature

257. Which of the following is a FALSE statement regarding a child diagnosed with cerebral palsy?
    a. The child will have delayed motor milestones.
    b. Hypertonia may be present.
    c. Hypotonia may be present.
    d. The child will have normal intellectual abilities.

258. Which of the following organs is NOT generally involved with cystic fibrosis?
    a. Liver
    b. Respiratory system
    c. Pancreas
    d. Reproductive organs

259. Which of the following statements is TRUE in comparing infants with Down syndrome to infants with no known abnormalities?
    a. Motor milestones are reached at the same time with both groups.
    b. Postural reactions are developed in the same time frame with both groups.
    c. Postural reactions and motor milestones are developed slower in patients who have Down syndrome, but with the same association as with normal infants.
    d. Postural reactions and motor milestones are not developed with the same association with patients who have Down syndrome as with normal infants.

260. The spastic a type of cerebral palsy usually results from involvement of which part of the brain?
    a. Corpus callosum
    b. Basal ganglia
    c. Motor cortex
    d. Cerebellum

261. Which of the following statements is true regarding myelodysplasia?
    a. Myelodysplasia is defined as defective development limited to the anterior horn cells of the spinal cord.
    b. Embryologically, myelodysplastic lesions can be related to either abnormal nervous system neurulation or canalization.
    c. Myelodysplasia is often associated with genetic abnormalities; however, there is no association with teratogens.
    d. Myelodysplasia refers to defects in the lower spinal cord only.

262. Which of the following statements is true regarding progressive neurologic dysfunction?
    a. Progressive neurologic dysfunction is common during periods of rapid growth but does not occur after skeletal maturity is reached.
    b. Deterioration of the gait pattern is one of the last symptoms to be detected.

   c. Symptoms include loss of sensation and/or strength, pain along a dermatome or incision, spasticity onset or worsening, and changes in bowel or bladder sphincter control.

   d. Development of scoliosis will always be rapid.

263. Development in children with cerebral palsy is characterized by which of the following?
   a. Failure to develop reciprocal patterns of muscle activation
   b. Appearance of fidgety movements as defined by Prechtl and colleagues at about 9 weeks of age
   c. Appearance of chorea at about 6 months of age
   d. Failure to develop binocularity of vision

264. Circling arm movements, finger spreading, and a poor repertoire of general movements are characteristic of which disorder?
   a. Down syndrome
   b. Muscular dystrophy
   c. Spastic cerebral palsy
   d. Dyskinetic cerebral palsy

265. A patient with Parkinson's disease taking levodopa/carbidopa might experience all of the following during therapy EXCEPT which?
   a. The "off" phase
   b. Dizziness
   c. Involuntary movements
   d. Marked bradycardia

266. Your patient is receiving antipsychotic drug therapy. During your therapy sessions you might notice a number of movement abnormalities—which one is the most severe?
   a. Tardive dyskinesia
   b. Tremor
   c. Akathisia
   d. Dystonia

267. Which of the following adverse reactions experienced during antiviral drug treatment might be encountered most frequently during therapy?
   a. Elevated blood pressure
   b. Aggressive and inappropriate behavior
   c. Neuralgia and myopathies
   d. Sedation and incoordination

268. Which of the following adverse reactions might be encountered during therapy sessions by a patient receiving anxiolytic drugs?
   a. Psychomotor impairment
   b. Erratic heart rates
   c. Frequent interruptions due to diarrhea
   d. Excessive sweating

269. A patient starting cholinergic agonist therapy for myasthenia gravis might have to interrupt the therapy session repeatedly because of which of the following?
    a. Abdominal cramps and diarrhea
    b. Intermittent tachycardia
    c. Joint stiffness and muscle cramps
    d. Extremely dry mouth

270. A patient has a tumor in the parietal lobe. The PTA anticipates problems with which of the following?
    a. Muscle strength
    b. Perception of spatial relationships
    c. Sensation and motor function
    d. Vision

271. What are the components of upper motor neuron syndrome?
    a. Fasciculations, spasticity, hyperreflexia
    b. Spasticity, rigidity, hyporeflexia
    c. Spasticity, positive Babinski's sign, rigidity
    d. Spasticity, hyperreflexia, positive Babinski's sign

272. A PTA working in an early intervention program is providing intervention for an infant diagnosed with Erb's palsy. This condition most often involves what nerve roots?
    a. C2-3
    b. C3-4
    c. C5-6
    d. C8-T1

273. A patient with Erb's palsy will have paralysis of all of the following muscles EXCEPT which?
    a. Flexor carpi ulnaris
    b. Rhomboids
    c. Brachialis
    d. Teres minor

274. A patient cannot find his dentures when they are on his crowded bedside table. His visual acuity tests at 20/20 with the Snellen eye chart. The PTA suspects which of the following problems?
    a. Figure-ground discrimination
    b. Body scheme awareness
    c. Agraphia
    d. Vertical orientation

275. Morton's neuroma is usually located between which metatarsal heads?
    a. First and second
    b. Second and third

c. Third and fourth
d. Fourth and fifth

276. Which impairment occurs in carpal tunnel syndrome?
    a. Atrophy of the hypothenar eminence
    b. Paresthesias over the dorsal aspect of the hand
    c. Decreased resisted thumb abduction
    d. Decreased resisted forearm pronation

277. Your patient complains of neck pain and peripheral symptoms.
    Radiographs revealed narrowing of the C4-5 intervertebral foramen.
    Which nerve root would most likely be involved?
    a. C5 nerve root
    b. C4 nerve root
    c. C6 nerve root
    d. Sensory branch of C 4

278. An infant with Erb's palsy presents with the involved upper extremity
    in which of the following positions?
    a. Hand supinated and wrist extended
    b. Hand supinated and wrist flexed
    c. Hand pronated and wrist extended
    d. Hand pronated and wrist flexed

279. A PTA is scheduled to treat a patient with cerebral palsy who has been
    classified as a spastic quadriplegic. What type of orthopedic deformity
    should the assistant expect to see in the patient's feet?
    a. Talipes equinovalgus
    b. Talipes equinovarus
    c. Hindfoot valgus
    d. Abnormally large calcaneus

280. Which complication of spinal cord injury is more likely to occur in
    children and teenagers than in adults?
    a. Hypercalcemia
    b. Autonomic dysreflexia
    c. Spasticity
    d. Deep vein thrombosis

281. Deficiencies of what vitamin are usually associated with connective
    tissue disorders?
    a. Vitamin A
    b. Vitamin B
    c. Vitamin C
    d. Vitamin D

282. A cancerous tumor at the hip joint most often refers pain to what part of the body?
    a. Lower and upper back
    b. Sacroiliac joint and knee
    c. Knee and foot
    d. Lumbar area and foot

283. What joint is the most common for patients with hemophilia to experience hemarthrosis?
    a. Shoulder
    b. Hip
    c. Wrist
    d. Knee

284. A patient with hemophilia presents to physical therapy after a recent episode within the quadriceps. Which of the following exercises is most appropriate to begin during the first session of physical therapy?
    a. Resistive terminal knee extension
    b. Quadriceps sets
    c. Exercise bike
    d. Full squats

285. Which of the following will have the most profound impact on physical work capacity?
    a. 1 week of bed rest
    b. 2 weeks of bed rest
    c. 3 weeks of bed rest
    d. 3 decades of aging

286. Women double their rate of musculoskeletal injury during what time?
    a. Pregnancy
    b. Menopause
    c. Adolescence
    d. Ovulation

287. Which of the following is TRUE regarding differences between adults and children during exercise?
    a. The child has a larger heart size than the adult.
    b. The child has a larger stroke volume than the adult.
    c. Children should be watched closely for poor form and posture during exercises.
    d. A child's heart rate is lower during maximal exercise than the adult.

288. Which of the following is FALSE regarding loss of muscle mass?
    a. The greatest decline of muscle mass for women occurs with inactivity, acute illness, and after age 70 years.
    b. The greatest decline of muscle mass in men occurs with inactivity, acute illness, and after age 70 years.

c. Males appear to be more vulnerable to loss of lean tissue than females.

d. Muscle mass is lost at a rate of 4 % to 6% per decade starting at age 40 years in women and age 60 years in men.

289. Loss of muscle function as we age can be attributable to all of the following EXCEPT which one?
   a. Decreased glucose uptake
   b. Decreased total fiber
   c. Decreased muscle fiber size
   d. Decreased high-threshold motor units

290. What is the most common type of scoliosis?
   a. Idiopathic
   b. Osteopathic
   c. Myopathic
   d. Neuropathic

291. Leg pain that increases with lower extremity elevation is associated with which of the following?
   a. Arterial insufficiency
   b. Venous insufficiency
   c. Neuropathic disease
   d. Congestive heart failure

292. Venous insufficiency is usually NOT caused by which of the following?
   a. A seated occupation
   b. Valvular incompetence
   c. Obesity
   d. Smoking

293. The most common cause of venous ulcer recurrence is which of the following?
   a. Weight gain
   b. Nonadherence to compression therapy
   c. Trauma
   d. Poor surgical techniques

294. Partial-thickness burns differ from superficial burns in which of the following ways?
   a. Partial-thickness burns are less painful than superficial burns.
   b. Partial-thickness burns do not blister, and superficial thickness burns commonly blister.
   c. Partial-thickness burns affect the dermis, and superficial burns affect the epidermis.
   d. Partial thickness burns do not require dressings, and superficial burns do require dressings

295. You see a patient with full-thickness burns to his arms and hands. Which of the following would you expect to happen during the first few weeks after the burn injury?
    a. The patient will be treated with intravenous fluids, wound care, and physical therapy and be scheduled for skin grafting surgery.
    b. The patient will be treated on an outpatient basis and followed for 2 to 6 weeks to see if the wounds heal.
    c. Physical therapy will not be consulted to see this patient until the surgeons have decided whether to perform skin grafting.
    d. The burns wounds will render physical therapy treatment of the patient ineffective secondary to severe pain and edema.

296. Which type of burn would heal in approximately 21 days with little or no scarring with proper medical management?
    a. Superficial burn
    b. Superficial partial-thickness burn
    c. Deep partial-thickness burn
    d. Full-thickness burn

297. Which is NOT a phase of wound healing?
    a. Inflammatory phase
    b. Proliferative phase
    c. Scar phase
    d. Remodeling phase

298. What is the immediate response of the blood vessels to injury?
    a. Vasoconstriction
    b. Vasodilation
    c. Increased capillary permeability
    d. There is no action by the blood vessels in the immediate time after a wound

299. Aggressive contraction of a wound occurs during what phase of wound healing?
    a. Inflammatory phase
    b. Proliferative phase
    c. Maturation phase
    d. Remodeling phase

300. Which of the following is NOT generally a cause of a venous stasis ulcer?
    a. Primary loss of vascular flow to the area
    b. Varicose veins
    c. Venous hypertension
    d. Obstruction of the venous system

301. Which of the following is NOT generally associated with an arterial wound?
    a. Irregular shape of the wound
    b. Wound is deep with a pale wound base
    c. Pain
    d. Moderate exudate

302. What type of ulcer is generally located on the plantar surface of the foot?
    a. Arterial wound
    b. Venous ulcer
    c. Neuropathic ulcer
    d. Pressure ulcer

303. What stage of pressure ulcer is characterized by full-thickness skin loss and extensive tissue destruction?
    a. Stage I
    b. Stage II
    c. Stage III
    d. Stage IV

304. A PTA is treating a patient with significant burns over the limbs and upper trunk. Which of the following statements is false about some of the changes initially experienced after the burn?
    a. This patient initially experienced an increase in the number of white blood cells.
    b. This patient initially experienced an increase in the number of red blood cells.
    c. This patient initially experienced an increase in the number of free fatty acids.
    d. This patient initially experienced a decrease in fibrinogen.

305. What are the four stages, in time order, of wound healing after surgery?
    a. Coagulation, inflammatory phase, granulation phase, scar formation and maturation
    b. Inflammatory phase, coagulation, scar formation and maturation, granulation phase
    c. Scar formation and maturation, granulation phase, coagulation phase, and inflammatory phase
    d. Inflammatory phase, granulation phase, coagulation, scar formation and maturation

306. A patient is taking tetracyclines for an infection. The PTA needs to be the most careful in doing which of the following?
    a. Not exposing the patient to excessive light or ultraviolet light therapy
    b. Only exercising the patient moderately
    c. Avoiding use of the warm therapeutic pool
    d. Having the patient get up very slowly from a lying position

307. Signs and symptoms of hypertrophic burn scar include all of the following EXCEPT which?
    a. Increasing itching and redness in a healed burn
    b. Increasing difficulty in achieving a full stretch of the burned area
    c. Fever and malaise
    d. Raised edges around a newly healed graft

308. A PTA is assessing a wound in a patient with the following signs: the right foot has a toe that is gangrenous, the skin on the dorsum of the foot is shiny in appearance, and no calluses are present. The patient has what type of ulcer?
    a. Venous insufficiency ulcer
    b. Arterial insufficiency ulcer
    c. Decubitus ulcer
    d. Trophic ulcer

309. Which of the following activities would have a detrimental effect on the immune system?
    a. Marathon running
    b. Running 5 kilometers
    c. Riding an exercise bike for 30 minutes
    d. Playing a baseball game

310. Individuals with what disease are at risk for splenic rupture?
    a. Infectious mononucleosis
    b. Herpes simplex virus type 1
    c. Herpes simplex virus type 2
    d. Varicella-zoster virus

311. Which of the following populations is at the lowest risk for influenza-related complications?
    a. Individuals older than 65 years
    b. Patients with diabetes
    c. Patients with Crohn's disease
    d. Patients with chronic pulmonary or cardiovascular disease

312. Release of epinephrine into the bloodstream has what effect on the body?
    a. Dilates peripheral blood vessels
    b. Catabolizes fats
    c. Causes hypotension
    d. Decreases blood glucose levels

313. Which of the following is a normal response to aging by the endocrine system?
    a. Blood supply is increased to the pituitary gland.
    b. The thyroid gland becomes larger.

c. The adrenal glands will have more fibrous tissue.

d. The thyroid gland becomes more elevated.

314. Which of the following is associated with carpal tunnel syndrome and endocrine disorders?

a. Unilateral symptoms

b. Thinning of the transverse carpal ligament

c. Vitamin B_6 deficiency

d. Diabetes

315. Which of the following is the typical presentation of type 1 diabetes?

a. Onset of the disease is gradual.

b. It occurs mostly in obese individuals.

c. Insulin production is above normal.

d. It occurs mostly in individuals younger than 20 years.

316. Which of the following is NOT a normal complication of type 1 diabetes?

a. Decreased use of glucose by the body

b. Increased fat mobilization

c. Nerve tissue disorders

d. Impaired protein use

317. Flapping tremor can be observed in several conditions. Which of the following conditions is NOT normally associated with flapping tremor?

a. Diabetes

b. Liver failure

c. Respiratory failure

d. Heart failure

318. Where is the site of referred pain from the hepatic and biliary systems?

a. Right hip

b. Left hip

c. Right shoulder

d. Left shoulder

319. Which of the following is true regarding aging and the hepatic system?

a. The liver increases in size and weight with advancing age.

b. There is increased blood flow to the liver as we age.

c. Aging has little effect on the gallbladder size or function.

d. The pancreas will increase in size as we age.

320. Which condition/dysfunction is NOT associated with jaundice?

a. Blood transfusion

b. Excessive drug intake

c. Alcohol-related hepatitis

d. Rheumatoid arthritis

321. One of the first symptoms of liver cirrhosis could be which of the following?
    a. Neuropathy in the glove-and-stocking distribution
    b. Bilateral swelling of the bilateral feet and ankles
    c. Bilateral swelling of the bilateral hands
    d. Complaints of left shoulder pain

322. Which of the following is TRUE of diabetic neuropathies?
    a. Generally do not follow a length-dependent pattern of distribution
    b. Are generally mononeuropathies
    c. Are considered acquired demyelinating mononeuropathies
    d. Generally present with sensory and motor signs and symptoms

323. Which of the following is NOT a risk factor associated with neuropathic ulcers in patients with diabetes?
    a. History of amputation
    b. Female gender
    c. Long-standing history of diabetes
    d. Foot deformities

324. Which of the following is TRUE of type 1 diabetes?
    a. It is the most common form of diabetes in older adults.
    b. There is a progressive decline in beta cell production of insulin.
    c. It was previously termed juvenile diabetes.
    d. There is a gradual decrease in responsiveness of all cells to insulin.

325. Which of the following foot deformities commonly associated with diabetes is defined as extension of the metatarsophalangeal joint of the digit combined with flexion of the proximal interphalangeal joint?
    a. Pes equinus
    b. Hallux limitus
    c. Hallux valgus
    d. Hammertoes

326. What is the usual pattern of reflex involvement in patients with diabetic neuropathy?
    a. Lower extremities more involved than upper extremities and distal reflexes more involved than proximal reflexes
    b. Upper extremities more involved than lower extremities and proximal reflexes more involved than distal reflexes
    c. The right side of the body more involved than the left side of the body
    d. The left side of the body more involved than the right side of the body

327. A patient is using a medication for a thyroid condition. Which of the following could be the result of overdosing with the drug and should be mentioned to the physician?
    a. Tachycardia and restlessness when using propylthiouracil
    b. Tachycardia when using a T4 medication
    c. Weight loss when using propylthiouracil
    d. Bradycardia when using a T4 medication

328. Which of the following statements about immune disorders is true?
    a. The progression of the disease will not change the clinical presentation of signs and symptoms.
    b. Early diagnosis is not likely to alter the course of the disease.
    c. Direct access will increase the likelihood that a physical therapist might be the first provider to identify potential autoimmune disorders.
    d. The risk factors for immune disorders are clearly understood and will assist in differential diagnosis.

329. Which of the following characteristics describes adrenergic receptors?
    a. Are subdivided into four major categories
    b. Include the muscarinic and nicotinic receptors
    c. Include the alpha and beta receptors
    d. When blocked, can cause dry mouth, decreased salivation, blurry vision, and constipation

330. A client with diabetes is exercising vigorously in an outpatient clinic. The patient informs the PTA that she received insulin immediately before the exercise session. If the patient goes into a hypoglycemic coma, which of the following is NOT a likely sign?
    a. Pallor
    b. Shallow respiration
    c. Bounding pulse
    d. Dry skin

331. After arriving at the home of a home health patient, the primary nurse informs the PTA that he has activated emergency medical services. The nurse found the patient in what appears to be a diabetic coma. Which of the following is most likely NOT one of the patient's signs?
    a. Skin flush
    b. Rapid pulse
    c. Weak pulse
    d. High blood pressure

332. A PTA is treating a patient in an outpatient facility. The patient has recently been diagnosed with type 1 insulin-dependent diabetes mellitus. The patient asks the PTA about the differences between type 1 insulin-dependent diabetes mellitus and type 2 non–insulin-dependent diabetes mellitus. Which of the following statements is true?
    a. There is usually some insulin present in the blood in type 1 and none in type 2.
    b. Ketoacidosis is a symptom of type 2.
    c. The age of diagnosis with type 1 is usually younger than the age of diagnosis with type 2.
    d. Both conditions can be managed with a strict diet, only without taking insulin.

333. Which of the following is an immediate effect of ionizing radiation on the cardiovascular and pulmonary symptoms?
    a. Radiation pneumonitis
    b. Radiation fibrosis
    c. Lymphedema
    d. Coronary artery disease

334. During normal venous function, which of the following activities would have the highest venous pressure in the lower extremities?
    a. Standing
    b. Walking across level surfaces
    c. Walking up stairs
    d. Running

335. A patient presents to outpatient physical therapy with complaints of lower extremity pain. The patient complains of diffuse leg pain that increases with ambulation and is made better with a few minutes of rest. What is the most likely cause of this patient's pain?
    a. Venous insufficiency
    b. Arterial insufficiency
    c. Renal insufficiency
    d. Cardiac insufficiency

336. Respiratory syncytial virus is the most common cause of hospitalization because of respiratory illness in which of the following patient populations?
    a. Frail elderly patients
    b. Middle-aged men
    c. Middle-aged women
    d. Very young patients

337. If dyspnea is relieved by leaning forward on the arms to lock the shoulder girdle, then the dysfunction is primarily within which body system?
    a. Cardiac
    b. Pulmonary

c. Muscular

d. Central nervous system

338. A PTA is treating a patient who is taking cardiac medication in the home health setting. What are the effects of an angiotensin-converting enzyme inhibitor on the heart and cardiovascular system?
    a. Prevents constriction of blood vessels and retention of sodium and fluid
    b. Constricts arterioles and increases retention of sodium and fluid
    c. Alters conduction patterns in the heart
    d. Prevents blood clot formation

339. Which of the following clinical symptoms is associated with orthostatic hypotension in the geriatric population?
    a. Tachypnea
    b. Altered vision
    c. Hypervigilance
    d. Dyspnea

340. What type of cardiomyopathy is the most common cause of sudden death in young competitive athletes?
    a. Delayed-onset cardiomyopathy
    b. Dilated cardiomyopathy
    c. Hypertrophic cardiomyopathy
    d. Restrictive cardiomyopathy

341. What type of cough indicates airway irritation?
    a. Nonproductive cough
    b. Dry cough
    c. Productive cough with purulent sputum
    d. Productive cough with nonpurulent sputum

342. Gasping inspiration followed by short expiration describes which of the following altered breathing patterns/sounds?
    a. Crackles/rales
    b. Apneustic
    c. Stridor
    d. Wheezing

343. Which of the following is true regarding aging and the renal system?
    a. There is a gradual increase of blood flow to the kidneys.
    b. There is a reduction of nephrons.
    c. There is a decrease in volume of urine.
    d. There is a tendency toward lesser renal vasoconstriction.

344. Which patient population is at risk for a urinary tract infection due to the dilation of the upper urinary system?
    a. Young females
    b. Females in a long-term care setting
    c. Middle-age females
    d. Pregnant women

345. What patient population is most likely to exhibit mental status changes with a urinary tract infection?
    a. Young females
    b. Young males
    c. Middle-age females
    d. Elderly females

346. Which of the following types of renal calculi is caused by recurrent bacterial urinary tract infections?
    a. Calcium stones
    b. Struvite stones
    c. Uric acid stones
    d. Cystine stones

347. Which of the following would be an uncommon site for extraskeletal calcification associated with end-stage renal disease?
    a. Coronary arteries
    b. Large intestines
    c. Lungs
    d. Skin

348. Which of the following types of urinary incontinence is marked by a sudden unexpected urge to urinate and then the uncontrolled loss of urine?
    a. Functional incontinence
    b. Stress incontinence
    c. Hyperreflexive bladder
    d. Overflow incontinence

349. Which of the following is NOT a normal degenerative change of the male reproductive system?
    a. The testes become larger.
    b. The seminiferous tubules thicken.
    c. The prostate gland enlarges.
    d. Sclerotic changes occur in the local vasculature.

350. Which of the following surgical interventions for benign prostatic hyperplasia require the client to wear a catheter for 1 to 3 weeks afterward?
    a. Transurethral prostatectomy
    b. Transurethral incision prostate
    c. Transurethral ethanol ablation of the prostate
    d. Water-induced thermal therapy

351. Which of the following is NOT a side effect of the prescription of estrogen after menopause?
   a. Breast cancer
   b. Fractures
   c. Heart disease
   d. Stroke

352. An 80-year-old woman complains of daily urinary accidents. She says that when she gets the urge to urinate, she simply cannot get to the bathroom in time. She has had a total hip replacement, 6 months ago. What "type" of incontinence would this patient most closely match?
   a. Urge incontinence
   b. Stress incontinence
   c. Functional incontinence
   d. Mixed incontinence

353. In a patient who has a uterine or bladder prolapse, which of the following findings do you expect?
   a. Decreased pelvic floor tone and strength, elongated pelvic floor muscles
   b. Increased pelvic floor tone, good pelvic floor strength
   c. Decreased pelvic floor tone and good pelvic floor strength
   d. Increased pelvic floor tone and poor pelvic floor strength

354. What structure is typically NOT compressed with an enlarged uterus (pregnancy)?
   a. Bladder
   b. Vulvar veins
   c. Breasts
   d. Inferior vena cava

355. Which of the following is NOT a strong predictor of persistent low back pain after pregnancy?
   a. Low body mass index
   b. High body mass index
   c. Early onset of pain during pregnancy
   d. Hypermobility of the spine

356. Your patient has complaints of loss of urine as soon as she has the urge to urinate. She also complains of deep pressure (NOT PAIN) in her lower pelvis area with prolonged standing. What kind of incontinence does this patient's symptoms most likely mimic?
   a. Stress incontinence
   b. Urge incontinence
   c. Mixed incontinence
   d. Functional incontinence

357. Serious side effects of nonsteroidal antiinflammatory drugs are usually NOT seen in which part of the body?
    a. Gastrointestinal tract
    b. Kidneys
    c. Cardiovascular system
    d. Skin

358. A 27-year-old man presents to physical therapy with a diagnosis of patella tendonitis. The patient explains that he has been "working out" for 5 to 6 hours per day for the past 2 to 3 weeks. The PTA notes an abnormal amount of facial acne and body hair. The therapist suspects drug abuse. What type of drug is this patient most likely abusing?
    a. Glucocorticoids
    b. Nonsteroidal antiinflammatory drugs
    c. Anabolic steroids
    d. Marijuana

359. A patient is receiving physical therapy while undergoing chemotherapy for a diagnosis of cancer. The patient has complained of fatigue throughout the course of therapy. Which of the following is incorrect advice to give this patient?
    a. The patient should be encouraged to increase physical activity.
    b. The patient should be instructed in low to moderate levels of aerobic exercise.
    c. The patient should be encouraged to sleep 10 hours per day.
    d. The patient should be encouraged to maintain compliance with a home exercise program.

360. Which of the following will be seen in patients with a high fever?
    a. Increased oxygen consumption
    b. Increased systemic vascular resistance
    c. Usually hypertension
    d. Decreased cardiac output

361. All of the following statements about the development of strength in children and adolescents are TRUE, EXCEPT which of the following?
    a. Multiple factors contribute to the development of strength, including gender, age, body size and type, muscle cross-sectional area, and proportion of fiber type.
    b. In girls, strength increases linearly until puberty and then increases sharply during adolescence because of hormonal influences.
    c. Changes in muscle function follow changes in muscle size, but qualitative changes also result from neural influences.
    d. Gender differences in strength are evident in children as young as 3 years old, with boys demonstrating greater strength than girls.

362. A combination of contractures in which of the following hip motions would lead to possible hip subluxation or dislocation in patients with myelomeningocele?
    a. Hip flexion, abduction, internal rotation
    b. Hip extension, adduction, internal rotation
    c. Hip flexion, adduction, internal rotation
    d. Hip flexion, adduction, external rotation

363. A 23-year-old L1 complete paraplegic is completing her outpatient rehabilitation. She asked the PTA if she would be able to have children. What is the appropriate answer by the therapist?
    a. Pregnancy is impossible after spinal cord lesion.
    b. Pregnancy should be encouraged after spinal cord lesion because there is no increased risk for complication.
    c. Pregnancy after spinal cord lesion is associated with complications, and the patient should follow up with her obstetrician.
    d. Pregnancy after spinal cord lesion should be discouraged because of the associated risks

364. Which of the following is TRUE regarding wound healing and nutritional status?
    a. Protein requirement increases 2 to 2½ times the baseline.
    b. Caloric needs for wound tissue remain the same as for healthy tissue.
    c. Loss of more than 10% of body weight slightly increases risk for pressure ulcers.
    d. There is minimal documentation to suggest patients with pressure ulcers require adequate nutrition.

365. What part of the gait cycle should be emphasized during gait training for an individual with venous insufficiency?
    a. Quadriceps contractions at midstance
    b. Gastrocnemius contractions at toe-off
    c. Dorsiflexor contractions at initial contact
    d. Gluteus medius contractions at early swing

366. Neuropathic ulcers are NOT associated with which of the following?
    a. Sensory and autonomic neuropathies
    b. Poorly fitting shoes with inadequate distribution of pressure during the gait cycle
    c. Diabetes
    d. Congestive heart failure

367. What is the most common neurologic complication after a burn injury?
    a. Decreased deep tendon reflexes
    b. Peripheral neuropathy
    c. Weakness related to decreased nerve conduction velocity
    d. Balance disorders related to vestibular dysfunction

368. There is evidence that physical activity will have several effects on the body. Which of the following is NOT an effect of physical activity on the body?
    a. Decreased blood pressure
    b. Inhibited endothelial function
    c. Decreased triglycerides
    d. Increased high-density lipoprotein

369. What muscles are most commonly affected in acute alcoholic myopathy?
    a. Gastrocnemius
    b. Forearm flexors
    c. Shoulder girdle
    d. Finger intrinsics

370. The PTA is beginning exercise intervention for a patient who is recovering from anorexia nervosa. At what body mass index can exercise begin with this patient?
    a. 12
    b. 15
    c. 17
    d. 19

371. Toxic polyneuropathy affects which of the following first?
    a. Heart and lungs
    b. Central nervous system
    c. Cranial nerves
    d. Distal limbs

372. If a female is a migraine sufferer, when will migraine headaches decrease during pregnancy?
    a. First trimester
    b. Second trimester
    c. Third trimester
    d. Delivery

373. Risk for which of the following musculoskeletal symptoms is NOT likely to rise with the onset of menopause?
    a. Hip fracture
    b. Carpal tunnel syndrome
    c. Osteoarthritis at the basilar joint of the thumb
    d. Adhesive capsulitis

374. What two body systems primarily regulate pH?
    a. Cardiovascular and respiratory
    b. Respiratory and renal
    c. Renal and cardiovascular
    d. Cardiovascular and neurologic

375. A patient who is taking combination contraceptive medication and also smoking must be warned that smoking increases the risk for which disorder?
    a. Thromboembolism
    b. Liver cancer
    c. Internal hemorrhaging
    d. Ovarian cancer

376. A patient taking combination contraceptive medication might experience all of the following EXCEPT which?
    a. Depressive episodes
    b. Weight gain
    c. Swelling of feet
    d. Joint or muscle pain

377. Which of the following are common signs and symptoms seen by a patient using over-the-counter diphenhydramine?
    a. Poor coordination and fatigue
    b. Increased blood pressure and irregular heart beat
    c. Excessive sweating and cold extremities
    d. Weight gain and ankle edema

378. A patient taking cancer chemotherapeutic drugs might experience all of the following adverse reactions EXCEPT which?
    a. Easy bruising and bleeding
    b. Fatigue and anemia
    c. Constipation with fecal impact
    d. Jaundice and hepatotoxicity

379. The patient has a dysfunction of the 10th rib but complains of nausea and fullness. What is this is an example of?
    a. Viscerovisceral reflex
    b. Viscerosomatic reflex
    c. Somatovisceral reflex
    d. Somatosomatic reflex

380. A patient who is 3 months pregnant asks advice on activities. Previous prepartum activities included rock climbing, soccer, and hiking. Which of the activities would you recommend?
    a. Rock climbing
    b. Soccer
    c. None of these activities—she's pregnant
    d. Hiking

381. Which of the following is the most likely reason for the change in posture associated with pregnancy?
    a. Ligament laxity
    b. Shift in the center of gravity
    c. Enlarging uterus
    d. Increased breast size

382. The Waddell tests are used to identify which of the following?
    a. Pain of a nonorganic origin
    b. Space-occupying lesions
    c. Balance and coordination functions
    d. History of alcohol or substance abuse

383. Which of the following is least likely in a woman in the 8th month of pregnancy?
    a. Center of gravity anteriorly displaced
    b. Heart rate decreased with rest and increased with activity (compared with heart rate before pregnancy)
    c. Edema in bilateral lower extremities
    d. Blood pressure increased by 5% (compared with blood pressure before pregnancy)

384. Which of the following circumstances would normally decrease body temperature in a healthy person?
    a. Exercising on a treadmill
    b. Pregnancy
    c. Normal ovulation
    d. Reaching age of 65 years or older

385. A PTA is speaking to a group of pregnant women about maintaining fitness level during pregnancy. Which of the following statements contains incorrect information?
    a. Perform regular exercise routines at least three times per week.
    b. Perform at least 15 minutes per day of abdominal exercises in supine position, during the second and third trimesters.
    c. Increase caloric intake by 300 calories per day.
    d. Exercise decreases constipation during pregnancy.

Answers

1. a. Crohn's disease affects the intestines and is therefore considered an organ-specific autoimmune disorder. The other choices are systemic autoimmune disorders.

2. d. The right upper quadrant is a common site of referred pain for liver cancer. The other choices could constitute worsening of the cancer or other symptoms. Any of the other symptoms would require the PTA to contact the supervising physical therapist or referring physician.

3. b. Belching, diarrhea, abdominal cramps, nausea, vomiting, and heartburn are gastrointestinal signs and symptoms associated with strenuous exercise.

4. d. Another cause of upper gastrointestinal bleeding could be use of nonsteroidal antiinflammatory drugs such as aspirin or ibuprofen.

5. b. The other choices listed can lead to increased gastric pressure, which is also a cause of gastroesophageal reflux disease.

6. d. Prilosec, Aciphex, Prevacid, and Nexium are medications that stop the chemical pump that transports acid into the stomach. This usually brings fast relief and healing of burns and erosions in the esophagus.

7. a. Perforation of the posterior duodenal wall causes steady midline pain in the thoracic spine from T6 to T1 with radiation to the right upper quadrant.

8. c. The other choices listed are characterized by diseased areas of intestine with normal intestine between (skip areas).

9. b. Sports hernias are a weakness in the posterior wall of the inguinal canal resulting in chronic activity-related groin pain but without a clinically detectable hernia. A femoral hernia is a protrusion of loop of intestine into the femoral canal, a tubular passageway into the thigh that carries nerves and blood vessels. Umbilical hernia occurs through a congenital defect in the abdominal muscle at the umbilical ring.

10. c. The liver is located in the right upper quadrant, making pain referral more common to the right shoulder. Coffee-ground emesis or melena is generally associated with gastrointestinal disorders because liver disease tends to create gray stools and dark urine.

11. b. Patients with anxiety usually present with hyperventilation, and strenuous exercise brings on Kussmaul's respiration. Patients with chronic fatigue syndrome present with hypoventilation. Cheyne-Stokes respiration is defined as a repeated cycle of breathing followed by shallow breaths or cessation of breathing.

12. b. Acute bronchitis is an inflammation of the trachea and bronchi that is of short duration and self-limited with few pulmonary signs. Chronic bronchitis is considered a chronic obstructive pulmonary disease.

13. a. Other signs include a persistent cough, diaphoresis, and intolerance to exercise. The rate of respirations also increases rather than decreases.

14. d. Head injury leads to increased intracranial pressure, which affects the respiratory centers of the brain. Bradypnea is common after a head injury. All the other choices cause tachypnea and could possibly lead to hyperventilation.

15. d. Deconditioning of the cardiopulmonary system impairs the transport of blood and oxygen to the body's tissues. This in turn leads to a decrease in oxygen to the skeletal muscle tissues. The musculoskeletal system is secondarily affected by the cardiopulmonary system.

16. d. Although there will be muscle weakness in any patient with deconditioning, endurance with functional activities is the primary impairment. Because of the deconditioning of the cardiopulmonary system, there will be significant limitation in the patient's functional activities.

17. d. Periods of decreased activity quickly result in the decline of maximum oxygen consumption rate and stroke volume. The other choices show decline after about 30 days of inactivity.

18. c. In chronic obstructive pulmonary disease, expiration is prolonged, producing ratios of 1:4 or 1:5.

19. d. Patients with chronic hyperinflation of the lungs present with barrel chest. There is usually thoracic kyphosis, reduced thoracic excursion, and reduced spinal flexibility associated with this disorder.

20. c. Crackles and wheezes are always considered abnormal. The other choices are normal when heard over a specific region of the thorax, but become abnormal when heard in a different region of the thorax.

21. c. Diastolic heart failure is more common in females and is more difficult to diagnose. Systolic heart failure is defined as an ejection fraction below 40%.

22. c. Heart failure is characterized by the inability of the heart to meet the demands of the body. Thus the patient will have decreased exercise or activities of daily living tolerance.

23. a. During stage 0 there is about 30% more fluid in the interstitium than normal. The patient could complain of limb heaviness and aching, but there is no measurable increase in limb girth.

24. d. Stage III lymphedema is characterized by a hardening of the tissues under the skin. This is accompanied by severe skin alterations and hyperkeratosis, which is a thickening of the outer layer of the skin.

25. b. Emphysema and chronic bronchitis are the two most common chronic obstructive pulmonary disease conditions and are often found together in the same patient.

26. c. When the right ventricle is not contracting efficiently, blood volume backs into the venous system and fluid collects in the liver, abdominal cavity, and legs. If the left ventricle does not function properly, an abnormal amount of blood volume remains in the lungs, which results in fluid collection.

27. c. The other three procedures listed are noninvasive procedures. A cardiac catheterization involves passing a catheter (a flexible tube) into an artery in the leg until it reaches the heart. The catheter can then be placed in the left chambers of the heart or in the coronary arteries or pulmonary veins.

28. c. Orthopnea, which is dyspnea in the recumbent position, is a typical symptom of chronic left heart failure. All of the other symptoms and signs are due to right heart failure.

29. a. Verapamil reduces contractility of the heart and increases coronary artery dilation, resulting in decreased cardiac workload and increased blood flow to the heart muscle.

30. c. Residual volume, the amount of air left in the lungs after a forceful expiration, increases with age.

31. c. Beta blockers block the beta receptors on the heart, block sympathetic nerve impulses, and reduce heart rate and contractility. The other drugs have no effects or might increase heart rate.

32. a. A beta agonist stimulates cardiac beta receptors, leading to an increase in heart rate and blood pressure.

33. c. Statin drugs inhibit HMG-CoA reductase and lower cholesterol levels most effectively (about 30 % or more), whereas the other drugs interfere with absorption and lipase activity.

34. d. All of the listed reactions can be observed with joint and muscle pain being the exception.

35. b. Although the use of an inhaler is user specific, it is generally recommended to have the patient inhale about 20 minutes before exercise, in particular in a cool environment, which seems to aggravate existing asthma.

36. b. All of the reactions can be expected, partly caused by blockade of beta receptors in the lungs and heart, along with drowsiness, perhaps by a central action. No muscle cramps and pain should be expected.

37. d. Beta-receptor blockade, peripherally and perhaps centrally, causes the blood pressure–reducing effects. Peripheral resistance is not reduced, but rather may be slightly increased (patient may complain about cold extremities).

38. c. Calcium channel blockers will cause all of the listed reactions, except tremors, by interfering with calcium fluxes in blood vessels and cardiac muscle.

39. a. Cardiovascular. All of the symptoms could potentially be related to musculoskeletal problems within the shoulder, but several factors make the cardiovascular system the best answer. The symptoms began insidiously, and many musculoskeletal shoulder issues can be traced back to a single incident or repetitive motion that results in damage to musculoskeletal tissue. The patient cannot remember an incident that triggered the symptoms. Most of the symptoms the patient is reporting can be attributed to the cardiovascular system. Lifting heavy objects, shoveling dirt, walking fast, high blood pressure, and shortness of breath are all symptoms indicative of cardiovascular system involvement. Therefore, the cardiovascular system is the best answer.

40. b. Pulmonary. Although some of the symptoms could be the result of musculoskeletal system involvement (i.e., rib fracture) or the cardiovascular system (left-sided pain), the best answer is the pulmonary system. The blood in the sputum is an indicator that the ribs may have punctured the lungs. This, coupled with the breathing problems, should move the pulmonary system up as your top hypothesis.

41. b. Aspirin and clopidogrel act as anticlotting/coagulant medications by prevent platelets from clumping together, thereby making it harder to form a clot.

42. d. Sublingual nitroglycerin acts very quickly to relieve anginal pain by relaxing blood vessels to allow more blood to flow to the heart. Nitroglycerin patches are used to prevent an angina attack, but sublingual nitroglycerin is most effective once an attack occurs.

43. a. Angina is caused by decreased blood flow to the heart, resulting in pain. Nitrates relax blood vessels, allowing more blood to flow to the heart and thereby decreasing pain.

44. a. Beta blockers block beta-1 and beta-2 receptors, resulting in decreased heart rate and dilation of blood vessels, which helps decrease hypertension. Unfortunately, they could also trigger an asthma attack in susceptible persons by blocking the beta-2 receptors in the lungs.

45. d. Short-acting beta agonists, also known as "rescue" meds, act very quickly by binding to the beta-2 receptors in the bronchioles and causing relaxation of the airways. They are indicated for asthma attacks and are not useful for long-term control of asthma symptoms.

46. c. Primary lymphedema is an inherited disorder resulting from abnormal formation of lymphatic vessels before birth. These malformations most commonly cause swelling that affects the feet and legs.

47. a. Easy bruising would not be expected, but dehydration with electrolyte changes, muscle cramping, and dyspnea is expected.

48. c. Normal PaO_2 ranges from 80 to 100 mm of Hg and is an important determinant of when it is safe to exercise a patient either with or without supplemental oxygen. PaO_2 is determined by examining the concentration of oxygen present in arterial blood. Understanding the parameters under which a patient may safely perform exercise is important.

49. b. Thromboembolus formation is a common complication of thrombophlebitis in lower leg veins. Thrombi can pass through the heart and obstruct major pulmonary arteries.

50. d. Apneusis can be described as an inspiratory cramp. Orthopnea is difficulty with breathing in a lying position. Eupnea is normal breathing. Apnea is the absence of breathing.

51. c. Mucoid sputum is clear or white and is not usually associated with infection. Thick sputum is referred to as tenacious. Foul-smelling sputum is called fetid and is often associated with infection.

52. b. Frothy sputum is thin and white or has a slight pink color. This type of sputum is commonly present with pulmonary edema. Purulent sputum resembles pus, with a yellow or green color. Mucopurulent sputum is yellow to light green in color. Rusty sputum is a rust-colored sputum often associated with pneumonia.

53. c. Rheumatoid arthritis is an autoimmune disease of the synovial tissue and joints. Systemic lupus erythematosus is also an autoimmune disease but can affect multiple organs. Sarcoidosis is characterized by granulomas that develop in the organs.

54. c. Herpes simplex virus type 2 is most often seen in the genitals, whereas varicella-zoster virus manifests in the distal sensory nerve distribution.

55. d. Clients with increased risk for cellulitis include older adults and people with lowered immune resistance from diabetes, malnutrition, steroid therapy, and the presence of wounds or ulcers.

56. c. The butterfly rash over the nose, cheeks, and forehead is commonly caused by exposure to sunlight. The rash is common over the nose and cheeks but can occur over the scalp, neck, upper chest, shoulders, extensor surface of the arms, and dorsum of the hand.

57. b. Sunburn causes a superficial burn, whereas a partial-thickness burn will be wet. Superficial burns and partial-thickness burns are painful, whereas full-thickness burns are not. Usually a full-thickness burn will present with the nerve endings destroyed. However, most full-thickness burns occur with superficial and partial-thickness burns in which nerve endings are intact and exposed.

58. a. Because the diabetic ulcer usually results from lack of sensation in the foot, the ulcer typically presents in areas of abnormal pressures. The plantar surface of the metatarsal heads, the toes, and the plantar area of the hallux are common areas for diabetic ulcers.

59. b. Choices a and d describe a venous insufficiency ulcer, whereas choice c describes a diabetic ulcer.

60. d. Skin breakdown commonly occurs over bony prominences such as the greater trochanter, ischial tuberosities, sacrum, heels, and possibly the cranium.

61. a. Because of the decrease in blood flow with an arterial wound, infection may not be as obvious as in a healthy individual. The body is not able to have an appropriate inflammatory response to infection because of arterial compromise.

62. b. The wound bed of a venous ulcer is red and usually shallow. An arterial ulcer often looks necrotic because of the lack of blood to the area. The margins to an arterial wound are often regular and distinct, leading to a "punched-out" appearance.

63. b. Kyphoscoliosis is a structural deformity classically characterized by anterior wedging of 5 degrees or more of three adjacent thoracic bodies and affecting individuals aged 12 to 16 years.

64. c. Choices a, b, and c are three common neural tube defects. Spina bifida occulta is incomplete fusion of the posterior vertebral arch, whereas myelomeningocele is a protrusion of the meninges and spinal cord.

65. d. In adults, the periosteum is firmly attached to the cortex and resists displacement. Infection disrupts and weakens the cortex, which predisposes the bone to pathologic fracture. Because sensory nerve endings are absent in cancellous bone, this process can progress without pain.

66. d. Back pain can be aggravated by motion but is present regardless of activity level in some individuals and throbbing at rest. It may radiate in a radicular distribution and is commonly accompanied by spinal tenderness and rigidity. Accessory motions of the spine are often difficult to perform.

67. c. The other choices are indicative of infection. Constant joint pain is indicative of infection, whereas mechanical loosening commonly causes pain with only motion or weight bearing. When both the distal and proximal components of a prosthetic joint demonstrate pathology on radiography, infection is more likely than mechanical loosening.

68. b. The other choices listed are all benign tumors of fibrous origin, cartilage, or bone.

69. a. The long bones such as the distal femur, proximal humerus, and proximal tibia have a relatively more active growth period than other bones making them vulnerable for osteosarcoma formation.

70. b. A Baker's cyst is a subtype of ganglion that often communicates within a joint space. A Baker's cyst is most often palpated behind the knee in older adults with osteoarthritis.

71. a. Vertebral compression fractures are the most common osteoporosis-related spinal fractures, presenting with clinical symptoms of back pain, posture change, loss of height, functional impairment, disability, and diminished quality of life.

72. d. The insufficient calcium absorption could occur because of either a lack of calcium or resistance to the action of vitamin D. The increased renal phosphorus losses can occur in association with renal and renal tubular insufficiency.

73. c. The most common presenting symptom is pain, which may be a headache or radicular, osteoarthritic, muscular, or other skeletal in origin. Direct pain from periosteal irritation of involved bones is deep and boring, worse at night, and reduced but not diminished with activity.

74. b. A stress fracture is caused by the bones' inability to withstand stress applied in a rhythmic, repeated, microtraumatic fashion. These types of stress fractures are found in track-and-field athletes, distance runners, and soldiers in training.

75. b. Osteochondritis dissecans is a disorder of one or more ossification sites with localized subchondral necrosis followed by recalcification. This condition affects the subchondral bone and layer or articular cartilage just above. The most common site of involvement is the medial femoral condyle.

76. c. Osgood-Schlatter syndrome results from the patella tendon pulling small bits of immature bone from the tibial tuberosity. It is most commonly seen in active adolescent boys 10 to 15 years of age but also can affect girls 8 to 13 years of age.

77. b. In grade II osteoarthritis, there is definite osteophyte formation with possible narrowing of joint space. Grade IV is the most severe arthritis with large osteophytes, marked joint space narrowing, severe sclerosis, and definite deformity of bone ends.

78. c. Choices a, b, and d are all indicative of rheumatoid arthritis. Rheumatoid arthritis is a systemic condition that affects all joints. Osteoarthritis affects mainly the weight-bearing joints. Inflammation is present in only 10% of the cases.

79. d. Boutonniere deformity is defined in choice b. Both swan-neck and boutonniere deformities are common with osteoarthritis.

80. c. A complication associated with brain injury is the formation of HO or abnormal bone growth around a joint.

81. c. Bone mass increases until about age 25 years when the epiphyses close, then peak mass is maintained until about age 45 to 50 years. Mass begins to decrease at that point.

82. c. Small-framed women of Asian and European descent have the greatest risk for developing osteoporosis.

83. d. All of the choices are manifestations of osteoporosis, but vertebral compression fractures are the most common.

84. c. Muscle loss generally occurs faster in the lower extremities than in the upper, and rate of loss depends on the muscle group. Changes in muscle strength after disuse wasting is called disuse atrophy.

85. b. Selection of interventions should be based on an accurate history. Patients may have had more success with one treatment than another in the past. This could give the therapist a clue to how to proceed with treatment.

86. d. Heberden's nodes are bony, hard areas of swelling over the distal interphalangeal joints common in osteoarthritis, not rheumatoid arthritis.

87. c. Rheumatoid arthritis is a systemic disease of unknown origin, and osteoarthritis is a chronic wearing of the articular surfaces of the joints. Ankylosing spondylitis is a chronic systemic inflammatory disorder.

88. a. Boutonniere deformity is associated with rheumatoid arthritis, but is not always present with rheumatoid arthritis. Chronic inflammation of the PIP joint with avulsion of the extensor hood leads to boutonniere deformity.

89. a. Polymyositis and dermatomyositis cause proximal muscle weakness. All of the conditions listed could cause proximal weakness, but among the choices, polymyositis is most likely to specifically target this area.

90. c. Gout is related to high uric acid levels in the blood (hyperuricemia). Uric acid levels are influenced by genetic and environmental factors, and not all people with hyperuricemia develop gout.

91. d. After articular cartilage is damaged and causes edema in the joint, the other choices occur.

92. a. Age, obesity, hip injury, developmental hip disorders, and genetic predisposition are all risk factors for the development of osteoarthritis. Male and female genders alone are not considered primary risk factors.

93. d. There are several types of intervertebral disk herniation. Choice a describes a herniated disk, choice b a vertical herniation, choice c an extruded herniation, and finally choice d a sequestered disk herniation

94. c. A transverse fracture occurs horizontally across the bone, and spiral fracture occurs in a circular motion along the axis of the bone. Compression fracture is usually seen in the lumbar spine and occurs when the bone is compressed beyond its limits of tolerance.

95. a. A greenstick fracture is more likely to occur in children than adults because the greenstick fracture occurs in a more elastic bone. Choices b, c, and d can occur in both adults and children.

96. d. Choices a, b, and c all would affect the healing process of a fracture.

97. d. The rate of fracture healing declines with age. Many medical conditions can also disrupt fracture healing in older adults.

98. c. Stress fractures are more common in females than males regardless of the activity. They are most common in females who participate in weight-bearing sports such as track and field, basketball, and soccer.

99. a. This loss of tensile strength results from the loss of ground substance and subsequent dehydration. These changes contribute to the formation of fibrous adhesions and increased friction between fibers. These factors lead to reduced tissue strength in the ligament.

100. a. As one ages, skeletal muscles show a decrease in the number of muscle fibers accompanied by an increase in connective and fatty tissues within the muscle.

101. b. Tendinopathies usually result in painful movements that are frequently seen in the patellar tendon at the knee in people who perform repeated jumping such as dancers, basketball players, and volleyball players.

102. a. Healing time is unchanged with this patient population.

103. c. The medial femoral condyle is the most common area, although it can occur in the femoral capital epiphysis.

104. c. The knee is most common with this diagnosis, followed by the ankles and elbows.

105. d. Pauciarticular juvenile rheumatoid arthritis occurs in 50% to 60% of the cases, followed by polyarticular, then systemic.

106. a. The healing phase of ligaments is divided into the following categories: inflammatory phase (first few days after injury), proliferative phase (1–6 weeks after injury), and remodeling phase (begins 7 weeks after injury).

107. b. A steroid injection can weaken tendons and ligaments, and thus the joint must be moved carefully.

108. d. Thyroid hormone is not used, but the parathyroid hormone is used in cases of certain calcium imbalances. All of the listed agents are used with bisphosphonates to be taken on an empty stomach and sitting or standing for at least 30 minutes.

109. d. Acetaminophen has analgesic and antipyretic but no antiinflammatory properties. It is not indicated in rheumatoid arthritis, which is an inflammatory condition, but can be used in osteoarthritis, which is not an inflammatory problem.

110. a. Some patients use certain aspects of spasticity to maintain balance, and weakening of this spasticity could interfere with their balance. Skeletal muscle relaxants (except botulinus toxin) weaken but do not paralyze muscles, and some may cause physical dependence, which prohibits abrupt cessation of their long-term use. Numerous studies have confirmed the effectiveness of skeletal muscle relaxants.

111. a. Torticollis involving the right sternocleidomastoid would cause right lateral cervical flexion and left cervical rotation.

112. c. This condition may be due to spasm or to abnormally short jaw muscles. There is an inability to open the jaw fully.

113. d. The condyle glides anterior translatory down the eminence (26–50 mm of opening) with the disk in the upper joint compartment. Occasionally, the disk is displaced anteriorly, and adhesions may occur that produce an anterior displaced disk without reduction (locked joint).

114. d. Ipsilateral rotation and contralateral translation describe lateral jaw movement.

115. a. Bilateral anterior translation describes jaw protrusion.

116. b. A combination of rotations occur during the first 26 mm, then anterior translation, describes wide jaw opening.

117. c. Opioids are a class of drugs that cause pain relief by binding to opioid receptors. Ibuprofen and aspirin are nonsteroidal

antiinflammatory medications, whereas acetaminophen is in a class of its own; however, none of these three medications binds to opioid receptors.

118. c. Drowsiness, blurred vision, and dry mouth are caused by the anticholinergic side effects that muscle relaxants possess. These side effects are also the ones patients complain about most often.

119. b. All nonsteroidal antiinflammatory drugs inhibit the enzyme cyclooxygenase, thereby decreasing the inflammatory reaction.

120. d. Celecoxib is unique from the other NSAIDs in that it specifically inhibits cyclooxygenase-2 (COX-2). One of the most worrisome side effects of NSAIDs is the potential for ulcers because nonselective COX-inhibiting NSAIDs block the production of prostaglandins that provide a protective effect against acids in the stomach. COX-2–specific NSAIDs do not inhibit the production of these protective prostaglandins.

121. d. Opioid analgesics stimulate opioid receptors leading to analgesia, sedation, miosis (vision problems in the dark because pupils cannot dilate), respiratory depression, and sometimes nausea (less in supine position) and constipation.

122. b. Whiplash injury includes hyperextension of cervical vertebrae that may tear the anterior longitudinal ligament that limits extension of the cervical spine. All of the other ligaments limit flexion of the cervical spine; accordingly, they may be torn in hyperflexion injuries.

123. d. Osteoporosis affects all bones of the body, but most commonly it produces symptoms in the major weight-bearing bones.

124. b. Osteoarthritis is induced by aging, trauma, and genetic factors. Hence, fibrillation, osteophytes, and decreased collagen II synthesis are the main features. In contrast, synovitis and inflammation occur in other forms, such as rheumatoid and giant villonodular arthritis.

125. b. Diffuse pain is a defining criterion of fibromyalgia. According to the American College of Rheumatologists 1990 criteria for the classification of fibromyalgia, widespread pain must be present for at least 3 months. Pain is considered widespread when all of the following are present: pain in the left side of the body; pain in the right side of the body; pain above the waist; pain below the waist; and axial skeletal pain. Pain in 11 of 18 tender point sites on digital palpation must also be present to establish the diagnosis of fibromyalgia.

126. a. A defect in the lamina of a vertebra usually occurs first. This defect is called spondylolysis. The vertebra may then slip because of shear forces; this slippage is called spondylolisthesis.

127. b. Rheumatoid arthritis is a systemic condition commonly involving joints bilaterally. Crepitus can be associated with osteoarthritis or rheumatoid arthritis, but rheumatoid arthritis is the most likely in this case.

128. b. Because juvenile rheumatoid arthritis attacks the joint as in adult rheumatoid arthritis, there are no neurologic signs or symptoms.

129. b. Osgood-Schlatter disease is an injury to apophyseal cartilage. It is not an inflammatory condition and occurs mainly in young boys.

130. a. The other choices are more probable in a tetraplegic child.

131. a. Damage to the right hemisphere or frontal lobe often causes a decrease in executive functions. Diffuse and/or global cortical damage results in poor complex problem solving, and diffuse cortical/subcortical damage results in slow information processing. Memory deficits usually arise from temporal lobe damage.

132. d. Deep brain stimulation uses a pacemaker-like device surgically implanted with the electrodes in the nuclei of choice and a pulse generator implanted in the chest. When a tremor begins, the client activates the low-voltage, high-frequency generator by passing a magnet over a generator implanted in the chest. Stimulation through the electrodes can be applied to the internal globus pallidus and the subthalamic nucleus or thalamus. Thalamic stimulation is most effective for tremor, with less effect on dyskinesia and rigidity.

133. b. Medial temporal lobe involvement can cause an acute disturbance in memory, particularly if it occurs in the dominant hemisphere. The individual also may demonstrate agnosia, which is difficulty in identification or recognition of faces, objects, mathematical symbols, or colors. Anomia is impaired ability to identify objects by name.

134. c. Tardive dyskinesia is characterized by repetitive, involuntary, and purposeless movements. The patient may demonstrate rapid movements of any extremity, including the tongue.

135. d. Choices a and b are both acute symptoms of radiation to the brain. Lhermitte's sign is generally described as a tingling or shocklike sensation passing down the arm or trunk when the neck is flexed. Radionecrosis is a serious long-term complication of radiation to the brain. Symptoms include headache, changes in cognition and personality, focal neurologic deficits, and seizures.

136. c. Neurologic manifestations of advanced HIV disease are numerous and usually involve the CNS. The CNS is more commonly attacked than the peripheral nervous system.

137. d. Facioscapulohumeral dystrophy is a mild form of muscular dystrophy beginning with weakness and atrophy of the facial muscles and shoulder girdle, usually manifesting in the second decade of life. Inability to close the eyes may be the earliest sign; the face is expressionless even when laughing or crying, forward shoulders and scapular winging develop, and the person has difficulty raising the arms overhead. Progression is descending, with subsequent involvement of either the distal anterior leg or hip girdle muscles.

138. a. Type I spinal muscular atrophy (Werdnig-Hoffmann) causes respiratory failure and early death in the first few years of life if respiratory support is not provided.

139. b. Erb-Duchenne palsy accounts for most cases of Erb's palsy. Whole-arm palsy affects C5 to T1, and Klumpke's palsy affects the lower C8-T1 nerve roots.

140. b. Secondary to the strength losses in the wrist flexors, long finger flexors, and hand intrinsics, there is a possibility for posterior dislocation of the radial head with Klumpke's palsy.

141. c. A lesion on the spinal cord would lead to a decrease in sensation on the same side of the lesion and decreased pain sensation on the contralateral side of the lesion. A lesion above the medulla would cause decreased touch and pain on the opposite side of the lesion.

142. b. The frontal lobe is the site of damage that will lead to personality changes, and myoclonus and cortical blindness are indicative of damage to the hippocampus.

143. a. Age-related reduction in adult brain weight represents loss of brain tissue. Nerve cell shrinking and decreased nerve conduction velocity with age are normal in the motor and sensory systems.

144. b. There are many types of meningitis. The most common form is viral meningitis, but the most severe form is bacterial meningitis.

145. c. The stretch or pressure on the meninges caused by meningitis will manifest with the cardinal sign of headache.

146. c. The CSF has about $\frac{1}{200}$ the amount of antibody as blood, and the number of white blood cells is very low compared with the blood. Vasculitis can lead to infarction and decreases in cerebral blood flow, causing a drop in the glucose level of the CSF.

147. c. Hyponatremia (low sodium ion levels in the blood) occurs about 30% of the time, with an average duration of 3 days, and can be managed by fluid restriction.

148. d. Encephalitis is an acute inflammatory disease of the parenchyma, or tissue of the brain, caused by a direct viral invasion or hypersensitivity initiated by a virus.

149. b. Signs and symptoms in encephalitis depend on the etiologic agent, but in general, headache, nausea, and vomiting are followed by altered consciousness. All of the choices listed are possible but will not be present in every case.

150. c. The other choices listed are indicative of upper motor neuron lesions associated with amyotrophic lateral sclerosis.

151. a. Throughout the course of the disease, eye movements and sensory, bowel, and bladder functions are preserved.

152. c. Alzheimer's disease is the most common cause of dementia overall. It is one of the principal causes of disability and decreased quality of life among older adults.

153. d. Acetylcholine is an important neurotransmitter in areas of the brain involved in memory formation, and loss of acetylcholine activity correlates with the severity of Alzheimer's disease.

154. b. Choices a, c, and d are considered normal signs of aging. There is an impaired sense of smell with dementia.

155. b. Secondary progressive MS describes an initial pattern of relapse and remission that changes into a steadily progressive pattern over time in more than 50% of the relapsing cases. There sometimes are continued relapses during this phase. This conversion generally occurs 5 to 10 years after the initial onset of relapsing symptoms.

156. b. Fatigue is typically present in the midafternoon and may take the form of increased motor weakness with effort, mental fatigue, and sleepiness. Fatigue related to multiple sclerosis presents as an overwhelming feeling of tiredness in those who have done little and are not depressed.

157. c. Tremor of Parkinson's disease often appears unilaterally and may be confined to one upper limb for months to even years. It is the most common initial manifestation of Parkinson's disease. It is first seen as a rhythmic back-and-forth motion of the thumb and finger, referred to as the pill-rolling tremor.

158. d. Choices a, b, and c are indicative of a possible severe course of multiple sclerosis. Sensory symptoms, infrequent attacks, full neurologic recovery after a relapse, and a low level of disability after 5 to 7 years may be associated with an improved prognosis.

159. c. Cerebral vascular disease, the primary cause of stroke, is caused by one of several pathologic processes involving the blood vessels of the brain. Hypertension is a risk factor for stroke and is not the primary cause.

160. b. The most common source of embolitic occlusion is the heart as a result of atherothrombotic disease. Atrial fibrillation is believed to cause thrombus formation in the fibrillating atrium.

161. b. It is not the size of the missile but its velocity that generally determines the extent of damage with traumatic brain injury. Loss of consciousness does not always occur, although there is generally an altered state of consciousness. Although contusion is the hallmark of traumatic brain injury, severe or even fatal damage to the brain can occur without contusion.

162. c. Contusions typically occur at the poles and on the inferior surfaces of the frontal and temporal lobes. Occipital blows are more likely to produce contusions than are frontal or lateral blows.

163. a. Although the oculomotor nerve works in conjunction with the trochlear and abducens nerve to move the eyeball to maintain gaze stability and scanning, damage to the abducens nerve itself will result in failure of the eye to abduct when the head is passively turned away from the side of the lesion.

164. d. With excessive verbal output, the patient provides too much information, and content may be overly detailed or redundant. Poor discrimination of appropriate topics for the social content describes inappropriate topic selection, and use of profanity or emotionally charged words that are inappropriate for social content is described as inappropriate word choice.

165. b. A concussion is an injury caused by a blow or violent shaking that results in the temporary loss of function. A laceration or maceration of the cord occurs with more severe injuries in which the glia is disrupted and the spinal cord tissue may be torn.

166. b. Central cord syndrome is a result of damage to the central aspect of the spinal cord, often caused by hyperextension injuries in the cerebral region. There is characteristically more severe neurologic involvement in the upper extremities than the lower extremities.

167. c. Heterotopic ossification is excessive bone formation in the soft tissue, and it can limit range of motion, cause pain, and impair seating and posture. It often develops near the large joints. It is always found below the level of lesion, and it begins to develop within the first year after injury.

168. c. Spastic cerebral palsy, particularly quadriplegia and spastic diplegia, accounts for the majority of cases.

169. b. In spastic monoplegia, only one limb is affected. Spastic hemiplegia refers to primarily one total side affected with the upper extremity more than the lower extremity. Spastic quadriplegia refers to the involvement of all four limbs, the head, and trunk.

170. c. Age does not affect the size or number of fascicles, but the perineurium and epineurium do thicken with age, and the endoneurium often becomes fibrosed with increased collagen.

171. b. The most common symptoms of motor nerve involvement include distal weakness and hypotonicity. Deep tendon reflexes are diminished or absent, and distal-most deep tendon reflexes will be affected first. In neuropathy, motor symptoms tend to occur first distally, whereas in myopathy, the weakness tends to be proximal.

172. b. Clinical signs of Charcot-Marie-Tooth disease include distally symmetrical muscle weakness, atrophy, and diminished deep tendon reflexes. Individuals will have high arch deformities and hammertoes.

173. d. Hyperglycemic neuropathy occurs in an individual with poorly controlled diabetes, and in those who have been newly diagnosed, rapidly reversible nerve conduction abnormalities have been reported. Symptoms disappear when the individual's blood sugar is controlled, although abnormalities in nerve conduction may persist. The other choices are considered generalized symmetrical polyneuropathies.

174. b. Demyelination, initiated at the known node of Ranvier, occurs because macrophages, responding to inflammatory signals, strip myelin from the nerves. After the initial demyelination, the body initiates a repair process.

175. b. Upper motor neuron lesions cause peripheral stretch reflexes to become hyperreactive.

176. b. Myasthenia gravis is a disease that involves improper transmissions of the nerve signal to the muscles, and muscular dystrophy is a hereditary disease. Carpal tunnel syndrome involves the median nerve at the wrist.

177. b. Patients taking more than four medications have an increased risk for falls, and a low score on the dynamic gait index corresponds to an increased risk for falls. A previous history of falls shows a pattern of behavior that the therapist should be concerned with.

178. c. The patient is experiencing nystagmus of the eye. This is sometimes normal at the end ranges of eye movements, but is abnormal in this situation. The assistant should allow the patient to sit down because there is an increased risk for falls while the patient is experiencing nystagmus. In saccades, the patient's eyes cannot track an object without the head.

179. b. Choice a refers to spastic, choice c ataxic, and choice d hypertonic cerebral palsy. Athetosis can impair postural control, increase latency of movement onset, and cause oral-motor dysfunction leading to dysphasia or dysarthria.

180. d. Botulinum toxin paralyses muscles by inhibiting the release of acetylcholine at the neuromuscular junction. If spasticity is reduced, often range of motion and function will increase in children with cerebral palsy.

181. a. Although the clinical manifestations of cerebral palsy often change over time, these changes are not due to additional brain damage. The clinical manifestations of cerebral palsy are likely to change over time because of medical interventions or increases in brain function.

182. d. Neonatal encephalopathy is a disturbed neurologic function in the earliest stage of life in the full-term infant. These infants have trouble initiating and maintaining respiration, have decreased muscle tone and reflexes, and often have seizures. In acute hypoxia there is lack of oxygen to the brain, and myelomeningocele is a disorder of the lower spinal cord.

183. c. Spastic hemiplegia affects the right or left side of the body, and spastic quadriplegia would involve the entire bodies as in choices b and d.

184. d. In this surgical procedure, certain selective sensory nerve roots in the lumbar and sacral region are transected. This intervention does lead to decreased spasticity, but also temporary or maybe even permanent muscle weakness. This surgical procedure has been made less popular over the years because of a greater selection of reversible pharmacologic interventions.

185. a. Cerebral palsy is a disorder of the brain characterized by abnormal tone in the musculature. Neonatal encephalopathy is a condition of decreased reflexes and decreased muscle tone at birth. These

infants also have difficulty breathing. A Chiari II malformation is an anomaly of the hind brain that results in sometimes life-threatening brainstem dysfunction.

186. c. Cerebral palsy is a disorder of the brain and is not associated with spinal cord malformation as is myelomeningocele. Choices a, b, and d are all possibilities with myelomeningocele. Cognitive delays are a result of hydrocephalus that occurs with 70% to 90% of children with myelomeningocele.

187. b. A left homonymous hemianopsia is a visual field deficit, and left hemiplegia is a decrease in strength on the left side. Left hemianesthesia would be defined as a decreased sensation on the left.

188. c. A diffuse area of energy could be associated with traumatic brain injury, but not stroke. Because usually a traumatic brain injury involves a closed force trauma, the brain could be injured by the point of initial contact, or from the opposite side of the brain coming in high-velocity contact with the skull. A stroke usually has a focal point of injury at a particular point in the brain.

189. c. In sensory neglect, the patient has decreased awareness of sensory stimulation on the side of the body. Decreased motor neglect is an inability to generate movement on the side of the neglect. This patient displays personal neglect and does not recognize the side of the body involved with the lesion. In spatial neglect, the patient does not recognize the space on the side of the body involved with the neglect.

190. a. As Huntington's disease progresses, athetosis, akinesia, and bradykinesia develop. Although the patient's reflexes may be hypertonic, spasticity is usually not a symptom of Huntington's disease.

191. d. Choice a refers to amyotrophic lateral sclerosis, choice b Parkinson's disease, and choice c multiple sclerosis.

192. c. Because most progressive central nervous system disorders will leave the patient with significant functional deficits, the respiratory system will eventually fail. The patient becomes progressively less ambulatory and does not stress the respiratory system adequately.

193. a. Most patients have this type of multiple sclerosis early in the course of the disease. Over time the disease either stays in this phase or moves to one of the other categories.

194. b. Along with tremor and rigidity, patients with Parkinson's disease show bradykinesia, impaired balance, and poor postural control. There is also usually a masklike expression in the face.

195. c. Alzheimer's disease and Huntington's disease both show significant cognition impairments early in the disease process. The later stages of Parkinson's disease and multiple sclerosis also have cognition deficits.

196. c. A neurotmesis is the complete laceration of a nerve. Surgical repair is necessary for possible regeneration of the nerve.

197. a. Because there is disruption in the peripheral nerve, there will be less reaction to a deep tendon reflex. This test is performed by tapping on tendons with a reflex hammer.

198. d. Disuse atrophy is common with muscle tissue. Nerve tissue is not susceptible to disuse.

199. b. Patients with Charcot-Marie-Tooth syndrome present with distal muscle weakness, structural foot abnormalities, soft tissue complications of calluses or ulcers, and electromyographic abnormalities. Absent or diminished deep tendon reflexes are also common. In patients with this diagnosis, symptoms typically begin in the teens or 20s and progress gradually over their lifetime.

200. c. Increased limb temperatures increase nerve conduction velocity. Choices a, b, and d are all associated with decreased nerve conduction velocities.

201. a. Although there is some sensory damage with Guillain-Barré syndrome, it primarily affects motor nerves.

202. b. CIDP develops slowly, with peak symptoms at about 8 weeks. Guillain-Barré syndrome typically has respiratory involvement, whereas the respiratory system is often not involved with CIDP. CIDP has a poor prognosis, and most patients do not fully recover.

203. a. Injuries above the cauda equina, which is approximately the L1-2 intervertebral space in adults, result in muscle weakness and paralysis, hypertonia, co-contraction, and hyperreflexia below the level of the lesion. Damage below the L1-2 intervertebral space results in damage to lower motor neurons only and muscle atrophy, flaccid paralysis, and fibrillations below the level of the injury.

204. d. Other reflexive movements involve the patient biting down when something is placed in the mouth, or closing the hand in response to stimulus to the palm. The other choices are learned responses.

205. c. This patient is considered to be in a minimally conscious state because he or she can follow commands and does have some reliability to the verbal responses. In a vegetative state, the eyes would

open spontaneously only, and in a coma, the eyes would not open to any stimuli.

206. a. Extension in the upper and lower extremities is described as a decerebrate posture. Both of these lesions are indicative of severe brain damage. Decerebrate posture is thought to be caused by deep bilateral cerebral lesions or compression of the brainstem.

207. a. The Charcot foot is an extreme example of neuroarthropathy and is characterized by a collapsed arch with a rocker-bottom shape and short foot length. The apex of the rocker bottom on the plantar surface of the foot is the most common site of ulceration.

208. a. The loss of sensation is the highest risk factor for neuropathic ulcers. Without sensation patients cannot feel the ischemia caused by improper footwear or bony abnormalities.

209. b. Neuropathic ulcers occur on weight-bearing surfaces or where the footwear would cause skin disruptions against the foot. Choices a, c, and d all fit this scenario. Arterial and venous ulcers sometimes occur above the ankle.

210. b. Exposure to chemicals is a concern with infants because the blood-brain barrier, which keeps the contaminants from reaching the central nervous system, is not yet developed, putting the infants at greater risk for neurologic impairments.

211. d. If a tumor is present in the superior temporal gyrus, the patient will often present with receptive dysphasia. Early hydrocephalus is a common sign of a midbrain tumor. Sixth cranial nerve involvement is indicative of a tumor in the pons.

212. c. Because astrocytomas in children are most common in the cerebellum, symptoms will manifest as unilateral cerebellar ataxia involving the limbs and trunk followed by signs of increased intracranial pressure.

213. a. Magnetic resonance imaging has evolved as the most informative brain imaging study because of its superior imaging capabilities and lack of artifact from the temporal bones. With the addition of gadolinium contrast enhancement, which distinguishes tumor from surrounding edema, magnetic resonance imaging detects tumors even a few millimeters in size.

214. c. There are several methods for emergency treatment of elevated intracranial pressure. Hyperventilation requires intubation and mechanical ventilation; however, the physician will be able to see the results of hyperventilation in seconds. Osmotherapy has an onset of minutes after initial dosage.

215. b. Back pain is the most common and prominent symptom of metastasis to the spinal column and cord and is present in 95% of cases. The other choices are usually present in some form, but back pain is the most common symptom.

216. b. Hypoxic-ischemic insult is the most common cause of neonatal convulsions, resulting from lack of oxygen to the brain during or before delivery. Seizures resulting from cerebral contusion are often a result of prolonged or traumatic labor. The other important cause of seizures arising in the early neonatal period is hypoglycemia, most often seen in babies who are small for gestational age.

217. b. In the tonic phase of a tonic-clonic seizure, the body becomes rigid, and the person has risk for falling. The clonic phase begins with rhythmic jerky contractions, especially in the extremities, and ends up with relaxation of all body muscles.

218. a. Many people with epilepsy experience a higher frequency of seizures with large doses of caffeine. Amphetamines and other stimulants should be avoided, as should some asthma drugs that can increase the incidence of seizure activity.

219. c. Vagal nerve stimulation can be provided through an implantable pulse generator. By stimulating the left vagal nucleus, an inhibitory projection influences the entire cerebral cortex. A 50% reduction in seizure with vagal nerve stimulation has been reported.

220. d. Simple partial seizures are associated with preservation of consciousness and unilateral hemispheric involvement. They may manifest as motor symptoms or somatosensory symptoms. Psychotic responses to seizure activity include hallucinations or illusions and a sudden sense of fears.

221. a. Atonic seizures, also known as drop attacks, are brief losses of consciousness and postural tone not associated with tonic muscular contractions. Atonic seizures occur most often in children with diffuse encephalopathies and are characterized by sudden loss of muscle tone that may result in falls with self-injury.

222. c. Examples of primary headaches are migraine headaches, tension headaches, and cluster headaches. Secondary headaches are caused by associated disease.

223. c. Nausea is not associated with tension headache, but reports of anorexia, mild photophobia, and phonophobia are common.

224. d. Although analgesics and nonsteroidal antiinflammatory drugs may decrease tension headache pain, overuse of these medications will cause rebound tension headaches. Estrogenic hormones may worsen tension-type headaches. Beta blockers are used to treat migraine headaches.

225. a. Cranial nerve V, or the trigeminal nerve, is associated with both sensory and motor functions in the face. The dural nerves that innervate the cranial vessels consist of fibers that are almost nociceptive in function, so stimulation of the cranial vessels causes pain.

226. c. If there is disk disease in the lower neck, compensatory movement in facet joints of the upper cervical spine will cause pain to travel along the C1-4 nerve to the interface of the trigeminal complex.

227. a. When there is disruption of the vestibular nerve on one side causing loss of tonic firing, it results in abnormal information relayed to the brain about the position or movement of the head. The brain, as it compares the two sides, then interprets the abnormal input as movement when the head is actually at rest.

228. d. A sensation of rotation may represent maladaptation of the input, reflecting a unilateral disorder. Orthostatic hypotension or vestibular/somatosensory system disruption is usually manifested by lightheadedness.

229. a. The sensation of vertigo will stop after 20 to 30 seconds in the static position with benign paroxysmal positional vertigo.

230. d. Unilateral vestibular neuronitis causes sudden onset of rotary vertigo, spontaneous horizontal nystagmus, nausea, and vomiting. Immediately after the onset of unilateral vestibular hypofunction there is intense disequilibrium.

231. b. The typical attack of hydrops related to Ménière's syndrome is experienced as an initial sensation of fullness of the ear, a reduction in hearing, and tinnitus. This is usually followed by rotational vertigo, postural imbalance, nystagmus, and nausea.

232. d. Malignant external otitis, an infection affecting older people with diabetes or immunosuppression, begins in the external auditory canal and spreads to the temporal bone. Permanent damage is possible when the infection causes damage to the structures of the labyrinth or the eighth cranial nerve.

233. d. Traumatic disorders such as a spinal cord injury or brain injury are most often caused by motor vehicle crashes and commonly involve clients in their teens to 30s. The other disorders are manifested most often from the 30s to the 60s.

234. b. Stroke refers to the neurologic problems arising from disruption of blood flow to the brain. This disruption may be caused by hemorrhage (bleeding) or blockage from a clot the results of an ischemia (decreased oxygen).

235. d. Tissue plasminogen activator has thrombolytic properties, whereas glutamate antagonists have neuroprotective properties. Calcium channel blockers have the ability to halt and reverse the cascade of events after ischemia.

236. a. Medications used after spinal cord injury prevent further damage to neural tissue and enhance repair and recovery. Depression is common after traumatic brain injury and spinal cord injury.

237. d. The most common symptoms of vestibular disorders are dizziness, unsteadiness, vertigo, and nausea.

238. c. Multiple sclerosis is the disease in which patches of demyelination in the nervous system lead to disturbances in the conduction of messages along the nerves.

239. b. Common symptoms include visual problems, sensory problems such as tingling and numbness, weakness, fatigue, problems with balance, and speech disturbances. The course of the early stages is unpredictable.

240. d. In secondary progressive multiple sclerosis, the disease progresses unremittingly and causes severe disability.

241. d. In relapsing-remitting multiple sclerosis, the disease seems to go into remission, and the patient is relatively symptom free, with no functional disabilities. This type of multiple sclerosis is also referred to as benign.

242. b. The classic triad of symptoms includes tremor, rigidity, and bradykinesia. Bradykinesia could be replaced by akinesia.

243. a. Parkinson's disease results from a deficiency of dopamine produced in a region of the brain called the substantia nigra. The specific cause of this depletion is unknown.

244. c. The tremor, rigidity, and bradykinesia have a great impact on the patient's ability to maintain balance and perform such activities as walking, stair climbing, and reaching. Patients tend to have a stooped posture, walk with short, shuffling steps, and lose reciprocal movements.

245. b. Currently no cure is available for this disease, and survival time is about 4 years from diagnosis to death.

246. c. Electroencephalography involves recording the electrical potential or activity in the brain by placement of electrodes on the scalp. This test is essential in diagnosis and management of seizure disorder. Electromyography involves recording the electrical activity in a muscle during a state of rest and during voluntary contraction. A nerve conduction velocity study involves recording the rate at which electrical signals are transmitted along peripheral nerves.

247. c. If the patient exhibits a diminished ability to receive and interpret verbal or written communication (receptive aphasia), or the patient has an impaired ability to communicate by speech (expressive aphasia), the therapist will have to use specific strategies to work with the patient successfully.

248. b. A child with a developmental delay has not obtained predictable movement patterns or behavior associated with children of a similar chronologic age.

249. d. Newborn infants may be born with positional deformities that are related to their position within the intrauterine environment. Congenital muscular torticollis is one condition that may be associated with these in utero constraints.

250. a. Congenital muscular torticollis refers to the posture of the infant's head and neck that results from shortening of one sternocleidomastoid muscle, which causes the head to tilt toward and rotate away from the shortened muscle.

251. a. The cause of juvenile rheumatoid arthritis is unknown, although genes associated with a variety of forms of the disease have been identified. Similar to other autoimmune disorders, juvenile rheumatoid arthritis appears to be a result of complex genetic and possibly environmental exposures.

252. a. The term clubfoot is derived from the position of the affected foot, which is turned inward and slanted upward.

253. b. Children with spina bifida and certain forms of cerebral palsy are more prone to developmental dysplasia of the hip and are monitored through regular physical examinations.

254. d. In Duchenne's muscular dystrophy, females do not manifest symptoms but are carriers of the disease, whereas males do manifest symptoms. Boys with Duchenne's muscular dystrophy usually develop normally until 3 to 5 years of age, when progressive lower extremity muscle weakness and wasting become apparent and are combined with enlarged yet weak calf muscles and tight heel cords.

255. a. Meningomyelocele is an open lesion with minimal to no skin protection covering the deeper nerve roots. This condition is the most severe of the spinal closure defects, with the potential for leaking spinal fluid and infection before surgical intervention and healing.

256. a. A child with Down syndrome is characterized by low muscle tone, flat facial profile, upwardly slanted eyes, short stature, varying levels of intellectual disability, slow growth and development, a small nose and low nasal ridge, and congenital heart disease.

257. d. Approximately one half to two thirds of children with cerebral palsy have intellectual disabilities. Early signs of cerebral palsy include poor sucking, irritability, hypertonia, hypotonia, or reduced movement quality.

258. a. Cystic fibrosis is a disorder of the exocrine gland function and involves the respiratory system, pancreas, reproductive organs, and sweat glands.

259. c. Postural reactions and motor milestone development occur in the same sequence as with normal infants, but the progression of an infant with Down syndrome is slower.

260. c. Involvement of the basal ganglia results in dyskinesia or athetosis. Cerebellar lesions produce ataxia, or unstable movement. The corpus callosum is not involved.

261. b. Myelodysplasia can involve the entire spine, not just the anterior cord. Teratogens are any agents that cause a structural abnormality during pregnancy. Excessive alcohol and drug intake has been shown to cause myelodysplasia. Although the lower spinal region is more likely to be effected in myelodysplasia, it can refer to defects in any part of the spinal column.

262. c. Exteriorization of neuralgic function can occur throughout life, and gait abnormalities are often the first complaint. Scoliosis can be slow in developing and should be monitored by the physical therapist.

263. a. Contractions of antagonistic muscle groups produce reciprocal patterns. This is not seen in children with cerebral palsy.

264. d. These movements remain until 5 months of age, when they become associated with a lack of movement of the extremities to midline.

265. d. Levodopa/carbidopa can cause all of the listed effects except bradycardia. Because of the off-phase effect, the patient may have to be scheduled at times when he or she is in the "on" phase.

266. a. All of these movement disorders can occur, but tardive dyskinesia is irreversible and may require an immediate change in the drug prescribed.

267. c. Neuralgia and myopathies are encountered during antiviral treatments, whereas all the other reactions are rare. For some drugs, it is important to ask the patient to drink a lot of water during strenuous exercise to prevent dehydration and drug precipitations in the kidney.

268. a. The most common adverse reactions are sedation, confusion, and psychomotor impairment.

269. a. Cholinergic agonists stimulate muscarinic receptors and cause diarrhea, sweating, salivation, bradycardia, decreased blood pressure, and miosis.

270. b. Perception of spatial relationships. The parietal lobes function to integrate sensory information for perception of spatial relations.

271. d. Spasticity, hyperreflexia, positive Babinski's sign. Fasciculation is also a sign of lower motor neuron disorders because it represents denervation hypersensitivity of the lower motor neuron. Upper motor neuron syndrome does not produce rigidity. Rigidity is a sign of basal ganglia disease. Hyporeflexia is a sign of lower motor neuron lesions.

272. c. An injury to the C5-6 nerve roots results in Erb's palsy. The flexor carpi ulnaris is innervated by C8-T1 nerve roots.

273. c. The most common injury of the brachial plexus is to the upper roots, C5 to C6, resulting in Erb's palsy.

274. a. The patient has difficulty finding an item within a crowded visual field; this is figure-ground discrimination. Agraphia is the inability to write. Vertical orientation and body scheme awareness relate to the patient's self-awareness.

275. c. A painful neuroma in the space between the third and the fourth metatarsal heads is called Morton's neuroma.

276. c. Atrophy of the hypothenar eminence is a sign of ulnar nerve lesion, whereas paresthesias over the dorsal aspect of the hand are symptoms of radial nerve lesion. Decreased resisted thumb abduction and forearm pronation are signs of median nerve lesion, but the motor branches of pronator teres and pronator quadratus arise before the median nerve enters the carpal tunnel.

277. a. It is well known that the C5 nerve root exits the C4-5 intervertebral space. The other choices exit above and below this level.

278. d. The involved upper extremity is in this position because of damage to the C5 and C6 spinal roots.

279. b. A person with spastic quadriplegia presents with talipes equinovarus. This term is synonymous with clubfoot. The hindfoot will be in varus, and the calcaneus will be abnormally small.

280. a. Although all of the choices do occur in children with a spinal cord injury, choice a is the most appropriate. During the first year of spinal cord injury, 40% of bone mineral density is lost through calcium excreted in the urine.

281. c. Vitamin C deficiency is often associated with many connective tissue disorders, including skin and gum lesions, impaired skin and wound healing, muscle weakness, and joint pain.

282. b. Cancerous tumors often refer pain to sites away from the actual location of the tumor. The hip joint refers pain commonly to the sacroiliac joint and knee.

283. d. Bleeding in the joints, or hemarthrosis, is one of the most common clinical manifestations of hemophilia, significantly affecting the synovial joints. The knee is the most frequently affected, followed by the ankle, elbow, hip, shoulder, and wrist.

284. b. When active bleeding stops, isometric muscle exercise should be initiated to prevent muscular atrophy. Quadriceps sets are the only exercise listed that are isometric in nature

285. c. Three weeks of bed rest has a more profound impact on physical work capacity than three decades of aging because of the significance in muscle atrophy and deconditioning of the cardiovascular and pulmonary systems.

286. d. Training and conditioning differently during different times of the month may help protect women from injury. The effectiveness of neuromuscular and proprioceptive training in preventing anterior cruciate ligament injuries in female athletes has been demonstrated.

287. c. The child has a smaller heart size than the adult; thus there is a smaller stroke volume. The child has a higher heart rate during submaximal and maximal exercise. Children should be monitored closely for correct form and posture during all aspects of a training program.

288. c. At all ages, females appear to be more vulnerable to loss of lean tissue than males.

289. a. Loss of muscle function appears to be due to decreased total fibers, decreased muscle fiber size, impaired excitation–contraction coupling mechanism, or decreased high-threshold motor units.

290. a. Idiopathic scoliosis has no known cause. It is present in 80% of all cases of scoliosis.

291. a. Elevation of the involved extremity with arterial insufficiency leads to an even further lack of blood flow to the area. There is pain in the tissues of the leg because of hypoxia.

292. d. The use of tobacco is the single most preventable risk factor for arterial disease. The other choices are consistent with vascular disease. Smoking contributes to atherosclerosis by promoting lipid accumulation in the vessels and plaque enlargement. Smoking also causes vasoconstriction and decreases oxygen-carrying capacity of red blood cells by loading them with carbon monoxide.

293. b. Most patients do not understand that even though their wound has healed, adherence to compression therapy will help alleviate recurrence of the wound. A total of 79% of those who did not adhere to compression therapy had wound reoccurrence compared with a 4% reoccurrence rate for those who continued with compression therapy.

294. c. Partial-thickness burns can be subclassified as superficial or deep partial-thickness burns. Superficial partial-thickness burns exhibit destruction of the epidermis and minimal damage to the superficial layers of the dermis. In deep partial-thickness burns, the epidermis and almost all of the dermis are destroyed.

295. a. Full-thickness burns are considered a severe injury. This patient would not survive without intravenous fluids and would not heal correctly without proper surgical management.

296. b. Superficial burns heal in 3 to 5 days, with superficial partial-thickness burns healing in an average of 21 days. Deep partial-thickness burns would take longer than 21 days, and full-thickness burns require surgical management, so the healing time is much longer.

297. c. Wound healing is commonly described in three phases: the inflammatory phase, the proliferative phase, and the remodeling phase. It is important that all phases of wound care occur simultaneously to some extent. For example, inflammation can occur while proliferative process is in progress.

298. a. With any injury comes an inflammatory phase during which repair of the tissue is initiated. Initial blood loss is decreased by the immediate vasoconstriction of the vessels. This vasoconstrictive response may last 5 to 10 minutes.

299. b. Wounds begin to contract slightly during inflammation; however, aggressive contraction at the wound commences during the proliferative phase. Fibroblasts, particularly myofibroblasts, have contractile capability.

300. a. Arterial insufficiency wounds are caused by a primary loss of vascular flow to an anatomic site, which leads to tissue death. The other choices are all causes of venous insufficiency

301. d. Wounds caused by arterial insufficiency are commonly found on the lower part of the leg, including the feet and toes. Because of the poor circulation to the wound, minimal, if any, exudate is seen.

302. c. Neuropathic ulcers are usually located on the plantar surface of the foot at pressure points or bony prominences.

303. d. Pressure ulcers are graded from stage I progressively to stage IV. A wound will begin at stage I with nonblanchable erythema of intact skin and progress to full-thickness skin loss with extensive tissue destruction in stage IV.

304. b. This patient is likely to experience a decrease in the number of red blood cells. All of the other statements are correct. Fibrinogen drops initially but then rises throughout recovery.

305. a. This is the correct order of incision or wound healing after surgery.

306. a. Tetracyclines cause mostly a toxic photosensitization and sunlight or ultraviolet light should be avoided. They should also not be given to children because of bone and teeth problems and should not be taken with antacids, which prevent their absorption.

307. c. Fever and malaise might be signs of infection or other medical complications. They are not signs of hypertrophic scarring.

308. b. These signs are characteristic of an arterial insufficiency ulcer. A venous ulcer often presents with the following symptoms: no pain around the wound, no gangrene, location typically on the medial ankle, pigmented skin around the ulcer, and significant edema. A trophic ulcer (also known as a pressure or decubitus ulcer) presents with decreased sensation, callused skin, and no pain and is located over bony prominences.

309. a. Strenuous/intense exercise or long-duration exercise such as marathon running is followed by impairment of the immune system. There are beneficial effects to the immune system with moderate exercise.

310. a. Infectious mononucleosis is an acute infectious disease caused by Epstein-Barr virus. The spleen may enlarge two to three times its normal size, causing left upper quadrant pain with possible referral to the left shoulder and left upper trapezius region. Individuals are at risk for splenic rupture, and care should be taken to avoid trauma.

311. c. Debilitated individuals have the greatest risk for influenza-related complications. These include individuals older than 65 years, residents of nursing homes, patients with chronic pulmonary or cardiovascular disease, and people with diabetes.

312. b. The release of epinephrine at sympathetic endings increases the rate and force of muscular contractions of the heart, constricts peripheral blood vessels, and raises blood glucose levels by the breakdown of fats. Epinephrine is released in the body's response to acute physical or emotional stress. Cardiac output and blood glucose levels are raised to prepare the body for immediate action.

313. c. The pituitary gland blood supply decreases with age, and the thyroid gland becomes relatively smaller and becomes lower lying with age.

314. c. Thickening of the transverse carpal ligament can occur with systemic disorders such as acromegaly or myxedema. Endocrine and metabolic conditions such as acromegaly, diabetes, pregnancy, and hypothyroidism can increase the chances of developing carpal tunnel system.

315. d. The other choices are typical of a patient with type 2 diabetes.

316. c. Nerve tissue, erythrocytes, cells of the intestines, liver, and kidney tubules do not require insulin for glucose transport and are affected the least if there is an insulin deficiency.

317. a. Flapping tremor is elicited by attempted wrist extension while the forearm is fixed. There is a rapid flexion and extension of the wrist to indicate a positive test. This neurologic abnormality is associated with uremia, respiratory failure, severe heart failure, and liver failure.

318. c. Referred pain from the hepatic and biliary systems can manifest in several areas. These areas include the area between the scapulae, right shoulder, right upper trapezius, right interscapular area, and right subscapular area.

319. c. The liver will decrease in size and weight with advancing age and have decreased blood flow. The pancreas undergoes structural changes such as fibrosis, fatty acid deposits, and atrophy.

320. d. Jaundice is clinically characterized by yellow discoloration of the skin, sclera, and mucous membranes. Jaundice occurs as a result of overproduction of bilirubin, deficits in the bilirubin metabolism, and presence of liver disease, or from obstruction of bile flow.

321. b. One of the most common symptoms associated with cirrhosis is ascites, an accumulation of fluid in the peritoneal cavity surrounding the intestines. This distinction often occurs very slowly over a number of weeks or months and may be associated with bilateral edema of the feet and ankles.

322. d. Diabetic neuropathies, no matter the advanced stage of the disorder, usually present with motor and sensory signs and symptoms. They do follow a length-dependent pattern of distribution. The toes are affected first, followed by the feet, and spreading up the legs. Because they affect several nerves, diabetic neuropathies are polyneuropathies.

323. b. The male gender is more predisposed to neuropathic ulcers secondary to diabetes. All of the other choices are high-risk factors.

324. c. In type 1 diabetes, there is autoimmune destruction of insulin-secreting beta cells in the pancreas. The onset of type 1 diabetes is generally during puberty but can begin as early as 9 months of age or as late as in the fifth decade. The other choices are indicative of type 2 diabetes.

325. d. Pes equinus is defined as a shortening of the Achilles tendon, and hallux limitus is limited range of motion of the great toe metatarsophalangeal joint. Hallux valgus is lateral deviation of the hallux in relation to the first metatarsal shaft.

326. a. Because of large motor nerve involvement, the lower extremities are generally more involved than the upper extremities. The distal reflexes are more involved than the proximal reflexes. The reflexes are usually equal bilaterally.

327. b. Tachycardia could be the result of taking too much thyroid hormone, and the patient may need a dose adjustment. Overdosing with propylthiouracil might cause lethargy and weight gain.

328. c. Direct access will increase the likelihood of therapists being the first provider for many conditions. Risk factor assessment is helpful in identifying immune problems, but the cause of and risk for many conditions are still unknown. Disease progression is common with different signs and symptoms, and early recognition of immune dysfunction can improve the course of the disease.

329. c. All the other characteristics are those of cholinergic receptors, with the exception of choice a, which is not a characteristic of any receptor group.

330. d. Dry skin is a sign of a diabetic coma.

331. d. A person in a diabetic coma has low blood pressure.

332. c. A person is usually diagnosed with type 1 diabetes at 25 years of age or younger. A person is usually 40 years of age or older when diagnosed with type 2 diabetes. Ketoacidosis is a symptom of type 1. Metabolism of free fatty acids in the liver causes this condition, which is an excess of ketones. Patients with type 2 diabetes may be able to control their condition with diet only (depending on the severity of the condition), but a patient with type 1 diabetes needs insulin.

333. a. Radiation pneumonitis is caused by significant interstitial inflammation creating a reduction of gas exchange. It usually occurs about 2 days to 3 months after completion of radiation therapy and typically resolves in 6 to 12 months. All of the other choices are delayed effects of ionizing radiation.

334. a. In the upright position, the blood pressure in the veins in the lower extremities is about 100 mm Hg. Contraction of the gastrocnemius muscle compresses and empties the deep veins, which promotes venous return and decreases venous pressure. Ambulatory pressure within the venous and capillary system is less than 20 mm Hg.

335. b. The patient is describing intermittent claudication. This is caused by ischemia from arterial involvement in the lower extremities. The pain results from a lack of oxygen to the lower extremity tissues. Venous insufficiency pain comes later in the progression of this disease and generally worsens when the limb is gravity dependent.

336. d. Respiratory syncytial virus causes annual outbreaks of pneumonia and other respiratory illnesses. It is the main cause of hospitalization of the very young.

337. b. Dyspnea relieved by any specific breathing patterns or body position is more likely to be pulmonary rather than cardiac in origin.

338. a. Choice c describes angiotensin II medications, whereas antiarrhythmics alter conduction patterns in the heart. Anticoagulants will prevent blood clot formation.

339. a. Orthostatic hypertension is often accompanied by dizziness, blurring or loss of vision, and syncope/fainting.

340. c. Dilated cardiomyopathy is characterized by fatigue, weakness, and angina like chest pain. Restrictive cardiomyopathy has clinical manifestations related to a decrease in cardiac output such as fatigue, shortness of breath, and peripheral edema.

341. d. A productive cough with purulent sputum may indicate infection, whereas a productive cough with nonpurulent sputum is nonspecific in indicating airway irritation.

342. b. Low-pitched sounds predominantly heard during inspiration are indicative of crackles or rales. A shrill harsh sound heard during inspiration is defined as stridor, and wheezing is a high-pitched continuous whistling sound with expiration.

343. b. Aging is accompanied by a gradual reduction of blood flow to the kidneys, coupled with a reduction of nephrons. As a result, the kidneys become less efficient at removing waste from the blood, and the volume of urine increases somewhat with age. A tendency toward greater renal vasoconstriction in the older adult is evident.

344. d. The increase in urinary tract infections in pregnant women is a result of dilation of the upper urinary system, reduction of the peristaltic activity of the ureters, and displacement of the urinary bladder.

345. d. Classic features of urinary tract infections in older children and adults include frequency, urgency, dysuria, nocturia, fever, chills, and malaise. Mental status changes, especially confusion or

increased confusion, are prominent features of urinary tract infections in the elderly population.

346. b. Calcium stones are the most common type of stone. Struvite stones are related to recurrent bacterial urinary tract infections with organisms that produce urease. Uric stones occur as a result of increased level of urate in the blood and uric acid crystals in the urine. Cystine stones are uncommon and are caused by the hereditary disorder cystinuria.

347. b. The most common sites of extraskeletal calcification include the coronary arteries, lungs, skin, peripheral arteries, joints, and cornea.

348. c. Functional incontinence occurs in people who have normal urine control but have difficulty reaching a toilet in time because of a muscle or joint dysfunction. Stress incontinence is the loss of urine during activities that increase intraabdominal pressure. Overflow incontinence is the constant leaking of urine from a bladder that is full but unable to empty.

349. a. The testes will become smaller in normal degenerative changes in the reproductive system.

350. d. Heated water is injected into a balloon inserted into the urethra. The heat destroys excess prostate tissue. This procedure is done on an outpatient basis, but a catheter must be worn for 1 to 3 weeks afterward.

351. b. Recently, estrogen and progestin were found to increase the risk for breast cancer, heart disease, stroke, and blood clots in women who took the medications after menopause. Estrogen replacement showed some benefit, but it was not enough to outweigh the risks.

352. c. Although this patient may have some symptoms that also match urge incontinence, the definition of functional incontinence is the following: Functional incontinence occurs when a person recognizes the need to urinate, but cannot physically make it to the bathroom in time because of limited mobility. Causes of functional incontinence include confusion; dementia; poor eyesight; poor mobility; poor dexterity; unwillingness to toilet because of depression, anxiety, or anger; or being in a situation in which it is impossible to reach a toilet.

353. a. Uterine prolapse occurs when pelvic floor muscles and ligaments stretch and weaken, providing inadequate support for the uterus. The uterus then descends into the vaginal canal.

354. c. Owing to the location of the baby, all but the breasts may be compressed at some point during a pregnancy.

355. a. Predictors of lower back pain after pregnancy include significantly earlier onset of pain during pregnancy, higher maternal age, higher body mass index, higher level of low back and pelvic pain during pregnancy and joint hypermobility.

356. b. Although this patient may also have some pelvic organ descent, her symptoms are most likely matching urge incontinence, which is defined as "involuntary loss of urine occurring for no apparent reason while suddenly feeling the need or urge to urinate. The most common cause of urge incontinence is involuntary and inappropriate detrusor muscle contractions."

357. d. The use of nonsteroidal antiinflammatory drugs is associated with a wide spectrum of side effects; however, most serious side effects are often seen in the gastrointestinal tract, kidneys, and cardiovascular system.

358. c. Side effects of anabolic steroids are often acne vulgaris and an increase in sexual drive, body hair, and aggressive behavior. There is also susceptibility to biceps and patella tendon strains. Therapists should always take a comprehensive history, looking for a possible anabolic steroid abuse.

359. c. Research has shown that people recovering from chemotherapy should not be instructed to rest but rather should increase physical activity within tolerances. Prolonged rest and decreased activity, coupled with sleep disturbances or too much sleep, can contribute to increased fatigue.

360. a. Fever raises the systemic metabolism and increases consumption of oxygen. As a result, a decrease in systemic vascular resistance occurs, thereby producing hypotension and an increase in cardiac output to increase flow of blood and the delivery of oxygen to organs.

361. b. Choice b is true regarding boys, not girls. The girls' strength curve continues linearly at puberty rather than sharply rising.

362. c. Because of the increased strength of these muscle groups compared with their counterparts, contractures in these planes are common in patients with myelomeningocele. Prolonged contractures would lead to possible subluxation or dislocation.

363. c. Although there are many risk factors associated with pregnancy, women with spinal cord injury can safely give birth to children. They should be followed closely by the obstetrician, who is familiar with the special needs of women with spinal cord injury.

364. a. The loss of more than 10% total body weight increases the risk for pressure ulcer formation by 74%. There is adequate documentation that patients need optimal nutrition status to allow the body to heal pressure ulcers. The caloric needs of wound tissue increase to 50% above baseline.

365. b. Consistent and forceful gastrocnemius contractions assist the pump mechanism to move venous blood back to the heart. Even though other choices are important, choice b is the only one with implications for venous insufficiency.

366. d. Neuropathic ulcers are associated with mechanical stress and sensory loss. This could be from peripheral vascular disease, diabetes mellitus, or other disorders of the central nervous system. Neuropathic ulcers are not generally associated with congestive heart failure.

367. b. Neuropathy is common in older adults who have suffered electrical burns and severe burns. Improper positioning or application of compression dressings can contribute to the neuropathy as the patient heals.

368. b. There is evidence that physical activity decreases blood pressure, improves lipid profile by decreasing triglycerides and total cholesterol while increasing high-density lipoprotein, improves insulin sensitivity, and enhances endothelial function, all of which contribute to decrease in cardiovascular risk.

369. c. Acute alcoholic myopathy is a syndrome of muscle pain, tenderness, and edema occurring after acute excesses of alcohol ingestion. The proximal muscles of the extremities, the pelvic and shoulder girdles, and the muscles of the thoracic cage are most commonly affected.

370. d. Exercise is not recommended if body mass index is less than 18. Strenuous exercise programs such as aerobics are not introduced until the person is at maintenance weight range, and then only if the condition is medically stable.

371. d. Toxic polyneuropathy affects the distal limbs first, reflecting the greater vulnerability of the longest nerve axons. Sensory disturbances are usually reported as a tingling or burning sensation distributed in a stocking-and-glove pattern.

372. b. In the first trimester of pregnancy, the number and severity of migraines rise. The headaches abate during the second trimester and then increase in the third trimester. Migraine can be triggered during delivery and may be more prevalent in the weeks and months following childbirth.

373. a. Carpal tunnel syndrome, osteoarthritis of the basilar joint of the thumb, and adhesive capsulitis are all likely to rise in incidence after menopause, primarily related to lower levels of estrogen.

374. b. By changing ventilation rate, the respiratory system compensates for an abnormal pH. The renal system contributes to pH regulation by altering the amount of hydrogen that passes through the urine and by synthesizing bicarbonate ion.

375. a. Contraceptive combination medications increase the risk for thromboembolism, which is markedly enhanced by smoking. All the others should not occur or should not be affected.

376. d. All of the listed reactions can occur, except joint or muscle pain.

377. a. Diphenhydramine is an antihistaminic that blocks histamine or histamine-1 receptors and is being used for allergic conditions (type 1 only). It can cause sedation, blurred vision, dry mouth and skin, contact lens intolerance, constipation, and urinary hesitancy (mostly by its anticholinergic actions, which are more pronounced in elderly people).

378. c. All the listed adverse reactions can result from suppression of platelet and red blood cell formation and liver damage (some drugs only), but gastrointestinal problems include diarrhea, which can often be severe.

379. c. It is possible to get these reflexes because the somatic and visceral afferents enter the spinal cord at the same level. Somatic sources that create visceral symptoms are known as somatovisceral reflexes

380. d. A review of current safe exercise guidelines would indicate avoiding exercises that risk direct trauma to the abdominal region. However, continuing an exercise program, in moderation, is highly recommended for the health of both the baby and mother during the pregnancy.

381. b. Although the other choices contribute to the changes in posture associated with pregnancy, the large shift of the center of gravity anteriorly has the greatest effect.

382. a. Waddell testing is used to identify patients suffering from pain of a nonorganic origin.

383. b. During pregnancy a woman normally experiences an increase in resting heart rate and a decrease in heart rate during exercise. This change is compared with the heart rate of the particular woman before pregnancy. The other answers are true about pregnancy.

384. d. The geriatric population usually has a decreased body temperature because of poor diet, decreased cardiovascular status, and decreased metabolic rates.

385. b. Supine positioning after the first trimester is associated with decreased cardiac output.

CHAPTER 3

Interventions

Questions

1. At what stage of HIV is it advisable for an individual to perform moderate or intense exercise?
   a. Early-stage HIV
   b. Advanced HIV
   c. Chronic HIV
   d. Disease that has progressed to AIDS

2. What is correct advice to give to a patient who is HIV infected?
   a. Exercise is a safe and beneficial activity for the HIV-infected person.
   b. Overtraining should be encouraged.
   c. Athletic competition is advisable for individuals with mild to moderate symptoms.
   d. Symptomatic patients should continue aggressive exercise.

3. A patient with a diagnosis of chronic fatigue syndrome begins outpatient physical therapy. Which of the following would be an inappropriate intervention on their first day of treatment?
   a. Treadmill walking uphill × 20 minutes
   b. Upper body ergometer × 5 minute
   c. Low-impact aquatic aerobics
   d. Recumbent stepper × 10 minutes

4. A patient in the acute stages of fibromyalgia begins physical therapy intervention. Which of the following would be an appropriate exercise prescription for this patient?
   a. Long low-load exercises of 30 minutes or more
   b. Short, intense exercise sessions
   c. 5 to 10 minutes of low-load exercise
   d. 30 minutes of upper body ergometer

5. An individual with hyperthyroidism is beginning outpatient physical therapy. What would you expect to observe clinically in this patient?
   a. Fatigue
   b. Heart rate of less than 80 beats/minute
   c. Proximal muscle spasticity
   d. Normal or enhanced cardiac output during exercise

6. Which of the following is TRUE regarding rehabilitation of a patient after parathyroidectomy?
   a. The patient should lie with the head down and feet elevated.
   b. Upper extremity exercise should begin immediately.
   c. Early ambulation is essential.
   d. Light-weight–resistive exercise is contraindicated.

7. Which of the following will occur with adhesive capsulitis associated with diabetes?
   a. Loss of external rotation and adduction
   b. Equal limitation in external rotation and internal rotation
   c. Limitation in hyperextension and internal rotation mostly
   d. Limitation in flexion and abduction only

8. Which of the following is correct advice for a patient with type 2 diabetes undergoing an exercise program?
   a. Exercise is a valuable treatment modality for type 2 diabetes.
   b. Hypoglycemia is a common problem for the individual with type 2 diabetes initiating an exercise program.
   c. Exercise can be initiated if blood glucose levels are 60 mg/dL or less.
   d. It is advisable to begin vigorous exercise 1 hour before attempting to sleep at night.

9. The home health PTA is currently treating a patient with a diagnosis of hepatic encephalopathy. The patient reports that yesterday he had unusual black/tarry stools. What should the PTA do after learning this information?
   a. Proceed with treatment
   b. Decrease intensity of treatment
   c. Contact the referring physician/supervising physical therapist
   d. Increase intensity of treatment

10. The PTA is providing intervention for a patient in the hospital diagnosed with acute pancreatitis. The patient asks the PTA what positions may relieve the abdominal pain. Which of the following is incorrect advice to give this patient?
    a. Lean forward while sitting.
    b. Sit straight up.
    c. Use the supine position with the legs extended.
    d. Lie on the left side in a fetal-flexed position.

11. A patient with diabetes is receiving physical therapy intervention. Which of the following would NOT be a focus of treatment?
    a. Lower extremity strengthening
    b. Upper extremity strengthening
    c. Altering the disease process
    d. Endurance training

12. Which of the following statements is TRUE about range of motion (ROM) of the diabetic foot?
    a. Limitations are of minor concern in the formation of a neuropathic wound.
    b. ROM limitations may cause abnormal peak pressures during gait and thereby contribute to ulcer formation.
    c. Measuring ROM during a foot examination is important only if there is an ulcer present.
    d. Only ankle dorsiflexion limitations affect the risk for ulceration.

13. A 14-year-old baseball player has type 1 diabetes and uses an insulin pump. His teammates want to know more about this condition. You inform them that all the following statements concerning insulin are true EXCEPT which one?
    a. It facilitates glucose transport out from the cell and into the blood.
    b. It is secreted from beta cells in pancreas.
    c. It decreases blood glucose levels.
    d. It may be present in decreased levels in those with type 2 diabetes mellitus.

14. To decrease the risk for hypoglycemia in a patient with type 1 insulin-dependent diabetes, which of the following is inappropriate?
    a. Eat or drink a snack high in carbohydrates 30 minutes before exercise.
    b. Exercise muscles that have not had an insulin injection recently.
    c. Eat a carbohydrate snack for each 30 to 45 minutes of exercise.
    d. Exercise at the peak time of insulin effect.

15. A PTA is discussing appropriate exercise parameters for a patient with type 2 diabetes. Which statement reflects inappropriate advice to the patient?
    a. Do not begin exercise if blood glucose is higher than 100 mg/dL.
    b. Be sure to stay adequately hydrated.
    c. Avoid insulin injections in the active extremities within 1 hour before exercise.
    d. Exercise at moderate intensity and use the Borg Scale of Perceived Exertion to help determine response to exercise.

16. What is the most important component of an exercise program to improve a patient's endurance after a period of deconditioning?
    a. Education
    b. A walking program
    c. Daily stretching exercises
    d. Constant monitoring by the PTA

17. A patient is just beginning exercise after a long bout with pneumonia. The PTA begins to walk the patient down the hall of an inpatient

facility. The patient's heart at rest was 86 beats/minute, and 2 minutes into the ambulation the PTA notices the heart rate is now 74 beats/minute. What is the appropriate course of action by the PTA?
a. Continue ambulation
b. Stop ambulation immediately and have the patient sit down
c. Increase the intensity of ambulation
d. Contact the supervising physical therapist

18. A patient is beginning an exercise program in outpatient physical therapy after a significant period of deconditioning. Of the choices that follow, which is the most important to include in this patient's deconditioning program?
a. A walking program
b. Stationary bike exercise
c. Warm-up and cool-down periods
d. A graded exercise test before initiating the program

19. A patient is beginning an exercise program. Assuming that the patient has not exercised in several years, what would be their target heart rate?
a. 30% to 40% of the estimated maximum heart rate
b. 40% to 50% of the estimated maximum heart rate
c. 55% to 65% of the estimated maximum heart rate
d. 65% to 75% of the estimated maximum heart rate

20. What should be the frequency of exercise for a severely deconditioned patient beginning therapy intervention?
a. 1 time per week
b. 3 times per week
c. 5 times per week
d. 7 times per week

21. What is the correct position for bronchial drainage of anterior segments of both upper lobes?
a. Left side lying
b. Sitting upright
c. Lying supine
d. Right side lying

22. What is a major benefit of diaphragmatic breathing?
a. Enhanced expansion and ventilation of the upper lobes
b. Improved airway clearance
c. Improvement in postural deficits of the thorax
d. Reduced dyspnea

23. What changes does pursed-lip breathing achieve?
a. Enhances airway clearance
b. Helps expand the alveoli

c. Reduces the physical work of expiration

d. Slows respiratory rate

24. Which of the following physical therapy interventions is most likely to help a patient with dyspnea?
    a. An aerobic exercise program
    b. Postural drainage
    c. A strength-training program
    d. Training with an assistive device

25. Strength in what muscle groups is needed most for effective coughing?
    a. Expiratory muscles of the thorax, and lumbar extensors
    b. Inspiratory muscles of the thorax, and abdominal muscles
    c. Expiratory muscles of the thorax, and abdominal muscles
    d. Inspiratory muscles of the thorax, and lumbar extensors

26. What is generally the first sign of respiratory distress with inadequate oxygenation during exercise?
    a. Cyanosis of the lips
    b. Flaring of the nostrils
    c. White nail beds
    d. Increased respiratory rate

27. Which of the following are considered primary accessory muscles of inspiration?
    a. Abdominals and back extensors
    b. Sternocleidomastoid and scalene muscles
    c. Sternocleidomastoid and lumbar extensors
    d. Scalene and upper trapezius muscles

28. What strategy for airway clearance is described by the following: The patient is instructed to take a medium breath then tighten the abdominal muscles firmly while forcibly exhaling with an open glottis. The patient should return to normal gentle breathing for approximately 30 seconds and then forcibly exhale with an open glottis?
    a. Forced expiratory technique
    b. Active cycle of breathing technique
    c. Autogenic drainage
    d. Coughing

29. A patient with cystic fibrosis recently was involved in a motor vehicle collision. The patient has increased intracranial pressure. Because of the advanced stage of cystic fibrosis, the patient requires postural drainage and chest physical therapy for the right middle lobe of the lung. What is the correct positioning for this intervention?
    a. Patient in left side-lying position with the foot of the bed elevated 14 inches
    b. Patient sitting

   c. Patient in left side-lying position on a flat bed
   d. Patient in left side-lying position with the foot of the bed raised 20 inches

30. When should PTAs use vibration to loosen secretions in the lungs of a patient with chronic obstructive pulmonary disease?
   a. Before inspiration
   b. During inspiration phase
   c. During expiration phase
   d. After expiration

31. What is the correct position to reduce dyspnea in patients with severe limitations of inspiratory pressure associated with chronic obstructive pulmonary disease?
   a. Standing
   b. Supine
   c. Prone
   d. Sitting with a forward flexed posture

32. In a patient with heart failure, which of the following would NOT be a reason to terminate the session?
   a. Symptomatic hypotension
   b. Acute onset of crackles in the lungs
   c. Controlled atrial fibrillation
   d. Symptoms of dyspnea and fatigue at rest

33. Which of the following is incorrect information regarding exercise intervention in a patient after heart transplantation?
   a. The patient should perform an adequate warm-up and cool-down.
   b. The patient should adhere to sternal precautions.
   c. Weight-bearing exercises may reduce the bone loss caused by needed medication.
   d. Target heart rate should be used for exercise.

34. Short bouts of moderate-intensity exercise are safe and effective for improving which of the following in patients with heart failure?
   a. Strength
   b. Quality of life
   c. Range of motion
   d. Power

35. Which type of exercise should be avoided by patients with heart failure?
   a. Isometric
   b. Aerobic
   c. Isotonic
   d. Range of motion

36. At what point on the angina scale should the patient stop exercising?
    a. Stage I
    b. Stage II
    c. Stage III
    d. Stage IV

37. Which of the following activities would have the highest MET range?
    a. Toileting
    b. Walking on level surfaces
    c. Vacuuming
    d. Shoveling snow

38. What are the three most important factors affecting the risk for exercising patients with heart failure?
    a. Age, intensity of exercise, and presence of ischemic heart disease
    b. Age, fluid retention levels, gender
    c. Patient participation level, age, intensity of exercise
    d. Presence of ischemic heart disease, age, and fluid retention levels

39. A patient with a functional capacity of less than 3 METs is beginning cardiac rehabilitation. About how long will the patient be able to tolerate exercise before resting?
    a. 5 minutes
    b. 15 minutes
    c. 20 minutes
    d. 30 minutes

40. Which of the following interventions is NOT indicated for patients receiving mechanical ventilation?
    a. Supine body positioning
    b. Functional and exercise training
    c. Deep-breathing exercises or other techniques to increase ventilation
    d. Stress and anxiety reduction techniques

41. In which of the following scenarios is it acceptable to continue functional exercises with a patient diagnosed with respiratory failure?
    a. Hypotension associated with diaphoresis
    b. Severe dyspnea
    c. Saturation less than 90% on supplemental O_2
    d. Angina scale rating 1/4

42. Which of the following muscles is considered a muscle of accessory expiration?
    a. Internal intercostals
    b. External intercostals
    c. Parasternal intercostals
    d. Scalenes

43. Which of the following interventions should NOT be used with manual lymphatic drainage?
    a. Compression bandaging or garments
    b. Exercise
    c. Skin care
    d. Pneumatic compression pumping

44. Six months after completing a course of complete decongestive physical therapy, a patient with secondary lymphedema after axillary lymph node dissection presents with 20-lb weight loss and a rapid 30% increase in the girth of her affected limb. Which of the following should you do?
    a. Increase the hours per day that she wears a compression garment
    b. Inform your supervising physical therapist or the patient's physician
    c. Recommend that the patient eat less protein
    d. Discontinue therapy and discharge the patient

45. Manual lymphatic drainage should NOT be performed on patients with which condition?
    a. Diabetes mellitus
    b. Congestive heart failure
    c. Hypertension
    d. A history of cancer

46. Which of the following is NOT a permanent precaution for a person with lymphedema?
    a. No blood pressure measurements on the involved extremity
    b. No cold packs to the affected extremity
    c. No needle sticks or blood draws to the affected extremity
    d. Immediate and careful treatment and follow-up of any break in the skin on the affected limb

47. In which of the following cases would it be NOT advisable to use compression therapy?
    a. A patient with a venous ulcer
    b. A patient with an ankle-brachial index of 1
    c. A patient with congestive heart failure
    d. A patient with venous insufficiency

48. Of the choices given, what is the correct frequency of aerobic exercise for an obese person to produce significant weight loss?
    a. 1 time a week
    b. 2 times a week
    c. 3 times a week
    d. 4 times a week

49. Which of the following laboratory values represents a contraindication to physical therapy intervention?
    a. Hemoglobin of less than 8 g/dL
    b. Hematocrit of 30% to 32%
    c. White blood cell count of 7500/mm³
    d. White blood cell count of 10,000/mm³

50. Which of the following is a postoperative factor that will influence the rate of recovery after chest surgery?
    a. Poor humidity to the lungs
    b. Reaction of lungs to anesthesia
    c. Atelectasis
    d. Drying of the pleura

51. What stage of cardiac rehabilitation occurs in the hospital?
    a. Phase I
    b. Phase II
    c. Phase III
    d. Phase IV

52. Generally how long does a phase II cardiac rehabilitation last?
    a. 2 weeks
    b. 4 weeks
    c. 6 weeks
    d. 10 weeks

53. At what stage of a seven-step inpatient rehabilitation program for myocardial infarction can a patient ambulate about 500 feet?
    a. Stage II
    b. Stage IV
    c. Stage V
    d. Stage VI

54. If a patient is in the prone position, what lobes of the lungs are being drained with postural drainage techniques?
    a. Both upper lobes
    b. Left upper lobe
    c. Right upper lobe
    d. Both lower lobes

55. During periods of intense physical activity, many physiologic adaptations occur, especially in the circulatory system. Which of the following occurs during increased physical exertion?
    a. Increased ventricular refilling, secondary to increased venomotor tone
    b. Decreased cardiac output
    c. Decreased stroke volume
    d. Increased cardiac cycle time

56. A patient is referred to physical therapy with a secondary diagnosis of hypertension. The physician has ordered relaxation training. The PTA first chooses to instruct the patient in the technique of diaphragmatic breathing. Which of the below is the correct set of instructions?
    a. Slow breathing rate to 8 to 12 breaths/minute, increase movement of the upper chest, and decrease movement in the abdominal region.
    b. Slow breathing rate to 12 to 16 breaths/minute, increase movement of the abdominal region, and decrease movement in the upper chest.
    c. Slow breathing rate to 8 to 12 breaths/minute, increase movement of the abdominal region, and decrease movement in the upper chest.
    d. Slow breathing rate to 12 to 16 breaths/minute, increase movement of the upper chest, and decrease movement in the abdominal region.

57. Which of the following statements is FALSE about cardiovascular response to exercise in trained and/or sedentary patients?
    a. If exercise intensities are equal, the sedentary patient's heart rate will increase faster than the trained patient's heart rate.
    b. Cardiovascular response to increased workload will increase at the same rate for sedentary as it will for trained patients.
    c. Trained patients will have a larger stroke volume during exercise.
    d. The sedentary patient will reach anaerobic threshold faster than the trained patient, if workloads are equal.

58. Which of the following is incorrect advice to give to a patient with a diagnosis of congestive heart failure that complains of shortness of breath and "smothering" while attempting to sleep?
    a. Sleep with the head on two or three pillows.
    b. Sleep without any pillows.
    c. Sleep in a recliner during exacerbations.
    d. During exacerbations, come a standing position for short-term relief.

59. A 53-year-old man with chronic obstructive pulmonary disease reports to an outpatient cardiopulmonary rehabilitation facility. Pulmonary testing reveals that forced expiratory volume in 1 second (FEV_1) and vital capacity (VC) are within 60% of predicted values. What is the appropriate exercise prescription?
    a. Exercise at 75% to 80% of the target heart rate three times per week.
    b. Begin exercise with levels of 1.5 METs and increase slowly three times per week.
    c. Exercise at 75% to 80% of the target heart rate seven times per week.
    d. Begin exercise with levels of 1.5 METs and increase slowly seven times per week.

60. A PTA is ordered by a physician to treat a patient with congestive heart failure in an outpatient cardiac rehabilitation facility. Which of the following signs and symptoms should the PTA NOT expect?
    a. Stenosis of the mitral valve
    b. Orthopnea
    c. Decreased preload of the right heart
    d. Pulmonary edema

61. Which instruction should be followed for strengthening exercises in persons with hemophilia?
    a. Begin as soon as a joint bleed is recognized.
    b. Never include isokinetic exercises.
    c. Increase exercises using high-repetition, low-load progressive resistance exercises.
    d. Only exercise joints that demonstrate muscle weakness.

62. A patient with cryoglobulinemia presents to outpatient physical therapy with complaints of lumber pain. Which of the following should the PTA avoid during intervention for this diagnosis?
    a. Moist heat packs
    b. Weight-bearing exercises
    c. Muscle energy techniques
    d. Cold pack application

63. The PTA is treating a patient with a history of coronary artery disease. During the treatment, the patient complains of recurring angina that increases when performing activities in standing. Which is the MOST appropriate course of action by the PTA?
    a. Stop treatment and contact the supervising physical therapist.
    b. Stop treatment until symptoms subside.
    c. Assist patient in taking medication for chest pain
    d. Perform treatment in a sitting position.

64. A patient who sustained a severe heart attack was categorized at a MET level of 2 to 3. The patient has completed the goal of doing homemaking activities, such as washing dishes and ironing. The PTA should progress intervention to include which occupational task?
    a. Driving an automobile
    b. Performing upper and lower extremity dressing
    c. Gardening in the yard
    d. Preparing 1 to 2 meals per day

65. A patient with emphysema complains of shortness of breath and generalized weakness in the upper extremities when performing daily chores. The PTA should encourage which of the following?
    a. Pursed lip breathing when working
    b. Gravity-assisted exercises before performing chores

    c. Use of oxygen with daily activities

    d. Avoidance of activities that consume a lot of energy

66. Persuading a sedentary patient to become more active, the PTA explains the benefits of exercise. Which of the following is an inappropriate list of benefits?

    a. Increased efficiency of the myocardium to obtain oxygen, decreased high-density lipoprotein (HDL) cholesterol, and decreased cholesterol

    b. Decreased low-density lipoprotein (LDL) cholesterol, decreased triglycerides, and decreased resting blood pressure

    c. Increased efficiency of the myocardium to obtain oxygen, decreased cholesterol, and decreased LDL

    d. Decreased resting blood pressure, decreased LDL, and increased HDL

67. The PTA is working in an outpatient cardiac rehabilitation facility. A 50-year-old healthy man inquires about the correct exercise parameters for increasing aerobic efficiency. Which of the following is the most correct information to convey to this individual?

    a. Exercise at 80% to 90% of maximal volume of oxygen utilization.

    b. Exercise with heart rate between 111 and 153 beats/minute.

    c. Exercise at about 170 beats/minute.

    d. Exercise at level 17 or 18 on the Borg Scale of Perceived Exertion.

68. What lobe of the lungs is the PTA attempting to drain if the patient is in the following position: resting on the left side, rolled ¼ turn back, supported with pillows, with the foot of the bed raised 12 to 16 inches.

    a. Right middle lobe, lingular segment

    b. Left upper lobe, lingular segment

    c. Right upper lobe, posterior segment

    d. Left upper lobe, posterior segment

69. The PTA works in a cardiac rehabilitation setting. Which of the following types of exercises is most likely to be harmful to a 64-year-old man with a history of myocardial infarction?

    a. Concentric

    b. Eccentric

    c. Aerobic

    d. Isometric

70. To determine whether an exercise session should be terminated, the patient is asked to assess level of exertion using the Borg Scale of Perceived Exertion. The patient rates the level of exertion as 9 on the scale of 6 to 19. A rating of 9 corresponds to which of the following?

    a. Very, very light

    b. Very light

c. Somewhat hard
d. Hard

71. A physician orders stage II cardiac rehabilitation for a patient. The orders are to exercise the patient below 7 METs. Which of the following is a contraindicated activity?
    a. Riding a stationary bike at about 5.5 mph
    b. Descending a flight of stairs independently
    c. Ironing
    d. Ambulating independently at 5 to 6 mph

72. A PTA is treating a patient with cystic fibrosis who has just walked 75 feet before experiencing significant breathing difficulties. In an effort to assist the patient in regaining her normal breathing rate, the PTA gives a set of instructions. Which of the following set of instructions is appropriate?
    a. Take a slow, deep breath through pursed lips and exhale slowly through your nose only.
    b. Take small breaths through your nose only and exhale quickly through pursed lips.
    c. Breath in through your nose and exhale slowly through pursed lips.
    d. Breath in through pursed lips and breath out slowly through pursed lips.

73. A PTA is treating a 65-year-old man with chronic obstructive pulmonary disease. The patient questions the benefits of the flow incentive spirometer left in the room by the respiratory therapist a few minutes ago. Which of the following is an appropriate response to the patient's question?
    a. It gives visual feedback on lung performance.
    b. You should use this for the rest of your life.
    c. You need to ask the respiratory therapist this question.
    d. It really doesn't do anything useful.

74. Which of the following exercises does NOT increase strength of the muscles of forceful inspiration?
    a. Active cervical flexion exercises
    b. Active glenohumeral extension exercises
    c. Shoulder shrugs
    d. Crunches

75. All of the following cardiopulmonary function variables will increase in children in response to training EXCEPT which?
    a. Heart volume
    b. Respiratory rate
    c. Stroke volume
    d. Tidal volume

76. Which is NOT a maternal response to mild to moderate exercise?
    a. Increased cardiac output
    b. Increased stroke volume
    c. Normal to increased heart rate
    d. Decreased respiratory rate

77. What is the most effective approach for treating calcification of tendons within the shoulder?
    a. Ultrasound
    b. Iontophoresis
    c. Electrical stimulation
    d. Surgery

78. Which of the following amputations will have the most edema postoperatively?
    a. Transfemoral
    b. Transtibial
    c. Transradial
    d. Transhumeral

79. Which of the following muscle groups is most important for increasing strength after a transtibial amputation?
    a. Knee extensors
    b. Knee flexors
    c. Hip abductors
    d. Hip adductors

80. A client with a diagnosis of stomach cancer is beginning a general strengthening program at outpatient physical therapy. Weight training has been prescribed by the supervising physical therapist. Which of the following is an appropriate program for this patient?
    a. Low repetition, high weight with a Borg Scale of Perceived Exertion rating of 14 or above
    b. High repetition, low weight with a Borg rating of 14 or below
    c. Low repetition, high weight with a Borg rating of 14 or below
    d. High repetition, low weight with a Borg rating of 14 or above

81. What is the youngest age that children can begin strength training safely?
    a. 5 years
    b. 8 years
    c. 12 years
    d. 15 years

82. A 70-year-old patient asks the PTA about beginning an exercise program. The PTA explains some of the benefits of exercise for this

individual. Which of the following is NOT a benefit of exercise for an individual in this age group?
a. Improved function
b. Improved balance
c. Improved insulin-stimulated glucose uptake
d. Improved nerve conduction velocity

83. With aging, what two joints are the most susceptible to proprioception decline?
a. Shoulder and wrist
b. Knee and shoulder
c. Ankle and wrist
d. Knee and ankle

84. A 15-year-old boy has just initiated a strength training program in a local gym. The client tells the PTA that he feels his strength has increased markedly over the first 3 to 4 weeks of this program. This initial gain is due to what phenomenon?
a. Increase of type I fibers
b. Improved neuromuscular recruitment
c. Increase of type II fibers
d. Increase in muscle mass

85. Which of the following is NOT a strength training benefit in the geriatric patient population?
a. Producing substantial increases in strength and power
b. Normalizing blood pressure in those with high normal values
c. Reducing insulin resistance
d. Increasing maximal oxygen uptake beyond normal

86. A 45-year-old man informs the PTA that he is beginning an endurance training program. The patient reports he is performing his program 2 days per week, at less than 50% maximal uptake, and for about 5 minutes. What is the correct advice to give this individual?
a. This is an adequate program to increase endurance.
b. The patient should maintain this current level for 2 weeks then increase his exercise intensity.
c. This exercise program is not adequate for increasing an individual's endurance.
d. The PTA is not qualified to comment on this individual's exercise program.

87. A patient is referred to physical therapy secondary to a diagnosis of infectious septic knee arthritis. What is the treatment of choice early in this patient's rehabilitation?
a. Weight-bearing exercises
b. Aggressive range of motion

    c. Splinting and simple range motion

    d. Isokinetic exercise

88. A patient has recently undergone surgery for an infection of the bursae in the hand. What is the appropriate course of rehabilitation for this patient?

    a. Splinting and gentle passive range of motion

    b. Early active range of motion exercise

    c. Therapy should be delayed for 2 weeks after surgery

    d. Ultrasound over the surgical site

89. Which of the following choices describes a rotationplasty?

    a. A custom-made rotating hinge prosthesis is implanted at the knee.

    b. The leg is amputated above the knee, and the tibia bone from the lower leg is inverted, making it possible for the ankle end of the tibia to be fused to the bottom of the femur.

    c. The tibia is resected, and the ankle joint is fused to the distal tibia at 180 degrees.

    d. The surgeon removes the affected bone in the femur, rotates the lower portion of the leg 180 degrees so that the foot faces in the opposite direction, and reattaches it to the upper femoral area.

90. Which of the following activities should be avoided by patients with a diagnosis of osteoporosis?

    a. Swimming

    b. Bowling

    c. Treadmill walking

    d. Low-intensity step aerobics

91. Which of the following is the least effective treatment for Osgood-Schlatter syndrome?

    a. Discontinuing the aggravating activity

    b. Icing the affected knee daily

    c. Stretching the hamstrings

    d. Immobilizing the knee

92. How long does morning stiffness associated with osteoarthritis typically last?

    a. 5 to 10 minutes

    b. 20 to 30 minutes

    c. 2 to 3 hours

    d. 4 to 6 hours

93. In which of the following muscle groups would you expect to find shortness or tightness in a patient with long-standing osteoporosis?

    a. Gluteals

    b. Hip flexors

c. Scapular retractors
d. Triceps

94. Which of the following exercise regimens is least effective for preventing excessive bone loss?
a. Resistance training
b. Stair climbing
c. Swimming
d. Soccer

95. Which impairment should cause the greatest concern for the patient with osteoporosis?
a. Decreased scapular strength
b. Increased deformity
c. Decreased balance
d. Decreased endurance

96. Which of the following would NOT be part of an immediate plan to manage a patient with an acute vertebral compression fracture?
a. Postural training
b. Log rolling in bed
c. Resistive exercise
d. Transcutaneous electrical nerve stimulation

97. Which of the following exercise programs would have the greatest effect on reducing the risk for new spine fractures in patients with osteoporosis?
a. Spinal extension exercise only
b. Spinal flexion exercise only
c. A combination program of spinal flexion and extension exercise
d. No exercise at all

98. Stability is increased by all of the following EXCEPT which?
a. Widening the base of support
b. Lowering the center of mass
c. Lowering the center of gravity
d. Narrowing the base of support

99. Carrying a backpack is likely to cause the body to compensate by which of the following?
a. Pulling the shoulders back
b. Extending the thoracic spine
c. Flexing the hips
d. Extending the lumbar spine

100. Which of the following is a nonmodifiable cause of poor posture?
a. Tight hamstrings
b. Weak iliopsoas

    c. Weak abdominals

    d. Scoliosis

101. What should be the initial intervention for a patient with postural defects?
    a. Biofeedback with a mirror
    b. Hamstring stretching
    c. Core strengthening program
    d. Hip flexor stretching

102. A patient presents with a 20-year history of tight hamstrings because of failed knee surgeries. What is the appropriate method to stretch these muscles?
    a. High-velocity training
    b. Low-load, long-duration stretching
    c. Low-load, short-duration stretching
    d. High-velocity, long-duration stretching

103. The ability of a muscle to perform repetitive activities over prolonged amounts of time without fatigue is known as what?
    a. Muscle power
    b. Muscle strength
    c. Muscle work
    d. Muscle endurance

104. Which training principle is associated with an adaptive response to increased training loads?
    a. SAID (specific adaptation to imposed demand) principle
    b. Specificity principle
    c. Overload principle
    d. Individuality principle

105. Resistance exercise will change which of the following muscle components?
    a. Change type I into type II fibers
    b. Change type II into type I fibers
    c. Increase the number of muscle fibers
    d. Increase the size of the muscle fibers

106. When does a muscle produce the most strength?
    a. At normal resting length
    b. At maximum shortened position
    c. At maximum lengthened position
    d. At the middle of its range of motion

107. A patient presents with full pain-free passive range of motion, but 50% active range of motion. What characteristic of muscle performance is inhibited?
    a. Muscle power
    b. Muscle endurance
    c. Muscle strength
    d. Muscle work

108. What activity would cause a patient to use his aerobic energy source?
    a. Running to first base
    b. Bicycle racing up a short hill
    c. Running a mile
    d. Returning a tennis serve

109. What would be the most effective exercise to return a baseball pitcher to active baseball play?
    a. Push-ups
    b. Chin-ups
    c. Biceps curls
    d. Isokinetic strengthening

110. Interventions that can be effective for managing symptoms and loss of function associated with inflammatory arthritis should NOT include which of the following?
    a. Joint protection
    b. Patient education
    c. Aggressive passive range of motion
    d. Aquatic therapy

111. Exercise will NOT have which of the following effects on children with arthritis?
    a. Decreased disease activity and severity
    b. Increased number of affected joints
    c. Increased mobility and strength
    d. Increased aerobic fitness

112. What would be a good recommendation for rest for a patient with an exacerbation of juvenile rheumatoid arthritis?
    a. 12 hours of sleep and 1 hour of rest per day
    b. 8 hours of sleep and 1 hour of rest per day
    c. 10 hours of sleep and 2 hours of rest per day
    d. 8 hours of sleep and 2 hours of rest per day

113. A PTA examines a patient with osteoarthritis who reports difficulty performing household tasks due to stiffness and aching in the fingers.

The PTA notes that the finger joints are stiff and not inflamed and includes superficial heating and exercises to decrease stiffness in the plan of care. Which of the following would be the ideal way to follow this plan of care?

a. Perform range-of-motion (ROM) exercises followed by a hot pack.
b. Apply paraffin to decrease the stiffness, then conduct ROM exercises.
c. Teach daily active ROM exercises to be done at the end of each day.
d. Teach home use of paraffin.

114. A patient with arthritis has stiff finger joints that are inflamed and warm. The PTA selects joint rest as part of the plan of care. Which of the following would be the ideal way to follow this plan of care?

a. Begin an aquatics program.
b. Increase the resistance and decrease the number of repetitions of the patient's exercise program.
c. Select a splint that supports the involved joints.
d. Instruct the patient to perform several repetitions of their active range of motion daily.

115. A PTA is working with a patient with frozen shoulder syndrome. The data from the initial evaluation revealed the following passive range-of-motion impairments of the left shoulder: external rotation 10 degrees, flexion 60 degrees, and abduction 40 degrees. The physical therapist states in the plan of care that ultrasound and mobilization will be used to increase the range of motion (ROM). The most important aspect of this patient's home program is which of the following?

a. ROM exercises
b. Strengthening exercises
c. Cryotherapy
d. Understanding and following joint protection principles

116. Which of the following motions would be most likely to increase cartilage health of a knee joint?

a. Running
b. Swimming
c. Cycling on an exercise bike
d. Performing straight leg raises

117. Which grade of tendonitis can be defined as the patient having pain with training that does NOT dissipate between training sessions along with significant pain at the insertion of the tendon?

a. Grade 1
b. Grade 3
c. Grade 4
d. Grade 5

118. A patient presents with an order from the physician for outpatient physical therapy. The diagnosis is tensor fascia lata tendonitis. Which of the following would NOT be an appropriate treatment for a patient with this diagnosis?
   a. Stretching of the iliotibial band
   b. Gluteus medius strengthening
   c. Adductor magnus strengthening
   d. Decreasing the patient's activity

119. Weakness in which of the following muscle groups would cause a patient to have Trendelenburg gait?
   a. Knee extensors
   b. Knee flexors
   c. Hip abductors
   d. Hip adductors

120. A patient with an acute inflammation of osteoarthritis begins physical therapy. What would NOT be an appropriate intervention at this point of the patient's stage of recovery?
   a. Low-intensity exercise bike
   b. Cryotherapy
   c. Treadmill walking uphill
   d. Aquatic exercises

121. A 65-year-old patient with a diagnosis of lumbar spinal stenosis presents with a forward-stooped posture and progressive chronic low back pain that extends down both legs, increases with prolonged standing and bending backward, and is relieved by sitting. The PTA's plan of care includes flexion exercises. What is the best intervention for this patient?
   a. Pelvic tilt and knee-to-chest exercises
   b. A walking program
   c. Prone press-up exercises
   d. Instructing the patient in a stretching program

122. Which of the following would most likely be an effective intervention to decrease low back pain in a woman in her seventh month of pregnancy?
   a. Sacroiliac belt
   b. Lumbar flexion exercises
   c. Lumbar extension exercises
   d. Posture correction

123. Using the McKenzie classification for spinal disorders, a patient is classified with an extension dysfunction syndrome. What is the suggested intervention to decrease this patient's symptoms?
   a. End-range flexion exercises
   b. Postural correction

   c. End-range extension exercises

   d. Repeated extension exercises

124. A patient with lumbar pain and radiculopathy into the left lower extremity presents to physical therapy seeking treatment. Repeated lumbar flexion increases the patient's pain into the left lower extremity, and repeated lumbar extension decreases this pain. What is the appropriate exercise intervention for this patient?
   a. End-range flexion exercises
   b. Stretching exercises for the adherent nerve root
   c. Correction of lateral shift then extension exercises
   d. Repeated extension exercises

125. What is the appropriate course of action for the following scenario? A 35-year-old man presents to physical therapy after a recent motor vehicle collision. He reports persistent pain beginning in the lumbar area and extending into the thoracic spine. He complains of bilateral lower extremity numbness and shows a significant restriction in lumbar flexion.
   a. Lumbar extension range of motion
   b. Hamstring stretching
   c. Lumbar flexion range of motion
   d. Immediate referral to a physician

126. Which of the following would constitute a positive straight leg raise test?
   a. The patient is placed supine, and the PTA passively lifts the leg; the patient has pain in the cervical area.
   b. The patient is placed prone, and the PTA passively flexes the knee; the patient has pain in the anterior thigh.
   c. The patient is placed supine, and the PTA passively lifts the involved lower extremity; the patient's symptoms reoccur in the involved lower extremity.
   d. The patient is prone, and the PTA moves the involved knee into passive flexion; the patient has pain along the posterior thigh.

127. What two muscles must work together through co-contraction to maintain spinal stability?
   a. Iliopsoas and multifidus
   b. Rectus abdominis and multifidus
   c. Transversus abdominis and multifidus
   d. Transversus abdominis and lateral oblique

128. Which of the following exercises is an example of a passive range-of-motion technique to increase ankle dorsiflexion if the patient has limited weight bearing?
   a. Standing calf stretch against the wall
   b. Supine heel slides on the wall

c. Long-sitting towel calf stretch

d. Sitting calf raises

129. Which form of muscle stretching is most likely to cause pain or muscle and tendon soreness in sedentary individuals?

a. Ballistic

b. Static

c. Passive

d. Proprioceptive neuromuscular facilitation

130. After total elbow arthroplasty, which movement of the elbow is the hardest to regain and maintain?

a. Flexion

b. Extension

c. Supination

d. Pronation

131. A particular total shoulder replacement procedure does not require the repair of the supraspinatus muscle; only the subscapularis is violated. How does this affect the initial stages of rehabilitation?

a. No precautions necessary

b. Limited passive external rotation and active internal rotation per surgeon

c. Limited passive internal rotation and active external rotation per surgeon

d. Limited passive external rotation

132. After a posterior approach total hip arthroplasty, which of the following precautions is NOT required to prevent dislocation?

a. Limiting flexion of the hip to less than 90 degrees

b. Limiting hip adduction

c. Limiting hip internal rotation

d. Limiting hip external rotation

133. After a right total hip arthroplasty, your patient exhibits a Trendelenburg gait. You notice that her hip drops on the left side. To correct this, you must do which of the following?

a. Strengthen the right hip abductors

b. Strengthen the left hip adductors

c. Strengthen the left hip abductors

d. Strengthen the right hip adductors

134. After total knee arthroplasty, what is the optimal amount of flexion range of motion needed for a patient to rise comfortably from a chair?

a. 90 degrees

b. 75 degrees

c. 105 degrees

d. 95 degrees

135. What is the most important factor in normalizing gait after a total knee arthroplasty?
   a. Obtaining more than 95 degrees of flexion
   b. Full extension
   c. Normal (5/5) quadriceps strength
   d. Normal (5/5) hip abduction strength

136. Patients with which disease processes tend to achieve the most active range of motion after total shoulder arthroplasty?
   a. Rotator cuff tear
   b. Rheumatoid arthritis
   c. Osteoarthritis with functioning rotator cuff and deltoid
   d. Osteoarthritis with a nonfunctioning deltoid

137. The patient underwent right total hip replacement 2 days ago and asks when she can drive again. What is the appropriate response?
   a. She can return to driving in 2 to 3 weeks.
   b. She can return to driving in 4 to 6 weeks.
   c. She can return to driving in 6 to 8 weeks.
   d. She should ask for the physician's permission to return to driving.

138. Which of the following activities should NOT be recommended for someone 6 months after a successful total hip replacement?
   a. Ballroom dancing
   b. Golf
   c. Swimming
   d. Basketball

139. When is the greatest risk for dislocation of a total hip arthroplasty?
   a. The first week postoperatively
   b. Three weeks postoperatively
   c. Six weeks postoperatively
   d. Twelve weeks postoperatively

140. Which of the following patella motions is essential to maximize knee flexion range of motion after a total knee arthroplasty?
   a. Full superior glide of the patella
   b. Full inferior glide of the patella
   c. Full lateral glide of the patella
   d. Full medial glide of the patella

141. Patella mobilization is very important after total knee arthroplasty. Where is scar tissue most likely to develop that would limit range of motion after a total knee arthroplasty?
   a. Quadriceps tendon
   b. Intracondylar notch

    c. Suprapatellar pouch
    d. Lateral retinaculum

142. Which of the following exercises should be avoided after total knee arthroplasty?
    a. Aquatic therapy
    b. Straight leg raises
    c. Hamstring curls
    d. Deep squats

143. A patient underwent an uncomplicated total shoulder arthroplasty secondary to osteoarthritis 1 week ago. He presents today in the outpatient physical therapy clinic for initiation of rehabilitation. Which of the following exercises would be appropriate for rehabilitation?
    a. Biceps curls with a 5-pound weight
    b. Aggressive overhead range-of-motion activities
    c. Passive external rotation to 75 degrees
    d. Shoulder pendulum exercises

144. In which of the following positions would the sheer forces of the glenohumeral joint be minimized during the initiation of active range of motion after total shoulder arthroplasty?
    a. Supine position
    b. Sitting position
    c. Standing position
    d. Prone position

145. How does controlled mobilization after a period of immobilization affect a healing ligament?
    a. Causes a loss of tensile strength
    b. Increases the amount of collagen in the ligament
    c. Reduces collagen fiber bundle diameter
    d. Delays functional recovery

146. Which interventions would be most appropriate to reduce inflammation in the early soft tissue postoperative rehabilitation period?
    a. Active exercise and motor level electrical stimulation
    b. Cryotherapy and compression
    c. Intermittent pneumatic compression and thermal (i.e., continuous) diathermy
    d. Moist hot pack and thermal ultrasound

147. The patient has recently undergone medial collateral ligament repair of the knee. Which of the following tests would be contraindicated during the examination at the patient's first physical therapy visit?
    a. Manual muscle testing
    b. Range-of-motion testing

    c. Limb circumference measurement

    d. One-leg standing test

148. Which phase of rehabilitation after soft tissue repair is often referred to as the maximum protection phase?
    a. Immediate postoperative phase
    b. Intermediate postoperative phase
    c. Advanced strengthening phase
    d. Return to activity phase

149. A patient is performing rehabilitation after a rotator cuff repair. The patient has no pain during activity, no edema, active and passive ranges of motion within normal limits, and 10% muscle strength difference compared with the uninvolved upper extremity based on isokinetic testing. What phase of rehabilitation is this patient most likely in?
    a. Immediate postoperative phase
    b. Maximum protection phase
    c. Intermediate postoperative phase
    d. Advanced strengthening phase

150. What type of meniscus tear has the least favorable outcome after meniscectomy?
    a. Posterior horn tear
    b. Bucket handle tear
    c. Anterior horn tear
    d. Circumferential tear

151. A patient has recently undergone lateral retinaculum release of the knee. Which of the following patella mobilizations should be avoided with this patient?
    a. Superior mobilizations
    b. Inferior mobilizations
    c. Lateral mobilizations
    d. Medial mobilizations

152. In which of the following surgical procedures should early range of motion be a goal?
    a. Thermal capsulorrhaphy of the shoulder
    b. Bankart repair of the shoulder
    c. Anterior cruciate ligament reconstruction
    d. Biceps tendon repair after a tendon rupture

153. Overstretching of what muscle group should be avoided to preserve a tenodesis grip?
    a. Long finger flexors
    b. Long finger extensors

    c. Biceps

    d. Wrist extensors

154. What is the appropriate position for the shoulders for a patient in the acute stage after a C6 complete lesion of the spinal cord?
    a. Abduction, flexion, internal rotation
    b. Adduction, slight flexion, neutral rotation
    c. Adduction, slight flexion, internal rotation
    d. Abduction, flexion, external rotation

155. How much hamstring length is considered appropriate to foster a normal long sitting position, assuming hamstring length is measured with a passive straight leg raise?
    a. 80 degrees
    b. 90 degrees
    c. 100 degrees
    d. 120 degrees

156. Which of the following is an inappropriate intervention to decrease tone in a patient's hypertonic muscles following an injury that leads to a vegetative state?
    a. Cryotherapy
    b. Prolonged muscle stretch
    c. Vibration
    d. Sitting postures

157. A patient recently had surgery on her right lower extremity. The orders include non–weight bearing on the right side. The supervising therapist's plan of care includes upper extremity strengthening. What specific upper body muscle strengthening will be most functional for this patient?
    a. Triceps and biceps
    b. Biceps and latissimus dorsi
    c. Triceps and latissimus dorsi
    d. Deltoid and triceps

158. The patient was observed to have excessive posterior pelvic tilt during the stance phase of gait. What is the least likely cause of this gait deviation?
    a. Inadequate lumbar flexibility
    b. Back pain
    c. Hip flexion contracture
    d. Postural malalignment

159. A patient shows poor hip flexion at initial contact. What muscles should be strengthened to alleviate this gait dysfunction?
    a. Luteus maximus
    b. Hamstrings

c. Plantar flexors

d. Iliopsoas

160. After recent stroke, a patient exhibits excessive knee flexion at initial contact. Which of the following is the least likely cause of this gait deviation?
    a. Knee extensor hyperactivity
    b. Pain
    c. Excessive ankle dorsiflexion
    d. Increased hamstring tone

161. Which of the following could be a cause of foot slap at initial contact into loading response?
    a. Ankle plantar flexion contracture
    b. Heel pain
    c. Weakness of ankle dorsiflexors
    d. Excessive knee flexion at the end of the swing phase

162. Which of the following is a likely cause of toe drag during the swing phase of gait?
    a. Inadequate hip extension
    b. Inadequate knee extension
    c. Weakness of the ankle dorsiflexors
    d. Weakness of the gluteus maximus

163. Which of the following gait deviations would be common for a patient who has a leg length discrepancy after a recent total hip replacement?
    a. Circumduction
    b. Gluteus maximus lurch
    c. Antalgic gait
    d. Trendelenburg gait

164. Which of the following would NOT be a cause of increased base of support during double stance phase of gait?
    a. Increase lower extremity tone
    b. Arthritic changes at the hip or knee
    c. Varus deformity at the knee
    d. Balance deficits

165. Which of the following is characterized by excessive hip and knee flexion during the swing phase of the gait cycle?
    a. Scissoring gait
    b. Steppage
    c. Ataxic
    d. Quadriceps avoidance pattern

166. What type of technique involves manual stretching of the tissue that surround muscle in the body?
    a. Myofascial release
    b. Massage
    c. Joint mobilization
    d. Functional training

167. A type of exercise in which the patient does NOT receive any support or resistance is an example of what type of exercise?
    a. Passive range of motion
    b. Active assistive range of motion
    c. Active free exercises
    d. Active resisted exercises

168. Which of the following is defined as the amount of work produced by the muscle in a given amount of time?
    a. Muscular strength
    b. Muscle endurance
    c. Muscle power
    d. Muscle repetition

169. If the goal of an exercise program is to increase endurance, which of the following programs would accomplish this task best?
    a. Low repetitions with heavy resistance
    b. Low resistance with high repetitions
    c. Explosive high intensity muscle activity
    d. Isokinetic programs

170. Which of the following is an example for an isotonic eccentric exercise for the biceps brachii muscle?   .
    a. Pushing against a wall
    b. Flexing the elbow with the dumbbell in the hand
    c. Extending the elbow with the dumbbell in the hand
    d. The down phase of a push-up

171. Why are closed kinetic chain exercises important for rehabilitation of the lower extremity?
    a. Because these exercises are easier to remember in a home exercise program for the patient
    b. Because these exercises are simpler
    c. Because these exercises are safer
    d. Because the lower extremity typically functions with the foot on the ground

172. A 13-year-old girl has fractured the left patella during a volleyball game. The physician determines that the superior pole is the location

of the fracture. Which of the following should be avoided in early rehabilitation?
a. Full knee extension
b. 45 degrees of knee flexion
c. 90 degrees of knee flexion
d. 15 degrees of knee flexion

173. Which of the following types of exercise is most likely to intensify delayed-onset muscle soreness (DOMS)?
a. Concentric
b. Eccentric
c. Isometric
d. DOMS will remain constant no matter the type of exercise.

174. A PTA is assisting a patient in gaining lateral stability of the knee joint. The assistant is using strengthening exercises to strengthen muscle groups that will increase active restraint on the lateral side of the joint. Which of the following offers the least amount of active lateral restraint?
a. Gastrocnemius
b. Popliteus
c. Biceps femoris
d. Iliotibial band

175. A patient is in an outpatient facility because of an injury sustained to the right knee joint. Only the structures within the synovial cavity were compromised during the injury. Knowing this information only, the PTA is NOT concerned with injury to which of the following structures?
a. Patellofemoral joint
b. Anterior cruciate ligament
c. Medial meniscus
d. Femoral condyles

176. Which of the following observations is NOT true in a patient without foot or ankle problems in the standing position?
a. The talus is situated somewhat medially to the midline of the foot.
b. In quiet standing, the muscles surrounding the ankle joint remain silent.
c. The first and second metatarsal heads bear more weight than the fourth and fifth metatarsal heads.
d. The talus transmits weight to the rest of the bones of the foot.

177. What are the signs and symptoms of a temporomandibular anterior displaced disk with reduction?
a. Crepitation with loss of opening
b. Clicking with opening
c. No clicking with loss of opening
d. Temporomandibular joint tenderness and loss of opening

178. Positioning of a patient in right side-lying position can create pressure on which of the following structures?
    a. Right ischial tuberosity
    b. Left greater trochanter
    c. Right lateral malleolus
    d. Occiput

179. Ideal postural alignment is influenced by appropriate muscle balance. What combinations of muscle imbalance would likely contribute to increased anterior pelvic tilt?
    a. Short hamstrings and elongated hip flexors
    b. Strong anterior abdominals and strong hip flexors
    c. Short hip flexors and lengthened anterior abdominals
    d. Strong anterior abdominals and strong hip extensors

180. A patient presents with anterior knee pain. Which of the following cannot be the source of that pain?
    a. Synovium
    b. Capsule
    c. Patella cartilage
    d. Patella bone

181. Anterior cruciate ligament (ACL) tears do NOT heal as well as medial collateral ligament (MCL) tears for which reason?
    a. The ACL is under greater tension.
    b. Synovial fluid inhibits ACL healing.
    c. The MCL is broad and flat, allowing better healing.
    d. There is more motion in the ACL.

182. Patellofemoral joint reactive forces are highest in what situation?
    a. Running
    b. Straight leg raises
    c. Prolonged sitting
    d. Plyometrics

183. Rotator cuff tear can be described as which of the following?
    a. Rare before 40 years of age
    b. Usually painful
    c. Progressing from the bursal side toward the articular side
    d. Requiring surgical repair

184. Foot drop after total hip arthroplasty most likely indicates which condition?
    a. Stroke
    b. Disk herniation
    c. Sciatic laceration
    d. Traction neurapraxia

185. Sever's apophysitis can be described as which of the following?
    a. Frequently occurring with Achilles tendinitis
    b. A result of leg length inequality
    c. Not an inflammatory condition
    d. Responding to ultrasound treatment

186. Pes planus can be described as which of the following?
    a. A painful condition
    b. Common in patients with hyperlaxity
    c. Requiring orthotics treatment
    d. Resulting in anterior knee pain if not corrected

187. A 10-degree hip flexion contracture produces what torque at the hip that increases demand on which muscle?
    a. Extension, quadriceps
    b. Flexion, biceps femoris
    c. Abduction, adductor magnus
    d. Flexion, iliopsoas

188. Fourteen weeks after surgical repair of the rotator cuff, a patient presents with significant deltoid weakness. Ranges of motion are within normal limits and equal bilaterally. Internal and external rotation strengths are equal bilaterally; flexion and abduction strength is significantly reduced. What is the most likely cause of this dysfunction?
    a. Poor compliance with a home exercise program
    b. Tightness of the inferior shoulder capsule
    c. Surgical damage to the musculocutaneous nerve
    d. Surgical damage to the axillary nerve

189. A patient has recently undergone an acromioplasty. What is the most important goal in early rehabilitation?
    a. Regaining muscle strength
    b. Return to activities of daily living
    c. Endurance and functional progression
    d. Return of normal range of motion

190. Which of the following are true for the child versus the adult?
    a. Children have less tolerance for exercise in the heat.
    b. Children have similar nutritional requirements.
    c. Children need more hydration in all situations.
    d. Children should follow the same weight-training routines.

191. Excessive femoral anteversion in children may result in all of the following EXCEPT which?
    a. Toeing-in during gait
    b. Increased hip internal rotation range of motion
    c. Increased external rotation range of motion
    d. Decreased external rotation range of motion

192. Your patient has a lesion of the left superior gluteal nerve. When your patient is in left unilateral stance, what may you observe?
    a. Right ASIS higher than left ASIS
    b. Right ASIS anterior to left ASIS
    c. Trunk side-bending to the left
    d. Lumbar spine side bent to the right

193. Standing on the left leg and flexing your right hip up requires you to use all the following muscles EXCEPT which?
    a. Right lumbar rotators
    b. Left gluteus minimus
    c. Right quadratus lumborum
    d. Left gluteus medius

194. What is a smaller than normal angle of inclination at the hip is called?
    a. Anteversion
    b. Retroversion
    c. Coxa vara
    d. Coxa valga

195. Hip extension may be limited by all of the following tissues EXCEPT which?
    a. Iliofemoral ligament
    b. Iliopsoas muscle
    c. Ischiofemoral ligament
    d. Gluteus minimus, posterior fibers

196. An angle of 170 to 175 degrees in the frontal plane taken on the lateral side of the knee is considered which of the following?
    a. Excess genu valgum
    b. Excess genu varum
    c. Normal
    d. Coxa vara

197. Where is the pes anserine insertion palpable and which tendons does it include?
    a. Medial tibia; semimembranosus, semitendinosis, gracilis
    b. Lateral tibia; biceps femoris, semitendinosus, iliotibial band
    c. Medial tibia; sartorius, gracilis, semitendinosus
    d. Medial femur; biceps femoris, semitendinosus, iliotibial band

198. As the knee extends and the patella moves superiorly in the trochlear groove, how does the sulcus angle change and what how does this affect patellofemoral joint stability?
    a. increases, less stable
    b. decreases, less stable
    c. increases, more stable
    d. decreases, more stable

199. The glenoid faces what direction?
    a. Lateral, inferior, and posterior
    b. Lateral, superior, and anterior
    c. Medial, superior, and anterior
    d. Medial, inferior, and posterior

200. During normal scapulohumeral rhythm, which of the following occurs?
    a. The scapula upwardly rotates 60 degrees, and the humerus abducts 120 degrees.
    b. The scapula upwardly rotates 2 degrees for every 1 degree of humeral abduction.
    c. The scapula abducts 60 degrees and upwardly rotates 120 degrees.
    d. The scapula upwardly rotates 120 degrees, and the humerus abducts 60 degrees.

201. Anterior glenohumeral dislocations are often accompanied by which of the following?
    a. Stretched subscapularis
    b. Hill-Sachs lesion
    c. Fracture of the greater tubercle
    d. Rotator cuff full-thickness tears

202. Which of the following is FALSE regarding biomechanics of persons with patellofemoral pain?
    a. Weakness of the hip abductors, external rotators, and extensors is frequently present.
    b. Excessive hip internal rotation or hip adduction is frequently present.
    c. Patella alta increases patellar instability.
    d. Increased trochlear groove depth increases patellar instability.

203. What is the MOST common myofascial pain syndrome of the low back?
    a. Piriformis
    b. Quadratus lumborum
    c. Iliopsoas
    d. Tensor fascia latae

204. While assessing the standing posture of a patient, the PTA notes that a spinous process in the thoracic region is shifted laterally. The therapist estimates that T2 is the involved vertebra because it is at what approximate level?
    a. Inferior angle of the scapula
    b. Superior angle of the scapula
    c. Spine of the scapula
    d. Xiphoid process of the sternum

205. While ambulating a patient who has had a stroke (the right side is the involved side), the PTA notes increased circumduction of the right lower extremity. Which of the following is an unlikely cause of this deviation?
    a. Increased spasticity of the right gastrocnemius
    b. Increased spasticity of the right quadriceps
    c. Weak hip flexors
    d. Weak knee extensors

206. The PTA is treating a 52-year-old woman after right total hip replacement. The patient complains of being self-conscious about a limp. She carries a heavy briefcase to and from work every day. The PTA notes a Trendelenburg gait during ambulation on level surfaces. What advice can be given to the patient to minimize gait deviation?
    a. Carry the briefcase in the right hand.
    b. Carry the briefcase in the left hand.
    c. Do not carry a briefcase at all.
    d. It does not matter in which hand the briefcase is carried.

207. Which of the following actions places the greatest stress on the patellofemoral joint?
    a. When the foot first contacts the ground during the gait cycle
    b. Exercising on a stair-stepper machine
    c. Running down a smooth decline of 30 degrees
    d. Squats to 120 degrees of knee flexion

208. While observing the ambulation of a 57-year-old man with an arthritic right hip, the PTA observes a right lateral trunk lean. Why does the patient present with this gait deviation?
    a. To move weight toward the involved hip and increase joint compression force
    b. To move weight toward the uninvolved hip and decrease joint compression force
    c. To bring the line of gravity closer to the involved hip joint
    d. To take the line of gravity away from the involved hip joint

209. Which of the following is observed by the PTA if a patient is correctly performing an anterior pelvic tilt in standing position?
    a. Hip extension and lumbar flexion
    b. Hip flexion and lumbar extension
    c. Hip flexion and lumbar flexion
    d. Hip extension and lumbar extension

210. At what point in the gait cycle is the center of gravity the lowest?
    a. Double support
    b. Terminal swing
    c. Deceleration
    d. Midstance

211. What is the most likely cause of anterior pelvic tilt during initial contact (heel strike)?
   a. Weak abdominals
   b. Tight hamstrings
   c. Weak abductors
   d. Back pain

212. A posterior-lateral herniation of the lumbar disk between vertebrae L4 and L5 most likely results in damage to which nerve root(s)?
   a. L4
   b. L5
   c. L4 and L5
   d. L5 and S1

213. While observing the gait pattern of a patient, the PTA notes significant posterior trunk lean at initial contact (heel strike). Which of the following is the most likely muscle that should be focused on during the exercise session to minimize this gait deviation?
   a. Gluteus medius
   b. Gluteus maximus
   c. Quadriceps
   d. Hamstrings

214. While observing the gait pattern of a patient, the PTA notes that the pelvis drops inferiorly on the right during the midswing phase of the right lower extremity. The patient also leans laterally to the left with the upper trunk during this phase. Which of the following is the most likely cause of this deviation?
   a. Weak right gluteus medius
   b. Weak right adductor longus
   c. Weak left gluteus medius
   d. Weak left adductor longus

215. When ambulating on uneven terrain, how should the subtalar joint be positioned to allow forefoot rotational compensation?
   a. Pronation
   b. Supination
   c. Neutral position
   d. The position of the subtalar joint does not influence forefoot compensation.

216. A PTA works on gait training for a patient in a long-term care facility with bilateral knee flexion contractures at 30 degrees. Which of the following indicates to the PTA that the patient will have a forward trunk lean during gait?
   a. The patient's line of gravity is anterior to the hip.
   b. The patient's line of gravity is anterior to the knee.

c. The patient's line of gravity is posterior to the ankle.

d. The patient's line of gravity is posterior to the hip.

217. What motion takes place at the lumbar spine with right lower extremity single-limb support during the gait cycle?
    a. Left lateral flexion
    b. Right lateral flexion
    c. Extension
    d. Flexion

218. In the terminal swing phase of gait, what muscles of the foot and ankle are active?
    a. Extensor digitorum longus
    b. Gastrocnemius
    c. Tibialis posterior
    d. Flexor hallucis longus

219. When the knee is at its maximal amount of flexion during the gait cycle, which of the following muscles are active concentrically?
    a. Hamstrings
    b. Gluteus maximus
    c. Gastrocnemius
    d. Flexor hallucis longus

220. When comparing the gait cycle of young adults to the gait cycle of older adults, what would a PTA expect to find?
    a. The younger population has a shorter step length.
    b. The younger population has a shorter stride length.
    c. The younger population has a shorter period of double support.
    d. The younger population has a decrease in speed of ambulation.

221. A springy block end feel in a joint is indicative of which of the following?
    a. Normal end feel
    b. An inflamed capsule
    c. A meniscal tear
    d. An unstable joint

222. Which grasp is often used to control tools or other objects?
    a. Hook grasp
    b. Power grasp
    c. Lateral pinch
    d. Tip pinch

223. A tennis player receives a surgical repair of the annular ligament. Where should the PTA expect to note the most edema?
    a. Radial ulnar joint
    b. Olecranon bursa

    c. Ulnohumeral joint

    d. Lateral triangle

224. Which muscle does NOT flex the knee and extend the hip?
    a. Semitendinosus
    b. Hamstring portion of the adductor magnus
    c. Long head of the biceps femoris
    d. Semimembranosus

225. Which of the following is used to treat a patient referred to physical therapy with a diagnosis of Dupuytren's contracture?
    a. Knee continuous passive motion
    b. Work simulator set for squatting activities
    c. Hand splint
    d. A 2-lb dumbbell

226. A PTA is treating a patient with balance deficits. During treatment the PTA notes that large-amplitude changes in center of mass cause the patient to lose balance. The patient, however, can accurately compensate for small changes nearly every time a change is introduced. What muscles most likely need to be strengthened to help alleviate this dysfunction?
    a. Tibialis anterior, gastrocnemius
    b. Peroneus longus and brevis, tibialis posterior
    c. Rectus abdominis, erector spinae
    d. Iliopsoas, gluteus maximus

227. A patient is referred to physical therapy with a history of temporomandibular joint pain. The PTA notices that the patient is having difficulty closing his mouth against minimal resistance. With this information, which of the following muscles would NOT be a target for strengthening exercise to correct this deficit?
    a. Medial pterygoid muscle
    b. Temporalis
    c. Masseter
    d. Lateral pterygoid muscle

228. A high-school athlete is considering whether to have an anterior cruciate ligament (ACL) reconstruction. The PTA explains the importance of this ligament, especially in a person who is young and athletic. Which of the statements below is correct in describing part of the function of the ACL?
    a. The ACL prevents excessive posterior roll of the femoral condyles during flexion of the femur at the knee joint.
    b. The ACL prevents excessive anterior roll of the femoral condyles during flexion of the femur at the knee joint.

    c. The ACL prevents excessive posterior roll of the femoral condyles during extension of the femur at the knee joint.

    d. The ACL prevents excessive anterior roll of the femoral condyles during extension of the femur at the knee joint.

229. Which tendon is most commonly involved with lateral epicondylitis?
    a. Extensor carpi radialis longus
    b. Extensor carpi radialis brevis
    c. Brachioradialis
    d. Extensor digitorum

230. A patient who has suffered a zone 2 rupture of the extensor tendon of the third digit presents to physical therapy. This patient had a surgical fixation of the avulsed tendon. During the period of immobilization, which of the following deformities is most likely to develop?
    a. Boutonnière deformity
    b. Claw hand
    c. Swan-neck deformity
    d. Dupuytren's contracture

231. Which of the following muscle tendons most commonly subluxes in patients who suffer from rheumatoid arthritis?
    a. Flexor digitorum profundus
    b. Extensor carpi ulnaris
    c. Extensor carpi radialis longus
    d. Flexor pollicis longus

232. A PTA is scheduled to work with a patient diagnosed with a chronic condition of hammertoes. Where should the PTA NOT expect to find callus formation?
    a. The distal tips of the toes
    b. The superior surface of the interphalangeal joints
    c. The metatarsal heads
    d. The inferior surface of the interphalangeal joints

233. Each of these factors influences the probability of scoliosis curve progression in the skeletally immature patient EXCEPT which?
    a. Magnitude
    b. Gender
    c. Race
    d. Age

234. The child with clubfoot will have what feature?
    a. A larger than normal calcaneus
    b. Forefoot valgus
    c. Significant tibial shortening
    d. Fixed equinus

235. In a child, what is the most common site of transient synovitis, slipped epiphysis, and septic arthritis?
    a. Shoulder
    b. Hip
    c. Knee
    d. Ankle

236. All of the following are common in children who have slipped capital femoral epiphysis EXCEPT which?
    a. Knee pain
    b. Obesity
    c. No history of trauma
    d. Negative findings on a frog-leg lateral radiograph

237. Which of the following conditions are NOT implicated in overuse injuries in youth?
    a. Training errors
    b. Musculotendinous imbalances
    c. Anatomic malalignment of the lower extremity
    d. Constant practice on turf (grass)

238. What is a temporomandibular reciprocal click?
    a. Clicking that occurs during the end of opening
    b. Clicking that occurs during the beginning of opening
    c. Clicking that occurs during the middle of opening
    d. Clicking that occurs during opening and closing

239. In the single-leg stance, when the contralateral hip drops because of weakness, it is considered which of the following?
    a. A compensated hip varus
    b. An uncompensated Trendelenburg
    c. A compensated Trendelenburg
    d. An uncompensated hip varus

240. During ambulation, a PTA notices that the patient is exhibiting genu recurvatum during the stance phase of the gait cycle. Of the choices listed below, the MOST LIKELY cause for the observed gait deviation is which?
    a. A tight gluteus maximus
    b. Tight hip flexors
    c. A tight gastrocnemius–soleus complex
    d. Tight ankle dorsiflexors

241. A PTA is treating a patient who has bilaterally "weak" knee and hip extensors. The patient is most likely to have the greatest difficulty performing which of the following functional activities?
    a. Transferring from a wheelchair to a mat
    b. Rolling from supine to side lying

   c. Transferring from sitting to supine

   d. Transferring from sitting to standing

242. The PTA is scheduled to work with a patient diagnosed with a boutonnière deformity. With this injury, in what position does the involved finger usually present?

   a. Flexion of the proximal interphalangeal (PIP) joint and flexion of the distal interphalangeal (DIP) joint

   b. Extension of the PIP joint and flexion of the DIP joint

   c. Flexion of the PIP joint and extension of the DIP joint

   d. Extension of the PIP joint and extension of the DIP joint

243. A 30-year-old woman who had a full-term infant 4 weeks ago presents to physical therapy with diastasis recti. The separation was measured by the physician and found to be 3 cm. Which of the following exercises is most appropriate to minimize the separation?

   a. Sit-ups while using the upper extremities to bring the rectus abdominis to midline

   b. Bridges while using the upper extremities to bring the rectus abdominis to midline

   c. Dynamic lumbar stabilization exercises in quadruped position

   d. Gentle head lifts in supine position while using the upper extremities to bring the rectus abdominis to midline

244. Proper supportive positioning of an infant with osteogenesis imperfecta is important for all reasons EXCEPT which?

   a. Keeping extremities immobilized to prevent fractures

   b. Protection from fracturing

   c. Minimizing joint malalignment and deformities

   d. Promotion of muscle strengthening

245. A gross motor program for a school-aged child with osteogenesis imperfecta should NOT include which of the following?

   a. Muscle strengthening

   b. Aerobic conditioning

   c. Protected ambulation

   d. Keeping extremities immobilized to prevent fractures

246. Which of the following is the only appropriate exercise in the third trimester of pregnancy?

   a. Single-leg balance activities

   b. Quadruped (crawling position) with hip extension

   c. Bilateral straight leg raise

   d. Bridging

247. During normal gait, in single-limb stance, which of the following occurs?

   a. Center of mass is at its highest point.

   b. Potential energy is at a low point.

    c. Kinetic energy is at its highest point.

    d. Magnitude of the ground reaction force is always greater than body weight.

248. A PTA is treating a patient with a Colles fracture. The patient's forearm has been immobilized for 3 weeks and will require 4 additional weeks in the cast before the patient can begin functional tasks. What should be an initial focus of treatment?

    a. Passive range of motion of the wrist

    b. Placement of the extremity in a sling

    c. Movement of the joints surrounding the fracture

    d. Avoiding treatment until the cast is removed

249. During a treatment session, the PTA observes that the patient can flex the affected shoulder through its full range of motion while side lying. The PTA should progress to activities that places the extremity in what position?

    a. A gravity-assisted position

    b. A gravity-eliminated position

    c. A neutral position

    d. An antigravity position

250. Which activity of daily living would the PTA caution a patient with a recent hip replacement to avoid?

    a. Tying shoes

    b. Pulling up pants

    c. Putting on shirt

    d. Bathing the back

251. During a treatment session, the PTA simulates the need for the client to walk up stairs to a kitchen with a painful and weak left leg. In what way should the patient be instructed to move?

    a. Left leg up to the next step with the cane

    b. Right leg up to the next step with the cane

    c. Right leg up and then the left leg and cane

    d. Left leg up and then the right leg and cane

252. You are working with a 53-year-old client who has had a stroke, leaving him with right hemiparesis. The patient is lying on a therapy mat, and you are performing passive range of motion (ROM) to her left arm. Once you have the patient's arm in 90 degrees of flexion, she complains of some discomfort and pain. What would be the best course of action?

    a. Continue as tolerated because passive ROM must be maintained.

    b. Begin the ROM again and make sure the scapula is gliding.

    c. Continue and do not go past the point of pain.

    d. Consult an orthopedic specialist.

253. The BEST strategy to use with a contracted joint that has a soft end feel is which?
    a. Perform tendon-gliding exercises.
    b. Apply low-load, long duration stretch.
    c. Use a quick stretch technique.
    d. Perform active range of motion.

254. For the best protection of lumbar mechanics, how should the driver's car seat be positioned?
    a. As far from the steering wheel as possible
    b. With the front of the seat lower than the back of the seat
    c. With the entire seat bottom level with the floor of the car
    d. As close to the steering wheel as practical

255. A pitcher is exercising in a clinic with a sports cord mounted behind and above his head. The pitcher simulates the pitching motion using the sports cord as resistance. Which proprioceptive neuromuscular facilitation diagonal is the pitcher using to strengthen the muscles involved in pitching a baseball?
    a. D1 extension
    b. D1 flexion
    c. D2 extension
    d. D2 flexion

256. What is the best way to first exercise the postural (or extensor) musculature when it is extremely weak to facilitate muscle control?
    a. Isometrically
    b. Concentrically
    c. Eccentrically
    d. Isokinetically

257. A 42-year-old receptionist presents to an outpatient physical therapy clinic complaining of low back pain. The supervising therapist decides that postural modification needs to be part of the treatment plan. What is the best position for the lower extremities while the patient is sitting?
    a. 90 degrees of hip flexion, 90 degrees of knee flexion, and 10 degrees of dorsiflexion
    b. 60 degrees of hip flexion, 90 degrees of knee flexion, and 0 degrees of dorsiflexion
    c. 110 degrees of hip flexion, 80 degrees of knee flexion, and 10 degrees of dorsiflexion
    d. 90 degrees of hip flexion, 90 degrees of knee flexion, and 0 degrees of dorsiflexion

258. A patient is positioned in the supine position. The involved left upper extremity is positioned by the PTA in 90 degrees of shoulder flexion. Resistance is applied into shoulder flexion, then quickly into

shoulder extension. No movement takes place. The PTA instructs the patient to "hold" when resistance is applied in both directions. Which of the following proprioceptive neuromuscular facilitation techniques is being used?
a. Repeated contractions
b. Hold–relax
c. Rhythmic stabilization
d. Contract–relax

259. A 32-year-old man is referred to physical therapy with the diagnosis of a recent complete anterior cruciate ligament tear. The patient and the physician have decided to avoid surgery as long as possible. The PTA provides the patient with a home exercise program and instructions about activities that will be limited secondary to this diagnosis. Which of the following is the best advice?
a. There are no precautions.
b. The patient should avoid all athletic activity for 1 year.
c. The patient should avoid all athletic activity until there is a minimum of 20% difference in the bilateral quadriceps muscle as measured isokinetically.
d. The patient should wear a brace and compete in only light athletic events.

260. A 20-year-old man with anterior cruciate ligament reconstruction with allograft presents to an outpatient physical therapy clinic. The patient's surgery was 5 days ago. The patient is independent in ambulation with crutches. He also currently has 53 degrees of active knee flexion and 67 degrees of passive knee flexion and lacks 10 degrees of full knee extension actively and 5 degrees passively. What is the most significant deficit on which the PTA should focus treatment?
a. Lack of active knee extension
b. Lack of passive knee extension
c. Lack of active knee flexion
d. Lack of passive knee flexion

261. A PTA is teaching a class in geriatric fitness and strengthening at a local gym. Which of the following is NOT a general guideline for exercise prescription in this patient population?
a. To increase exercise intensity, increase treadmill speed rather than the grade.
b. Start at a low intensity (2–3 METs).
c. Use machines for strength training rather than free weights.
d. Set weight resistance so that the patient can perform more than eight repetitions before fatigue.

262. A 76-year-old woman received a cemented right total hip arthroplasty 24 hours ago. The surgeon documented that he used a posterolateral

incision. Which of the following suggestions is inappropriate for the next 24 hours?
a. Avoid hip flexion above 30 degrees.
b. Avoid hip adduction past midline.
c. Avoid any internal rotation.
d. Avoid abduction past 15 degrees.

263. A patient is being treated in an outpatient facility after receiving a meniscus repair to the right knee 1 week ago. The patient has full passive extension of the involved knee but lacks 4 degrees of full extension when performing a straight leg raise. The patient's active flexion is 110 degrees and passive flexion is 119 degrees. What is a common term used to describe the patient's most significant range-of-motion deficit? What is a possible source of this problem?
a. Flexion contracture, quadriceps atrophy
b. Extension lag, joint effusion
c. Flexion lag, weak quadriceps
d. Extension contracture, tight hamstrings

264. A PTA is attempting to increase a patient's functional mobility in a seated position. To treat the patient most effectively and efficiently, the following should be performed in what order?
1. Weight shifting of the pelvis
2. Isometric contractions of the lower extremity
3. Trunk range of motion exercises
4. Isotonic resistance to the quadriceps
a. 1, 2, 3, 4
b. 2, 3, 1, 4
c. 4, 3, 2, 1
d. 3, 2, 1, 4

265. A PTA is speaking to a group of avid tennis players. The group asks how to prevent tennis elbow (lateral epicondylitis). Which of the following is incorrect information?
a. Primarily use the wrist and elbow extensors during a backhand stroke.
b. Begin the backhand stroke in shoulder adduction and internal rotation.
c. Use a racket that has a large grip.
d. Use a light racket.

266. Which of the following is an inappropriate exercise for a patient who received an anterior cruciate ligament reconstruction with a patella tendon autograft 2 weeks ago?
a. Lateral step-ups
b. Heel slides
c. Stationary bike
d. Pool walking

267. A PTA is speaking to a group of receptionists about correct posture. Which of the following is incorrect information?
    a. Position computer monitors at eye level.
    b. Position seats so that the feet are flat on the floor while sitting.
    c. Position keyboards so that the wrists are in approximately 20 degrees of extension.
    d. Take frequent stretching breaks.

268. Which degree of strain in the following joints would normally take the longest amount of time to rehabilitate?
    a. Grade I medial collateral ligament of the knee injury
    b. Grade I anterior cruciate ligament injury
    c. Grade II ulnar collateral ligament of the elbow injury
    d. Grade III anterior talofibular ligament injury

269. A PTA is treating an automobile mechanic. The patient asks for tips on preventing upper extremity repetitive motion injuries. Which of the following is incorrect advice?
    a. Use your entire hand rather than just the fingers when holding an object.
    b. Position tasks so that they are performed below shoulder height.
    c. Use tools with small straight handles when possible.
    d. When performing a forceful task, keep the materials slightly lower than the elbow.

270. A patient is 6 weeks post acromioplasty and is showing difficulty performing shoulder flexion and scaption exercises correctly. The patient shows shoulder "hike" above 70 degrees of shoulder flexion. Which of the following interventions would most quickly improve this problem?
    a. Eccentric elbow flexion
    b. Heavy resistance supraspinatus exercise
    c. Gravity resistance supraspinatus exercise
    d. Upper trapezius strengthening

271. Shoulder range of motion is restricted in a patient 8 weeks after rotator cuff repair. Internal rotation and horizontal adduction are the most restricted motions. Which portion of the shoulder capsule should be stretched or mobilized?
    a. Anterior
    b. Posterior
    c. Inferior
    d. Superior

272. A patient who underwent shoulder acromioplasty 6 days ago presents with pain and limited use for the involved upper extremity during

activities of daily living. What is the most appropriate advice to decrease this patient's pain while at home?
a. Discontinue use of sling and ice at home.
b. Use sling during waking hours and ice throughout the day.
c. Begin progressive resistance exercises at home.
d. Discontinue use of sling and use a moist heat pad at home.

273. A patient complains of pain in the ear. What structure does NOT refer to the ear?
a. Sternocleidomastoid trigger point
b. Deep masseter trigger point
c. Anterior digastric trigger point
d. Temporomandibular joint

274. What symptoms are indicative of a temporomandibular dysfunction problem?
a. Limited range of motion or altered mechanics
b. Tinnitus and hyperacusia
c. Dizziness and spinning
d. Retroorbital headache and sinus pain

275. What is a reasonable rehabilitation goal for active opening after arthroscopy of the temporomandibular joint for an anterior disk displacement without reduction?
a. Opening to 58 mm
b. Opening to 28 mm
c. Opening to 38 mm
d. Opening to 48 mm

276. What is the best evidence-based intervention for a painful anterior displaced disk with reduction in the temporomandibular joint?
a. Exercises that avoid painful click such as hinge axis and midline opening
b. Aggressive mobilization to reduce the clicking
c. Wide opening exercises to reduce the clicking
d. Ice and no exercise

277. Your patient has limited knee flexion in pre-wing phase of gait. What do you suspect?
a. Hamstring weakness
b. Plantar flexor spasticity
c. Plantar flexor weakness
d. Dorsiflexor weakness

278. A patient demonstrates excessive hip adduction in swing phase of gait. What are the hypothesized causes for this deviation?
a. Adductor hypertonicity of the swing leg
b. Quadriceps weakness of the swing leg

    c. Plantar flexor weakness of the swing leg

    d. Gluteus medius hypertonicity of the swing leg

279. A PTA is scheduled to work with a 72-year-old woman who has suffered a recent stroke. The supervising physical therapist has requested the PTA to focus on pregait activities. Which of the proprioceptive neuromuscular facilitation (PNF) diagonals best encourages normal gait?

    a. D1

    b. D2

    c. PNF is contraindicated

    d. Pelvic PNF patterns only

280. In which type of cognitive deficit should the PTA use repetition to teach the patient new activities?

    a. Decreased executive functions

    b. Poor complex problem solving

    c. Slowed information processing

    d. Memory deficits

281. At what stage of amyotrophic lateral sclerosis would a patient begin to use adaptive equipment to facilitate activities of daily living (ADLs)?

    a. Stage I

    b. Stage II

    c. Stage III

    d. Stage IV

282. Which of the following would be an effective intervention strategy for patients diagnosed with Alzheimer's disease?

    a. Exercise outdoors

    b. Use several different therapists in the patient's exercise session

    c. Perform multiple exercises with each session

    d. Perform short, simple, repetitive exercises

283. Why do many clients with Duchenne's muscular dystrophy exhibit increased lumbar lordosis?

    a. Quadriceps weakness

    b. Hip abductor weakness

    c. Abdominal and hip extensor weakness

    d. Tight iliopsoas muscles

284. Which of the following choices is indicative of class B impairment according to the American Spinal Injury Association (ASIA)?

    a. Complete: injury with no sensory or motor function preserved in segment S4-S5

    b. Incomplete: sensory but no motor function preserved below the neurologic level; sensory level extends through segment S4-S5

   c. Incomplete: motor function preserved below the neurologic level, with the majority of key muscles below the neurologic level having a muscle grade of less than 3

   d. Incomplete: motor function preserved below the neurologic level, with the majority of key muscles below the neurologic level having a muscle grade of greater than or equal to 3

285. The level of motor innervation according to the American Spinal Injury Association is determined by the most distal key muscle with what grade or better (with the segment above being a grade 5)?
   a. Grade 2
   b. Grade 2+
   c. Grade 3
   d. Grade 3+

286. When the descending tracts are involved with spinal cord injury, what will be the clinical presentation?
   a. Immediate spasticity and hyperreflexia below the level of injury
   b. Immediate flaccidity and hyperreflexia below the level of injury
   c. Immediate spasticity and loss of reflexes below the level of injury
   d. Immediate flaccidity and loss of reflexes below the level of injury

287. What is a common site for pressure ulcers as an individual with a spinal cord injury begins to use a wheelchair for mobility?
   a. Ischium
   b. Sacrum
   c. Scapula
   d. Heel

288. Which of the following is indicative of asymmetrical tonic neck reflex?
   a. Turning the head to the right elicits right upper extremity extension and left upper extremity flexion
   b. Turning the head to the left elicits right upper extremity extension and left upper extremity flexion
   c. Turning the head to the right elicits right lower extremity flexion and left lower extremity extension
   d. Turning the head to the left elicits left lower extremity flexion and right lower extremity extension

289. Abnormal spasticity in what two muscle groups will lead to hip dislocations in patients with cerebral palsy?
   a. Hip extensors and abductors
   b. Hip flexors and abductors
   c. Hip extensors and adductors
   d. Hip flexors and adductors

290. Which of the following is a true statement regarding muscle dysfunction in cerebral palsy?
   a. Both hypertrophy and atrophy can be present in a child diagnosed with cerebral palsy.
   b. There is an increase in number of sarcomeres per muscle fiber.
   c. Muscle will grow faster than bone.
   d. There will be a decrease in fat and fibrous tissue and an increase in blood flow to muscles.

291. Why do children with cerebral palsy adopt a wide-based sitting posture?
   a. With wide-based sitting, the upper extremities are more involved than the lower extremities.
   b. With wide-based sitting, the lower extremities are more involved than the upper extremities.
   c. It increases the ability to turn and rotate in the sitting position.
   d. Wide-based sitting allows the child with poor trunk control to maintain the posture.

292. Which of the following is an effect of moderate hypotonia in a child with cerebral palsy?
   a. Truncal kyphosis
   b. Contractures of the hip and knee flexors
   c. Flexed, adducted, pronated upper extremity
   d. Using arms for sitting balance

293. A client is receiving Botox injections into the gastrocnemius muscle secondary to spasticity associated with cerebral palsy. In general, when will the symptoms of muscle spasms decrease?
   a. Immediately after injection
   b. In 1 to 2 days
   c. In 3 to 7 days
   d. In 7 to 10 days

294. What is the ambulation potential of a patient with cerebral palsy that has the presence of primitive reflexes beyond age 2 years?
   a. Poor
   b. Fair
   c. Good
   d. Excellent

295. Therapy intervention for children with cerebral palsy that is solely aimed at motor outcomes can be characterized as which of the following?
   a. Is appropriate for this patient population
   b. Has worse outcomes than programs based on cognition
   c. Should be used at the discretion of the supervising therapist only
   d. Is a poor predictor of functional outcomes

296. The majority of children diagnosed with spastic cerebral palsy present with which of the following?
    a. Low muscle tone throughout the course of the pathology
    b. Increased muscle tone throughout the course of the pathology
    c. Spasticity early in the first year of life and later development of low muscle tone
    d. Low muscle tone early in the first year of life and later development of spasticity

297. Which of the following is true after orthopedic surgery and casting for a patient with cerebral palsy?
    a. There is no need to inspect for skin breakdown at the edges of the cast.
    b. The family should wash and dry the skin at the edge of the cast frequently.
    c. The patient should not begin therapy intervention for 4 weeks after surgery.
    d. The skin inside the edges of the cast should be kept moist.

298. Appropriate positioning in a wheelchair has been shown to improve several aspects of a child's functional ability with cerebral palsy. Which of the following will NOT be accomplished with appropriate positioning?
    a. Increase in vital capacity
    b. Improved performance on cognitive testing
    c. Increase in extensor tone
    d. Smoother and faster reach

299. Which of the following clients with cerebral palsy would benefit the most from a hinged ankle-foot orthosis?
    a. A beginning stander
    b. Nonambulator
    c. Ambulator with excessive ankle pronation
    d. Client with some, but limited, functional mobility

300. Which of the following sensations has the slowest nerve conduction velocity?
    a. Proprioception
    b. Pressure
    c. Temperature
    d. Pain

301. Prolonged compression of a nerve that produces an area of infarction and necrosis is defined as which of the following?
    a. Neurapraxia
    b. Myelinopathy
    c. Axonotmesis
    d. Neurotmesis

302. Which of the following is a common clinical manifestation of ulnar nerve palsy?
    a. Flattening of the thenar eminence
    b. Claw-hand deformity
    c. Ulnar deviation of the hand when the wrist is flexed
    d. Impaired sensation along the thumb and first digit

303. A patient presents to outpatient physical therapy with a diagnosis of thoracic outlet syndrome. Which of the following treatments would be inappropriate for this individual?
    a. Forceful stretching to mobilize the first rib
    b. Postural and breathing exercises
    c. Strengthening exercises for the shoulder girdle musculature
    d. Moist heat to the upper trapezius

304. Which of the following is correct advice for a PTA to give a patient with a diagnosis of post-polio syndrome that is beginning an outpatient physical therapy intervention program?
    a. The patient should exercise to the point of fatigue at the first visit.
    b. The patient should stop exercise if pain or weakness increases.
    c. The patient should focus on lower extremity aggressive exercise.
    d. Functional exercises should be of maximal intensity.

305. Which of the following is the least common symptom of a paraneoplastic neuropathy?
    a. Weakness
    b. Burning and aching
    c. Numbness
    d. Paresthesia

306. At what stage of the complex regional pain syndrome is the skin thin, shiny, cyanotic, and dry?
    a. Acute
    b. Dystrophic
    c. Atrophic
    d. Subacute

307. A patient presents with pathology restricted to a peripheral nerve injury distally in one upper extremity. Is this patient at increased risk for loss of balance?
    a. Yes, peripheral nerve injury affects strength, and an intact motor system is necessary for normal postural control.
    b. No, the impairments are restricted to the distal upper extremity, which is minimally involved in normal postural control.
    c. Yes, the peripheral nerve injury affects sensation, and an intact sensory system is necessary for normal postural control.
    d. No, pathologies that affect central systems have more influence on normal postural control than those affecting peripheral systems.

308. Which of the following best describes the disease process for a patient with permanent bilateral vestibular loss?
    a. Because of the importance of the vestibular system in balance, the patient will need to be supported when upright.
    b. After an initial period of disability, the patient will adapt sufficiently to rely on other sensory systems for balance information when upright.
    c. One of the other sensory systems will take over the role of the vestibular system in mediating conflicting information during balance activities.
    d. The patient will no longer be able to keep the head oriented or turn appropriately for auditory input.

309. A patient has fallen twice recently: once when carrying a large box upstairs and once when trying to get to the bathroom at night without turning on the light. A Romberg test is positive, and the PTA determines that the patient's balance dysfunction is due to sensory deficits and reliance on vision to compensate. Which of the following would be the most important intervention to keep this patient safe and decrease risk of falls?
    a. Have her strengthen her lower extremities.
    b. Instruct her to keep a night light on.
    c. Practice walking with eyes closed.
    d. Instruct her to use a walker for community ambulation.

310. Appropriate physical therapy intervention to decrease standing loss of balance in a patient who has hemiparesis following a stroke would best incorporate which of the following?
    a. Facilitation to improve strength and timing of symmetrical ankle and hip strategies
    b. Exercises to habituate response to head turning
    c. Facilitation on the paretic side in sitting while patient shifts weight to the nonparetic side
    d. Practice the Clinical Test of Sensory Integration and Balance several times

311. Appropriate physical therapy intervention to decrease dizziness in a patient with benign paroxysmal peripheral vertigo would best incorporate having the patient do which of the following?
    a. Habituate responses by practicing the rotary chair test.
    b. Roll over several times in bed to get the otoconia to reposition.
    c. Practice switching gaze from objects to the right and then to the left for improved control without dizziness.
    d. Perform the Brandt-Daroff exercises.

312. Which of the following choices would be an example of the motor system assisting in balance control?
    a. Determination of body position
    b. Adjust body position

    c. Receive information from the vestibular system

    d. Receive information from the visual system

313. In quiet standing, which postural strategy is used primarily?
    a. Ankle strategy
    b. Hip strategy
    c. Stepping strategy
    d. Change in support strategy

314. A PTA is performing beginning treatment of an older adult who complains of several recent falls. What postural strategy should the PTA most likely be focused on to decrease this patient's risk for falls?
    a. Change in support strategy
    b. Stepping strategy
    c. Hip strategy
    d. Ankle strategy

315. A PTA begins intervention on a patient who recently suffered a stroke. A chart review finds that the cerebellum was affected by the stroke. What limitations could the PTA be expected to see with this patient?
    a. Visual field deficits
    b. Vertigo
    c. Slowed or involuntary movement
    d. Ataxia

316. Which of the following is progression from small to large base of support?
    a. Tandem stance, normal stance, single-leg stance
    b. Normal stance, tandem stance, single-leg stance
    c. Single-leg stance, tandem stance, normal stance
    d. Single-leg stance, normal stance, tandem stance

317. Which of the following exercises would most likely trigger the hip postural sway strategy during treatment?
    a. Have the patient stand on a firm flat surface.
    b. Have the patient stand on an irregular surface such as a balance/wobble board.
    c. Have the PTA push the patient in several different directions while in standing position.
    d. Have the patient stand on a smooth surface with eyes closed.

318. What is the primary focus of a fall prevention program?
    a. Restoring normal strength
    b. Restoring normal range of motion
    c. Preventing injury from falls
    d. Improving independence with an assist device

319. Which of the following is the correct progression of motor development according to Rood?
    a. Stability, mobility, combined mobility, and skill
    b. Skill, combined mobility, stability, and mobility
    c. Mobility, stability, combined mobility, and skill
    d. Mobility, skill, stability, and combined mobility

320. Which stage of motor development could be defined as "the ability to maintain weight-bearing postures against gravity"?
    a. Mobility
    b. Stability
    c. Combined mobility
    d. Skill

321. In normal growth and development, by what age can most children sit without upper extremity support?
    a. 4 months
    b. 5 months
    c. 6 months
    d. 8 months

322. In normal growth and development, when can most infants roll from supine to prone?
    a. 4 months
    b. 5 months
    c. 8 months
    d. 9 months

323. An example of an activity-focused intervention is which of the following?
    a. Range of motion
    b. Strength training
    c. Stair climbing
    d. Aerobic conditioning

324. Which of the following interventions would be considered an impairment-focused intervention for a child with cerebral palsy?
    a. Constrained induced movement therapy
    b. Using adaptive equipment for feeding
    c. Using a standing frame for pregait activities
    d. Electrical stimulation

325. Which of the following techniques would be most appropriate for facilitating initiation of movement in a paretic upper extremity?
    a. Slow reversals
    b. Alternating isometrics
    c. Rhythmic initiation
    d. Agonistic reversals

326. Which of the following feedback and practice paradigms is most effective for promoting motor learning?
    a. Practice one task repeatedly with feedback given every trial
    b. Practice one task repeatedly with feedback given every other trial
    c. Practice a variety of tasks with feedback given every trial
    d. Practice a variety of tasks with feedback given every other trial

327. A PTA points out the next patient to be seen for the day has a left upper extremity flexion synergy. What is the most likely presentation of this patient's left upper extremity?
    a. Shoulder abduction, elbow flexion, forearm supination
    b. Shoulder adduction, elbow flexion, forearm supination
    c. Shoulder abduction, elbow extension, forearm supination
    d. Shoulder abduction, elbow flexion, forearm pronation

328. Which of the following interventions is based on the inhibition of abnormal synergies and tone and the facilitation of normal movement patterns with the ultimate goal of optimizing function?
    a. Neurodevelopmental treatment
    b. Proprioceptive neuromuscular facilitation
    c. Constraint-induced movement therapy
    d. Body weight supported

329. Which of the following is NOT a core principal of proprioceptive neuromuscular facilitation (PNF)?
    a. Normal coordinated activities are accomplished through complex movement patterns that do not occur in straight planes.
    b. The stretch reflex is most effectively elicited when the extremity is elongated in a specific diagonal.
    c. The muscular response is more coordinated and forceful when resisted within a specific diagonal.
    d. Tone must be normalized before initiating PNF.

330. A PTA is providing beginning treatment for a patient after a recent traumatic brain injury. The patient is learning to bring a spoon to his mouth for eating. The PTA places ice cream on the spoon, and the patient brings it to his mouth for the first time to eat the ice cream. What type of feedback is this patient experiencing?
    a. External feedback
    b. Augmented feedback
    c. Knowledge of results feedback
    d. Intrinsic feedback

331. During treatment, a PTA begins with the patient in sitting. The PTA then sits in front of the patient. The PTA's hands are positioned diagonally from the patient's trunk to the back. The hands then give the patient a forward cue up and the abdominal musculature is also cued.

What intervention is being utilized by the PTA using and what motion is being facilitated?

a. Neurodevelopmental treatment, posterior pelvic tilt
b. Neurodevelopmental treatment, anterior pelvic tilt
c. Proprioceptive neuromuscular facilitation, anterior pelvic tilt
d. Proprioceptive neuromuscular facilitation, posterior pelvic tilt

332. Which of the following muscle groups is the most important to strengthen in order to increase sit-to-stand ability after stroke or traumatic brain injury?

a. Hip flexion
b. Knee extension
c. Plantar flexion
d. Abdominal strength

333. The PTA is using proprioceptive neuromuscular facilitation to facilitate rolling from side lying to prone by using mass flexion. What motions must the shoulder and pelvis make to accomplish this task?

a. Anterior shoulder depression and elevation at the pelvis
b. Posterior shoulder depression and depression at the pelvis
c. Anterior shoulder depression and depression at the pelvis
d. Posterior shoulder depression and elevation at the pelvis

334. Which of the following impairments would you most expect to be reported in the examination of a patient with Parkinson's disease?

a. Weak quadriceps muscles
b. Reduced arm swing and trunk rotation during gait
c. Reduced upper extremity sensation
d. Reduced lower extremity sensation

335. Which of the following is NOT TRUE regarding physical therapy and Parkinson's disease?

a. Physical therapy is needed because it can alter the disease process.
b. Physical therapy is needed to help the patient optimize movement skills.
c. Physical therapy is needed to assist with the prevention of secondary complications.
d. Physical therapy is needed to improve balance and decrease risk for falls.

336. A patient with multiple sclerosis has bilateral hamstring and gastrocnemius spasticity graded as 3 on the Modified Ashworth Scale. He complains of being tired during the exercise program you have developed for him. On his next scheduled treatment day, you would do which of the following?

a. Continue with the treatment plan, but change the treatment time to the late afternoon.
b. Continue with your prescribed exercise program, but have the patient exercise in a warmer room.

   c. Provide the patient with relaxation strategies and reduce the exercise intensity.

   d. Take the patient to the pool because temperatures greater than 90 degrees will be beneficial for him.

337. Of the following diseases, which is the least likely to show spasticity to passive stretch of a muscle?
    a. Huntington's disease
    b. Parkinson's disease
    c. Amyotrophic lateral sclerosis
    d. Multiple sclerosis

338. In which of the following patients should the PTA be concerned regarding overwork in aerobic conditioning?
    a. Patients with amyotrophic lateral sclerosis
    b. Patients with Parkinson's disease
    c. Patients with Alzheimer's disease
    d. Patients with Huntington's disease

339. Balance training should begin immediately after a patient is diagnosed with which of the following conditions?
    a. Huntington's disease
    b. Parkinson's disease
    c. Multiple sclerosis
    d. Alzheimer's disease

340. What is the natural progression of Frenkel's exercises?
    a. Standing, walking, sitting
    b. Lying, sitting, standing
    c. Walking, sitting, lying
    d. Lying, walking, sitting

341. In what sequence does return of sensation typically occur?
    a. Protective sensation, light touch, discriminative touch
    b. Light touch, discriminative touch, protective sensation
    c. Discriminative touch, protective sensation, light touch
    d. Protective sensation, light touch, discriminative touch

342. A patient with a surgical nerve repair was examined by the PTA. The plan of care includes nerve mobilization. Which of the following is consistent with this plan of care?
    a. Application of neuromuscular electrical stimulation to denervated muscle
    b. Application of nerve gliding techniques
    c. Application of an ice pack over the postsurgical incision to reduce edema
    d. Immobilization of one or more joints over which the repaired nerve crosses

343. What is a common gait deviation for patients with Charcot-Marie-Tooth disease?
    a. Trendelenburg gait
    b. Antalgic gait
    c. Forward flexed posture
    d. Foot drop, steppage gait

344. A patient with distal lower extremity weakness associated with poly-neuropathy will often complain of which of the following disturbances?
    a. Difficulty rising from a seated position
    b. Difficulty negotiating stairs
    c. Frequent tripping
    d. Difficulty getting into a car

345. Muscle weakness in the intrinsic foot muscles is responsible for what foot abnormality and what disease is this normally associated with?
    a. Pes cavus, alcoholic neuropathy
    b. Equinovarus, Charcot-Marie-Tooth
    c. Pes cavus, Charcot-Marie-Tooth
    d. Equinovarus, alcoholic neuropathy

346. A patient with Guillain-Barré syndrome is beginning outpatient physical therapy. After the first day's exercise session, the patient complains of muscle soreness in the quadriceps that lasted more than 24 hours. What is the appropriate action by the PTA?
    a. Change to a more eccentric strengthening program
    b. Decrease exercise intensity
    c. Increase exercise intensity
    d. Remain at the same exercise intensity

347. At what level of spinal cord injury should a patient be instructed on glossopharyngeal breathing?
    a. C4
    b. T2
    c. T6
    d. T8

348. Which of the following exercises is appropriate for a patient with a neuropathic ulcer?
    a. Step aerobics
    b. Closed-chain lower extremity exercises
    c. Treadmill
    d. Bicycle

349. The purpose of any off-loading device for a patient with a neuropathic ulcer is which of the following?
    a. To protect the dressing
    b. To allow the patient to ambulate without pain

   c. To distribute the plantar foot pressures and reduce stress at the wound site

   d. To avoid use of ill-fitting shoes

350. Carpal tunnel syndrome symptoms involve compression of what nerve at the wrist?

   a. Ulnar

   b. Radial

   c. Median

   d. Axillary

351. If the motor components of the visual-ocular system were damaged, which of the following would be true?

   a. Visual and vestibular controlled eye movements would be normal.

   b. Visual and vestibular controlled eye movements would be abnormal.

   c. Visually controlled eye movements would be normal, but vestibular dependent eye movements would be abnormal.

   d. Visually controlled eye movements would be abnormal, but vestibular dependent eye movements would be normal.

352. Which of the following head positions will place the posterior canal of the ear in the vertical position?

   a. The body is prone with the head turned to the side.

   b. The body is supine, and the head is flexed beyond neutral and rotated 45 degrees to the ipsilateral side.

   c. The body is prone, and the neck is extended to neutral and rotated 45 degrees to the contralateral side.

   d. The body is in supine, and the head is extended beyond neutral and rotated 45 degrees to the ipsilateral side.

353. Vigorous functional training of a client with spinal cord injury can begin when?

   a. When the client is admitted to the rehabilitation unit

   b. When medical and orthopedic clearance is obtained

   c. When the client is admitted to outpatient physical therapy

   d. When the client's spinal fractures have healed

354. Which of the following techniques emphasize a specific pattern of movement in the retraining process of damaged muscles?

   a. Brunnstrom's approach

   b. Neurodevelopmental treatment

   c. Constraint-induced movement therapy

   d. Proprioceptive neuromuscular facilitation

355. Which current intervention for patients with neurologic injuries involves facilitating automatic walking patterns using intensive task specific training while the body weight is supported?
    a. Constraint-induced movement therapy
    b. Locomotor training
    c. Task-oriented approach
    d. Neurodevelopmental treatment

356. When do most children begin to walk?
    a. 6 to 8 months
    b. 8 to 10 months
    c. 10 to 13 months
    d. 13 to 15 months

357. What are developmental milestones?
    a. Types of standardized tests for measuring progression of a pediatric client
    b. Intervention protocols
    c. Functional goals for a child
    d. The PTA's individual goals for a child

358. Which of the following is an inappropriate treatment for the prevention of idiopathic scoliosis curve progression?
    a. Bracing
    b. Stretching
    c. Electrical stimulation
    d. Family education

359. What is emphasized in using the dynamical systems theory when providing intervention for pediatric clients?
    a. The product of the movement
    b. Family intervention
    c. The process of moving
    d. Using a specific muscle to perform a specific task

360. What physical therapy intervention uses manual facilitation and inhibition techniques to present the child with a normal sensory experience?
    a. Dynamical systems theory
    b. Neurodevelopmental treatment
    c. Sensory integration
    d. Normal development theory

361. A patient asks the PTA whether she should be concerned that her 4-month-old infant cannot roll from his back to his stomach. What is the most appropriate response to the parent?
   a. This is probably nothing to be concerned about because, although it varies, infants can usually perform this task by 10 months of age.
   b. This is probably nothing to be concerned about because, although it varies, infants can usually perform this task by 5 months of age.
   c. Your infant probably needs further examination by a specialist because, although it varies, infants can usually perform this task at 2 months of age.
   d. Your infant probably needs further examination by a specialist because, although it varies, infants can usually perform this task at birth.

362. A PTA must have a clear understanding of the normal development of the human body to treat effectively and efficiently. Which of the following principles of treatment is incorrect?
   a. Early motor activity is influenced primarily by reflexes.
   b. Motor control develops from proximal to distal and from head to toe.
   c. Increasing motor ability is independent of motor learning.
   d. Early motor activity is influenced by spontaneous activity.

363. Which of the following statements about developmental motor control is incorrect?
   a. Isotonic control develops before isometric control.
   b. Gross motor control develops before fine motor control.
   c. Eccentric movement develops before concentric movement.
   d. Trunk control develops before distal extremity control.

364. Fine synergistic control of neck flexors and extensors in the upright position typically appears when?
   a. The second month
   b. The third month
   c. The fourth month
   d. The fifth month

365. Ballistic movements of arms and legs are characterized by which of the following?
   a. Reciprocal activation of antagonist muscles
   b. Coactivation of antagonist muscles
   c. Need for proprioceptive feedback during movement
   d. Visual guidance during movement

366. Successful head turning in prone with an erect head in typically developing children is characterized by which of the following?
   a. Hip extension, medial rotation, and abduction
   b. Cervical spine extension and rotation with weight bearing on upper abdomen

c. Shoulder flexion and abduction with weight bearing on elbows

d. Caudal weight shift with load bearing on lateral thighs and lower abdomen

367. Once a new motor skill is obtained, further development entails which of the following?
   a. Performance with more use of sensory feedback
   b. Constricting the degrees of freedom used when performing the skill
   c. Perfecting of postural control and transitions between postures
   d. Developing a single way of performing the skill

368. Which of the following is a typical accomplishment of a 3-year-old child?
   a. Manage buttoning well
   b. Alternate feet when ascending stairs
   c. Be unafraid of falling
   d. Show no dysmetria during block stacking

369. A patient whose seizures are controlled with an anticonvulsant should be treated in a room or an area with what characteristics?
   a. Devoid of bright flickering lights and repetitive, loud noises
   b. No electronic equipment near the patient
   c. Warm and somewhat humid
   d. Not frequented by many people

370. The PTA observes a patient with the latter stages of Parkinson's disease during ambulation. Which of the following characteristics is the PTA most likely observing?
   a. Shuffling gait
   b. Increased step width
   c. Wide base of support
   d. Increased cadence especially at the onset of gait

371. A patient presents to an outpatient facility with complaints of pain in the groin area (along the medial left thigh). With manual muscle testing of the involved lower extremity, a PTA determines the following: hip flexion = 4+/5, hip extension = 4+/5, hip abduction = 4+/5, hip adduction = 2+/5, hip internal rotation = 2+/5, and hip external rotation = 2+/5. Which nerve on the involved side is most likely injured?
   a. Lateral cutaneous nerve of the upper thigh
   b. Obturator nerve
   c. Femoral nerve
   d. Ilioinguinal nerve

372. A PTA is reviewing the chart of a 24-year-old woman with a diagnosis of L2 incomplete paraplegia. The physician noted that the left

quadriceps tendon reflex is 2+. What does this information relay to the PTA?
a. No active quadriceps tendon reflex
b. Slight quadriceps contraction with reflex testing
c. Normal quadriceps tendon reflex
d. Exaggerated quadriceps tendon reflex

373. Which of the following muscles would you NOT expect to be affected by a C6-C7 lesion?
a. Biceps brachii
b. Anterior deltoid
c. Infraspinatus
d. Triceps brachii

374. A 2-month-old infant is diagnosed with left congenital muscular torticollis that has resulted in plagiocephaly. This would result in which of the following?
a. Flattening of the left frontal and left occipital regions
b. Flattening of the right frontal and left occipital regions
c. Flattening of the right frontal and right occipital regions
d. Flattening of the left frontal and right occipital regions

375. A patient recently diagnosed with multiple sclerosis presents to a physical therapy clinic. The patient asks the PTA what she needs to avoid with this condition. Which of the following should the patient avoid?
a. Hot tubs
b. Slightly increased intake of fluids
c. Application of ice packs
d. Strength training

376. What is necessary for an infant to have mastered before sitting independently on propped upper extremities can be achieved?
a. Rolling prone to supine and supine to prone
b. Translation of grasped objects from hand to hand
c. Extending the head and neck in prone, and controlling the pelvis while using the upper extremities in supine
d. Crawling and creeping

377. Your patient was in a car accident and now has a herniated nucleus pulposus at vertebral level C5-6. She reports difficulty removing her shirt overhead. With nerve root injury at the level of C5-6, what part of the motion will most likely be problematic for your patient and why?
a. Grasping the shirt because of weakness of all finger flexors
b. Internally rotating the shoulder because of weakness of teres minor
c. Shoulder flexion because of weakness of deltoid
d. Cervical flexion to remove shirt because of weakness of deep neck flexors

378. Your patient has an involvement of the fifth lumbar nerve root on the left secondary to a lumbar disk protrusion. Which of the following is TRUE?
    a. The ankle jerk is diminished or absent.
    b. The patient has fatigueable weakness in the calf.
    c. Sensation was diminished between the first and second toes.
    d. Sensation was diminished on the plantar surface of the foot.

379. An 81-year-old woman with right-sided hemiparesis due to stroke is being treated by a PTA through home health services. The PTA is attempting to increase the functional reach of the right upper extremity. The patient currently has 120 degrees of active flexion. The PTA decides to use trunk mobility and stability facilitation techniques to help achieve the patient's functional goals. Which of the following skills need to be mastered by the patient to attain the ability to reach 2 feet in front of her wheelchair and 2 feet to the right of midline at 125 degrees of shoulder flexion with the right upper extremity?
    a. Weight shifting to the left buttock and right-sided trunk elongation
    b. Weight shifting to the left buttock and left-sided trunk elongation
    c. Weight shifting to the right buttock and right-sided trunk elongation
    d. Weight shifting to the right buttock and left-sided trunk elongation

380. A PTA working in early intervention is helping a parent to get the baby to hold and drink from a bottle. Based on typical development, the PTA should begin to introduce this skill at what age?
    a. 12 to 14 months
    b. 10 to 12 months
    c. 8 to 10 months
    d. 6 to 8 months

381. After 3 months of intervention, the PTA notices that the child is beginning to integrate the reflex that turns the head toward the child's extended arm while in prone. What is this reflex?
    a. Asymmetrical tonic neck reflex
    b. Symmetrical tonic neck reflex
    c. Moro reflex
    d. Tonic labyrinthine reflex

382. A child has poor ability to maintain trunk and neck extension. The PTA uses which of the following as the best technique to facilitate increased strength and control?
    a. Have child prone on a therapy ball and play with toys
    b. Have child supine on a platform swing while playing with toys
    c. Have child in side lying on a mat shield playing with toys
    d. Have child sit on physio ball while playing with toys

383. A PTA is working with a child who has cerebral palsy. The child has limited range of motion in bilateral upper extremities and is unable to reach out for objects. The PTA provides intervention that focuses on allowing the child to participate in play activities. What is the best position to place the child in?
    a. Side lying
    b. Prone
    c. Supine
    d. Sitting

384. As a home health therapist, you are treating a 55-year-old who has a very supportive spouse and a caregiver during the day who helps with self-care and other tasks needed in the home. The patient enjoys his children and grandchildren who live in the immediate area. The patient is currently in stage 3 of amyotrophic lateral sclerosis, with severe weakness of the ankles, wrists, and hands. The patient minimally ambulates and fatigues easily. What would be an appropriate intervention?
    a. Light strengthening program
    b. Helping prioritize activities and providing work simplification
    c. Learning how to cook three-course meals
    d. Worksite assessment

385. A 3-year-old has spina bifida and needs mobility augmentation to be able to move outdoors, in hallways, and in corridors. What mobility device could be recommended?
    a. Hand-propelled tricycle model
    b. Supine electric scooter
    c. Aeroplane mobility device
    d. Crocodile posterior walker

386. You are visiting the home of a client recently diagnosed with Alzheimer's disease. The environment is terribly cluttered and seems to add to the patient's current level of confusion. What would be an appropriate intervention for the PTA?
    a. Clean up the place by yourself, throw away a lot, and put everything else away properly to help organized the environment for the client.
    b. Leave it alone and just recognize that this is how the person will be living.
    c. Engage family members in helping the client to sort through some of the cluttered items and make some choices about what to and what not to keep.
    d. Encourage the family to hire a housekeeper, who will make sure that the environment is clean and tidy all the time.

387. To treat effectively most patients with Parkinson's disease, the PTA should emphasize which proprioceptive neuromuscular facilitation pattern for the upper extremities?
    a. D2 extension
    b. D2 flexion
    c. D1 extension
    d. D1 flexion

388. Which of the following is the most energy efficient and allows a T1 complete paraplegic the most functional mobility during locomotion?
    a. Manual wheelchair
    b. Electric wheelchair
    c. Bilateral ankle-knee orthoses and crutches
    d. Bilateral ankle-foot orthoses and crutches

389. To facilitate development of a functional tenodesis grip in a patient with spinal cord injury, what should the treatment plan include?
    a. Stretching of the finger flexors and finger extensors
    b. Stretching of the finger flexors
    c. Allowing the finger flexors and finger extensors to shorten
    d. Allowing the finger flexors to shorten

390. A PTA is treating a patient with an injury at the T8 level and compromised function of the diaphragm. If no abdominal binder is available, what is the most likely position of comfort to allow the patient to breathe most efficiently?
    a. Sitting position
    b. Semi-Fowler's position
    c. Upright standing position using a tilt table
    d. Supine position

391. A PTA is assisting a patient with an injury at the C5 level in performing an effective cough. The patient has experienced significant neurologic damage and is unable to perform an independent, effective cough. If the patient is in supine position, which of the following methods is most likely to produce an effective cough?
    a. The PTA places the heel of one hand just above the xiphoid process, instructs the patient to take a deep breath while pressing down moderately on the sternum, and instructs the patient to cough.
    b. The PTA places the heel of one hand, reinforced with the other hand, just above the xiphoid process; instructs the patient to take a deep breath; instructs the patient to hold the breath; and presses moderately as the patient coughs.
    c. The PTA places the heel of one hand on the area just above the umbilicus, instructs the patient to take a deep breath, applies

moderate pressure, and releases pressure just before the patient attempts to cough.

d. The PTA places the heel of one hand just above the umbilicus, instructs the patient to take a deep breath, and applies moderate pressure as the patient is instructed to cough.

392. A 60-year-old woman who has suffered a recent stroke has right-sided homonymous hemianopsia. Which of the following statements is true about placement of eating utensils in early rehabilitation?
a. The utensils should be placed on the left side of the plate.
b. The utensils should be placed on the right side of the plate.
c. The utensils should be placed on both sides of the plate.
d. The plate and utensils should be placed slightly to the right.

393. A PTA is observing a 5-day old infant with cerebral palsy. The infant has an abnormal amount of extensor tone. Which of the following is incorrect positioning advice for the family and nursing staff?
a. Keep the infant in supine position.
b. Keep the infant in prone position.
c. Keep the infant in right side-lying position.
d. Keep the infant in left side-lying position.

394. A PTA is treating a 76-year-old woman with left lower extremity hypotonia secondary to a recent stroke. Which of the following is an incorrect method to normalize tone?
a. Rapid irregular movements
b. Approximation
c. Prolonged stretch
d. Tactile cues

395. A PTA is attempting to open the spastic and flexed hand of a patient who has suffered a recent stroke. Which of the following does NOT inhibit hand opening?
a. Avoiding touching the interossei
b. Applying direct pressure to the thenar eminence
c. Hyperextending the metacarpophalangeal joint
d. Applying direct pressure to the hypothenar eminence

396. Which of the following is inappropriate for a PTA to perform for an infant with a gestational age of 27 weeks and Down syndrome?
a. Bottle feeding
b. Encouraging side-lying position
c. Tactile stimulation with the entire hand rather than the fingertips of the examiner
d. Prone positioning

397. Which of the following sources of stimulation is least effective in obtaining functional goals when treating an infant with decreased muscular tone?
    a. Vestibular
    b. Weight bearing
    c. Cutaneous
    d. Vibratory

398. A patient who has suffered a recent stroke is being treated by a PTA. The patient exhibits increased extensor tone in the supine position along with an exaggerated symmetrical tonic labyrinthine reflex. What position should be avoided if the PTA is attempting to initiate flexion movements of the lower extremity?
    a. Prone position
    b. Right side-lying position
    c. Supine position
    d. Left side-lying position

399. A patient presents to outpatient physical therapy with tarsal tunnel syndrome. What nerve is involved? Where should the PTA concentrate treatment?
    a. Superficial peroneal nerve, inferior to the medial malleolus
    b. Posterior tibial nerve, inferior to the medial malleolus
    c. Superficial peroneal nerve, inferior to the lateral malleolus
    d. Posterior tibial nerve, inferior to the lateral malleolus

400. Which of the following positions should be avoided in the right upper extremity with a patient who has a diagnosis of right hemiplegia secondary to a stroke?
    a. Prolonged shoulder adduction, internal rotation, elbow flexion
    b. Prolonged shoulder abduction, internal rotation, elbow flexion
    c. Prolonged finger and thumb flexion
    d. Prolonged wrist flexion, and finger adduction

401. A 35-year-old man has a diagnosis of right C5-6 cervical nerve root compression. He is being seen in physical therapy for gentle manual cervical traction. What position is ideal for traction with this patient?
    a. Upper cervical flexion and lower cervical extension
    b. Cervical lateral flexion to right
    c. Cervical extension
    d. Cervical flexion

402. During physical therapy sessions, the PTA protects tenodesis of the patient with diagnosis of C6 tetraplegia. What position must be maintained during upper extremity weight bearing and why?
    a. Maintain finger flexion with wrist extension to protect extrinsic wrist extensors
    b. Maintain wrist flexion to protect intrinsic finger extensors

    c. Maintain finger flexion to protect extrinsic finger flexors

    d. Maintain wrist extension to protect intrinsic finger flexors

403. Which is NOT a typical clinical finding of a patient with a brachial plexus injury?
    a. Decreased range of motion and contractures
    b. Decreased muscle strength
    c. Spasticity
    d. Altered sensation

404. Which of the following exercise programs is most appropriate for a 62-year old, postmenopausal female patient with multiple sclerosis with poor balance and decreased strength?
    a. Stretching, posture and balance program, and strengthening exercises as tolerated
    b. Stretching and progressive hill training on treadmill
    c. Warm-water aquatic therapy
    d. Progressive hill training on treadmill with plyometric training

405. A patient has experienced a grade 2 reaction to radiation in the axilla. Which of the following would be inappropriate treatment or advice for a patient with this diagnosis?
    a. Perform active and passive range motion from the shoulder
    b. Use skin cream on the area
    c. Use antiperspirants
    d. Wash the area daily with water and gentle soap

406. The PTA applies ice to a patient's hand. The patient has sudden blanching, cyanosis, and arrhythmia of the fingers. The ice pack is removed, and 10 to 15 minutes later, blood flow returns to the fingers. At this point the fingers become red and painful. What phenomenon does this patient present with, and what other condition will this patient most likely present with?
    a. Raynaud's phenomenon, systemic lupus erythematosus
    b. Raimiste's phenomenon, scleroderma
    c. Raynaud's phenomenon, scleroderma
    d. Raimiste's phenomenon, systemic lupus erythematosus

407. What is a contraindicated treatment for a patient with a localized cold injury?
    a. Rewarming the injured body part
    b. Pain control with medication
    c. Supporting the affected body part
    d. Massaging the affected body part

408. Paul has incomplete T10 paraplegia, classified as ASIA C, as the result of a stab wound. He is nearing the end of his inpatient rehabilitation stay and is preparing for the transition to home. The most likely technique that Paul will use for performing regular pressure relief will be which of the following?
    a. Use a tilt or recline wheelchair for position changes
    b. Use the push-up technique
    c. Transfer out of his chair and lie prone for 5 minutes
    d. Perform side-to-side leans using wrist extension to hook on the wheelchair push handle

409. What is the most appropriate advice to give to a patient with a complete T11 spinal cord injury to prevent pressure ulcers?
    a. Change position every hour in bed and every hour while seated.
    b. Change position every 2 hours in bed and 2 hours when seated.
    c. Change position every hour in bed and every 20 minutes when seated.
    d. Change positions every 2 hours in bed and every 20 minutes when seated.

410. In positioning protocols, which of the following would NOT be a reason to develop the skin protocols for patients with disorders of consciousness?
    a. Avoid development of pressure ulcers
    b. Mobilize lung secretions
    c. Avoid development of aspiration pneumonia
    d. Improve strength

411. Alleviating causative factors by altering seating and bed surfaces, protecting the skin, and frequently changing the patient's position are which of the following?
    a. Wound bed preparation
    b. Necessary only for stage III and IV pressure ulcers
    c. Part of standard care for all pressure ulcers
    d. Provided only by the primary caregiver

412. How much pressure is considered "standard" for compression to treat venous insufficiency?
    a. 20 to 28 mm Hg
    b. 30 to 40 mm Hg
    c. 10 to 15 mm Hg
    d. 9 to 12 mm Hg

413. The most important aspect of venous ulcer intervention is which of the following?
    a. Antibiotic therapy
    b. Topical steroids

    c. Compression therapy
    d. Surgery

414. A patient presents for physical therapy treatment of a wound on the lower leg over the medial malleolus. The wound is red with irregular margins, and the tissue around the wound is swollen. What type of insufficiency does this patient most likely have?
    a. Arterial insufficiency
    b. Venous insufficiency
    c. Renal insufficiency
    d. Cardiac insufficiency

415. A patient is being treated in outpatient physical therapy because of an arterial insufficiency ulcer. During the past 2 weeks, the wound size has increased. During today's treatment session, the PTA notes a foul odor and necrotic tissue in the wound. What is the appropriate course of action by the PTA?
    a. Initiate hydrotherapy
    b. Perform débridement
    c. Contact the supervising physical therapist
    d. Use a wet to dry dressing over the wound

416. What is the dressing of choice for arterial ulcers?
    a. Adherent dressings that keep the wound moist
    b. Nonadherent dressings that keep the wound moist
    c. Adherent dressings that keep the wound dry
    d. Nonadherent dressings that keep the wound dry

417. Instructions in self-care for the patient with a neuropathic ulcer include which of the following?
    a. Foot and skin protection
    b. Total contact casting
    c. Débridement
    d. Application of Unna boot

418. You are treating a 53-year-old patient with general weakness 2 weeks after a 22% total body surface area burn injury. What is the most likely cause of his weakness?
    a. Disuse and burn injury–related pain
    b. Disuse and increased catabolism secondary to the burn injury
    c. Disuse, bed rest, and wound contraction
    d. Disuse, fluid loss, and damaged nerves in the skin

419. In which position should the patient's shoulder rest after an axillary burn?
    a. 30 degrees of shoulder abduction and neutral rotation
    b. Functional position

   c. 180 degrees of shoulder abduction with 45 degrees of horizontal flexion

   d. 90 to 110 degrees of shoulder abduction with slight horizontal flexion

420. Anticontracture positioning is recommended for which of the following?
   a. Any contracting scar
   b. Only hypertrophic scaring
   c. Only full-thickness burns
   d. After the scar has completed forming and is "mature"

421. Range of motion for scar tissue lengthening is thought to be the most beneficial during which phase(s) of healing?
   a. Proliferation phase only
   b. Remodeling phase only
   c. Proliferation and remodeling phases
   d. Acute open wound phase and directly after grafting

422. Ambulation training is often started as soon as a patient with a burn is medically stable and able to follow directions. Early ambulation will not help achieve which of the following outcomes?
   a. Improved strength
   b. Increased lower extremity edema to improve healing
   c. Improved lower extremity strength
   d. Improved aerobic capacity

423. Which of the following types of wounds should be treated with a moisturizing lotion immediately after the burn?
   a. Superficial
   b. Superficial partial thickness
   c. Deep partial thickness
   d. Full thickness

424. What is the earliest point after surgery that the PTA could begin range-of-motion exercises for a patient's elbow after a skin graft to the biceps area?
   a. Immediately after surgery
   b. 12 hours
   c. 24 hours
   d. 48 hours

425. The patient begins outpatient physical therapy secondary to range-of-motion deficit into knee flexion after skin grafting of a burn on the anterior thigh. The PTA has chosen to use passive range of motion

as an intervention to increase this patient's functional ability. What would be an inappropriate end feel for this particular stretch into knee flexion?
a. Bone to bone
b. Leathery
c. Tissue stretch
d. Tissue approximation

426. How many hours a day should pressure support garments be worn to decrease scarring after a burn?
a. 6 hours
b. 12 hours
c. 18 hours
d. 23 hours

427. At what point of the wound healing phase can the PTA be the most aggressive with range of motion or exercise?
a. Inflammatory phase
b. Proliferative phase
c. Maturation phase
d. Healing phase

428. Which of the following is an area at risk for pressure ulcer development if the client stays in the seated position for an extreme amount of time?
a. Scapulae
b. Ischial tuberosities
c. Occiput
d. Malleoli

429. What type of wound should have a dressing that increases moisture at the wound site?
a. Arterial wound
b. Venous wound
c. Pressure wound
d. Avulsion injury

430. Compression therapy should be performed in an extremity with what type of wound?
a. Arterial wound
b. Neuropathic ulcer
c. Venous wounds
d. Pressure ulcer

431. A client has a full-thickness burn over the foot. The physician has ordered positioning to decrease range-of-motion loss. What is the correct position for this client's foot and ankle?
    a. Full dorsiflexion with toe extension
    b. Ankle neutral with flexion of the toes
    c. Full plantar flexion with full toe flexion
    d. Neutral ankle with neutral toes

432. A comatose client is in the acute portion of the hospital. The PTA decides to begin a turning schedule with the patient to prevent pressure ulcers. How often should the patient be turned?
    a. 30 minutes
    b. 1 hour
    c. 2 hours
    d. 3 hours

433. What is the most common hand deformity following burn injury in children?
    a. Hyperextension of fifth metacarpophalangeal
    b. Radial deviation of wrist
    c. Boutonnière deformity
    d. Palmar contracture

434. A 67-year-old man with a below-knee amputation presents to an outpatient clinic. His surgical amputation was 3 weeks ago, and his scars are well healed. Which of the following is incorrect information about stump care?
    a. Use a light lotion on the stump after bathing each night.
    b. Continue with use of a shrinker 12 hours per day.
    c. Wash the stump with mild soap and water.
    d. Use scar massage techniques.

435. A PTA is treating a 35-year-old man with traumatic injury to the right hand. The patient has several surgical scars from a tendon repair performed 6 weeks ago. What is the appropriate type of massage for the patient's scars?
    a. Transverse and longitudinal
    b. Circular and longitudinal
    c. Transverse and circular
    d. Massage is contraindicated after a tendon repair.

436. A PTA is treating an acute full-thickness burn on the entire right lower extremity of a 27-year-old man. What movements need to be stressed with splinting, positioning, and exercise to avoid contractures?
    a. Hip flexion, knee extension, and ankle dorsiflexion
    b. Hip extension, knee flexion, and ankle plantar flexion

   c. Hip extension, knee extension, and ankle dorsiflexion
   d. Hip flexion, knee extension, and ankle plantar flexion

437. Which of the following does not facilitate ambulation when the feet are burned?
   a. Constant movement, avoiding standing still
   b. Loosening or removing the bandages and wraps
   c. Establishing a clear goal for walking, such as to a favorite person or place
   d. Exercising before standing upright

438. What is the most correct ambient temperature for a room that normally has a predominant population of burn patients?
   a. 65° F
   b. 72° F
   c. 78° F
   d. 85° F

439. A patient is beginning cardiac rehabilitation after recent coronary artery bypass graft. Which of the following would be a clinical sign to discontinue or modify the patient's current exercise?
   a. Resting heart rate of 100 beats/minute
   b. Oxygen saturation of 98%
   c. Body temperature of 99.1° F
   d. Blood pressure during exercise of 280/120 mm Hg

440. Treatment of severe arterial insufficiency usually involves which of the following?
   a. Walking program
   b. Increase in dietary protein
   c. Surgical intervention
   d. Compression

441. A patient presents today with a metered-dose inhaler (MDI). What is the proper advice to give this patient on when to take this particular medication?
   a. 15 to 20 minutes before exercise
   b. 1 to 2 minutes before exercise
   c. During exercise
   d. 5 to 10 minutes after exercise

442. Which of the following activities is most likely to result in an episode of exercise-induced asthma?
   a. Soccer
   b. Baseball
   c. Gymnastics
   d. Running sprints

443. You are ambulating a patient who is recovering from pneumonia. Which of the following would NOT be a sign of a decreased O_2 saturation during gait?
    a. Cyanotic appearance
    b. Dyspnea
    c. Mental confusion
    d. Decreased respiratory rate

444. Which of the following is TRUE regarding exercise and blood pressure?
    a. Physical exertion increases blood pressure acutely and decreases resting blood pressure over time.
    b. Physical exertion decreases blood pressure acutely and decreases resting blood pressure over time.
    c. Physical exertion decreases blood pressure acutely and increases resting blood pressure over time.
    d. Physical exertion increases blood pressure acutely and increases resting blood pressure over time.

445. The PTA is beginning intervention for a patient who recently suffered a myocardial infarction. The PTA uses a pulse oximeter and finds oxygen saturation of 97%. What is the appropriate action by the PTA?
    a. Continue with treatment as normal.
    b. Contact the patient's physician immediately.
    c. Contact the supervising physical therapist immediately.
    d. Cancel today's intervention and monitor the patient for 2 hours.

446. What is the most common mode of exercise for severely deconditioned patients?
    a. Stationary bicycle
    b. StairMaster
    c. Walking
    d. Treadmill

447. What is the most common method for determining the goal for the intensity of an exercise?
    a. METs
    b. VO_2
    c. Ventilation rate
    d. Heart rate

448. What type of activity typifies 1 MET?
    a. Slow walking
    b. Fast walking
    c. Standing performing activities of daily living
    d. Sitting at rest

449. Using the Borg Scale of Perceived Exertion, what is the recommended level of exertion for a deconditioned patient beginning a conditioning program?
    a. 6 to 8
    b. 8 to 10
    c. 10 to 12
    d. 12 to 14

450. What is the heart rate reserve for a patient with a resting heart rate of 80 beats/minute and an estimated maximum heart rate of 170 beats/minute?
    a. 5 beats/minute
    b. 90 beats/minute
    c. 110 beats/minute
    d. 250 beats/minute

451. What is the recommended intensity and duration of an exercise in a circuit weight-training program?
    a. 5 to 10 lb for 15 repetitions
    b. 2 to 5 lb for 15 repetitions
    c. 40% to 60% of 1 repetition maximum for 12 to 15 repetitions
    d. 60% to 75% of 1 repetition maximum for 12 to 15 repetitions

452. What is the single most important factor for continuing an exercise program after a period of deconditioning?
    a. Heart rate response
    b. Patient motivation
    c. Decreasing VO_{2max}
    d. The amount of medication the patient is currently taking

453. The PTA is beginning to tailor an exercise program for a patient who has suffered from deconditioning. This particular patient has a body mass index of 33. How should the PTA proceed with this exercise program with this information only?
    a. Begin with strenuous aerobic exercise
    b. Begin with strenuous muscle strengthening exercises
    c. Begin with low-level endurance activities
    d. This patient should not participate in any strengthening program at this time.

454. Which of the following exercises will help an individual with dysphagia in swallowing?
    a. Head rotations right
    b. Head rotations left
    c. Head-lifting exercise
    d. Cervical flexion exercise

455. Weakness of what muscle can lead to a hiatal hernia?
    a. Rectus abdominis
    b. Scalene
    c. Intercostals
    d. Diaphragm

456. A client complains to the PTA of nocturnal gastroesophageal reflux. Which of the following is the best sleep position for this individual?
    a. Prone
    b. Supine
    c. Left side lying
    d. Right side lying

457. Which of the following positions is recommended after any type of gastrectomy?
    a. Head of bed raised 6 to 12 inches with knees slightly flexed
    b. Right side lying with a pillow between the knees
    c. Left side lying with a pillow between the knees
    d. Foot of bed raised 6 to 12 inches with the head on a pillow

458. Which of the following muscles are first affected with weakness associated with end-stage renal disease?
    a. Triceps
    b. Quadriceps
    c. Gastrocnemius
    d. Gluteus medius

459. Which of the following is a true statement regarding chronic kidney disease and exercise?
    a. It is best to exercise on nondialysis days.
    b. The most important independent quality-of-life predictor is the usual level of exercise activity.
    c. People on dialysis have a higher maximum MET level than the corresponding age-matched population.
    d. Individuals with chronic renal disease will benefit from stationary bicycle exercise at 80% to 90% of target heart rate.

460. A patient is beginning a pelvic floor–strengthening program secondary to urinary incontinence. Which of the following muscles is inappropriate to strengthen during this intervention?
    a. Gluteus medius
    b. Pelvic diaphragm
    c. Urogenital diaphragm
    d. External sphincter muscle

461. Pelvic floor reeducation is an appropriate treatment for which of the following types of prostatitis?
    a. Acute bacterial prostatitis
    b. Chronic bacterial prostatitis
    c. Chronic prostatitis and chronic pelvic pain syndrome
    d. Asymptomatic inflammatory prostatitis

462. Which of the following would be an inappropriate physical therapy intervention for a client with acute prostatitis?
    a. Straight leg raises
    b. Toe raises
    c. Stationary bicycle
    d. Hamstring strengthening

Answers

1. a. During asymptomatic HIV or early-stage HIV, metabolic parameters are within normal limits and no limitations are placed on the individual. However, during later stages of HIV, strenuous exercise is not recommended.

2. a. Symptomatic patients should avoid exhaustive exercise but may be able to continue under close supervision.

3. a. Chronic fatigue symptoms can be exacerbated by aggressive physical therapy. Patients should begin with low-level intermittent physical activity and progress to accumulate 30 minutes of exercise per day.

4. c. The patients with acute fibromyalgia will require short exercise sessions lasting possibly only 5 to 10 minutes. These sessions should be spread out throughout the day, but the therapist and patient should work toward a goal of 30 minutes of daily exercise.

5. a. Hyperthyroidism is associated with exercise intolerance and reduced exercise capacity. Cardiac output is either normal or enhanced during exercise in the hyperthyroid state. Proximal muscle weakness with accompanying myopathy is characteristic in these individuals. If the heart rate is more than 100 beats/minute, blood pressure and pulse rate should be monitored frequently.

6. c. After parathyroidectomy, the patient should use a semi-Fowler's position with support to the head and neck to decrease edema, which can cause pressure on the trachea. Upper extremity exercise is contraindicated early on in rehabilitation secondary to the location of the surgical procedure. Early ambulation is essential because weight bearing and pressure on the bones can speed up calcification. Light-weight lower extremity resistance exercises also can accomplish this same task.

7. b. The common patterns of adhesive capsulitis are limitations of external rotation followed by abduction. The normal presentation with diabetic clients is significant global tightness, with external and internal rotation being equally limited.

8. a. For anyone with diabetes, exercise should not be initiated if the blood glucose is 70 mg/dL or less. Vigorous exercise should not be undertaken within 2 hours of going to sleep at night because this is when exercise-induced hypoglycemia can occur with potentially fatal consequences. Exercise-induced hypoglycemia is a more common problem for patients with type 1 diabetes.

9. c. Black or tarry stools could be a sign of gastrointestinal bleeding that will result in protein accumulation in the gastrointestinal tract. The supervising physical therapist/referring physician should be notified of this condition.

10. c. Choices a, b, and d are all preferred positions to decrease abdominal pain. The patient also might consider using moist heat across the stomach to decrease muscular tension.

11. c. Physical therapy intervention should focus on improving functional limitations, not curing disease.

12. b. ROM limitations in any plane will cause abnormal pressures on the foot and lead to possible ulcer formation. ROM should be consistently measured on the foot of diabetic patients to possibly prevent ulcer formation.

13. a. Insulin works to decrease blood glucose levels by transporting glucose out of the bloodstream and into cells.

14. d. Exercising at the peak time of insulin effect causes hypoglycemia. Insulin causes the liver to decrease sugar production. The body needs increased levels of blood glucose during exercise.

15. a. Blood glucose levels should be between 100 and 250 mg/dl. The other instructions are all appropriate for the diabetic patient.

16. a. Understanding the psychological and physiologic benefits of exercise will help reinforce the patient's goal for treatment and assist the patient in adhering to the exercise program. The patient should also be taught the signs of fatigue and medical emergencies.

17. b. A drop below the resting heart rate or an increase of more than 20 to 30 beats/minute above the resting heart rate is an indication to stop the exercise session. Also a systolic blood pressure drop of more than 10 mm Hg below the resting rate should stop any exercise session. The patient should be monitored for a few moments, and if symptoms do not improve, then the therapist should contact other medical personnel.

18. c. During these phases, the activity level is slowly increased to the prescribed level, and then decreased from the prescribed level. This allows the cardiopulmonary and muscular symptoms the appropriate amount of time to respond to the prescribed level of intensity. Studies have shown a decrease in adverse cardiac events when a warm-up and cool-down period is used.

19. c. The American College of Sports Medicine recommends beginning an exercise program for unfit individuals at 55% to 65% of the estimated maximum heart rate or at 40% to 50% of the heart rate reserve.

20. d. When initiating an intervention program for a severely deconditioned patient, brief bouts of exercise every day have been shown to be the most tolerable. Frequency can be decreased and intensity increased as function progresses.

21. b. This position is optimum to allow gravity to assist in drainage of the anterior segments of the right or left upper lobe of the lung.

22. d. Diaphragmatic breathing exercises enhance diaphragm function throughout the inspiration and expiration cycle. This allows the patient to return to a more normal pattern of breathing and reduce shortness of breath.

23. d. Pursed-lip breathing appears to reduce respiratory rate and increase tidal volume. This technique is easy for patients to learn and should be taught to anyone complaining of shortness of breath.

24. a. Patients with dyspnea will benefit from consistent exercise. These patients will need to begin with low-intensity exercise and progress to a more intense program. Although an early aerobic exercise program might require the patient to use an assistive device, it is not necessary in an advanced program.

25. c. Strong contractions of these muscle groups will lead to a forceful cough. Inspiratory muscles will not affect coughing, and the abdominal muscles are more active in a cough than the lumbar extensors.

26. a. The bluish tinge could extend to the nail beds as well. Although these patients will sometimes have an increased respiratory rate, this is not the first sign of distress. Respiratory rate could increase with an increased intensity of exercise. Flaring of the nostrils could also occur with an increase in exercise.

27. b. During increased inspiratory workload, these muscles assist the diaphragm for inspiration. Patients with chronic lung disease often overuse these accessory muscles.

28. a. The forced expiratory technique employs a forced expiration or huff after a medium-sized breath. The relaxation between huffs helps relax the airway as secretions continue to be mobilized during deep breathing.

29. c. Because this patient has increased cranial pressure, the patient cannot tolerate the foot of the bed being raised. Although this is not the optimum position for right middle lobe drainage, it is the only position the patient can tolerate.

30. c. During the expiration phase of respiration, the air being exhaled from the lungs is more likely to carry secretions and debris from the lungs when the vibration technique is used. A successful treatment will result in coughing and evacuation of the secretions.

31. d. The forward-leaning posture results in a significant increase in maximum inspiratory pressures, thereby relieving the sensation of dyspnea.

32. c. Symptomatic hypotension could possibly mean pallor or excessive fatigue. Any acute onset of breath sounds in the lungs should be a prompt to end the session. Patients with shortness of breath at rest should not begin an exercise program. Many patients in this population will have controlled atrial fibrillation.

33. d. Because of abnormal heart rate response after transplantation, the Borg scale should be used for exercise prescription in this patient population.

34. b. Because heart failure is a disease that can lead to many complications, the goal of any rehabilitation program would be to improve quality of life. Overall activity tolerance would be seen with an increase in endurance, but not the other choices listed.

35. a. Because isometric exercises often increase blood pressure and heart rate quickly, they are not tolerated by patients with heart failure. All of the other exercises are appropriate within given guidelines.

36. c. At stage III, patients begin to complain of severe pain and will want to stop exercising. A patient who rates angina pain at either stage III or stage IV exercise should be stopped.

37. d. Shoveling snow has a MET range of approximately 6 to 7. The other choices have MET ranges of less than 5. Most activities of daily living have a MET range of less than 5.

38. a. Intense exercise for a patient with ischemic heart disease should be avoided. Older age should also be a precaution to ensure exercise safety.

39. a. Patients with a functional capacity of less than 3 METs generally tolerate multiple exercise bouts of 5 to 10 minutes. Patients at a 3 to 5 METs tolerate about 15 minutes, and those with greater than 5 METs can tolerate 20 to 30 minutes.

40. a. The prone position and the upright body position replicate normal cardiovascular and pulmonary function during most functional activities. Not all patients receiving mechanical ventilation will be able to tolerate a prone or upright position. Patients should be gradually moved into these positions throughout their stay in the hospital.

41. d. Choices a, b, and c are all reasons to stop exercise training in the patient with respiratory failure. An angina scale rating of 3/4 or 4/4 should stop or postpone intervention.

42. a. The other choices are considered accessory muscles of inspiration. The abdominals are also considered accessory muscles of expiration.

43. d. Manual lymphatic drainage uses light massage techniques to move lymphedema from the extremities. Pneumatic compression pumping uses pressures above the criteria for manual lymphatic drainage.

44. b. This patient could possibly have cardiac system involvement. Because the removal of fluid from the extremities would add fluid to the circulatory system, patients can have cardiac or renal overload. This patient possibly has either of these emergency situations, and the supervising therapist and/or physician should be notified immediately.

45. b. Manual lymphatic drainage should not be performed in pregnant women or in patients with acute kidney infection or renal failure, congestive heart failure, or deep vein thrombosis.

46. b. Because the chances of infection are increased in an extremity with a history of lymphedema, care should be taken to avoid skin disruptions on the affected extremity, including needle sticks. Cold packs can be used on an extremity with a history of lymphedema, but heat should be avoided.

47. c. All forms of compression are contraindicated in patients with congestive heart failure because of the risk for cardiovascular system overload. Compression is also contraindicated in patients with a possible deep vein thrombosis or when arterial revascularization has been performed on the involved lower extremity. Static compression therapy is contraindicated in patients with an ankle-brachial index of less than 0.5.

48. d. Aerobic exercise four times per week to produce significant weight loss is recommended because it provides the greatest caloric expenditure per minute of training.

49. a. Hemoglobin concentration is a measure of anemia. Exercise intervention should not be performed with a hemoglobin concentration lower than 8 g/dL.

50. c. Choices a, b, and d are all factors that will influence the recovery during the actual surgical procedure. Other postoperative factors are pain, shallow breathing, decreased coughing, and weakness.

51. a. Inpatient rehabilitation after a cardiac event is referred to as phase I or the acute phase. Outpatient rehabilitation is generally broken into phase II or III, and ongoing rehabilitation is phase IV.

52. d. During phase II, close physician management is always available. Depending on the severity of the problem, the patient will attend supervised training sessions three or four times a week for 10 to 12 weeks.

53. d. The seven-step inpatient rehabilitation program begins with stage I of active and passive range of motion in the bed, and progresses to stage VII, in which clients can ambulate up a flight of steps. Stage V is marked by ambulating 300 feet twice daily, whereas stages VI and VII generally show an ambulation of 500 feet.

54. d. There are various positions for postural drainage of secretions in the lung. Both lower lobes are drained with a prone technique.

55. a. Cardiac output and stroke volume both increase during exertion. Increased cardiac cycle time is just another way of saying the heart is beating slower, which is the opposite of what occurs with exertion.

56. c. Answer c provides correct instructions. The patient is often instructed to begin this technique in the supine position and progress to the sitting position. This technique should be practiced for about 5 minutes several times per day.

57. b. The sedentary patient's cardiovascular response increases faster than the trained patient's if the workloads are equal.

58. b. In complete supine position, patients with this diagnosis will have excess fluid move from the lower body to the chest cavity. This causes a decrease in heart and lung function and efficiency.

59. d. This patient has moderate lung disease. Because the intensity of exercise is low, frequency should be increased to five to seven times per week.

60. c. Patients with congestive heart failure often develop an enlarged heart because of the burden of an increased preload and afterload.

61. c. All exercises for this population should avoid the possibility of joint bleeding. High-velocity isokinetics or high-weight, low-repetition exercises are a contraindication. Provided there is no active bleeding, exercise to any joint is indicated.

62. d. In cryoglobulinemia, ischemia can be caused by abnormal blood proteins gelling at low temperatures. Moist heat will not affect this condition.

63. a. Angina is recurring chest pain and is an indication of coronary artery disease. An onset of angina during treatment should be considered an emergency, because of the possibility of a heart attack, and will need to be addressed by the physician.

64. d. MET refers to the amount of energy consumed at rest that is approximately equivalent to 3.5 ml of oxygen per kilogram of body weight per minute. Various tasks or activities require a certain amount of energy to perform. After performing homemaking activities, such as washing dishes and ironing, the next progression in homemaking tasks from the choices listed would be preparing a meal (MET level 3–4). Driving and dressing qualify as a MET level of 2 to 3; gardening has an MET level of 4 to 5.

65. a. Pursed-lip breathing technique is helpful when shortness of breath occurs. Technique: the person inhales deeply through nose, purses the lips as though whistling, and very slowly exhales through the lips.

66. a. There are many benefits of exercise. Decreased HDL in choice a makes this an inappropriate list of the benefits of exercise. HDL is considered "good" cholesterol. Exercise decreases LDL and increases HDL in the bloodstream.

67. b. Choice b has the patient exercising at 65% to 90% of his age-adjusted maximal heart rate. Choice c is the patient's age-adjusted maximal heart rate. Choice a is much too high a parameter. Exercise in the 65% to 90% of maximal VO_2 is much more appropriate. Patients should exercise at level 12 to 15 on the Borg scale.

68. a. Choice a is the correct postural drainage. Choice b is drained by resting on the right, ¼ turn to the back, and foot of the bed elevated 12 to 16 inches. Choices c and d are drained with patient in long sitting position or leaning forward over the pillow in sitting position.

69. d. Performing isometric exercises places too much load on the left ventricle of the heart for many cardiac patients.

70. b. A rating of 9 corresponds with "very light." A rating of 7 is "very, very light." A rating of 13 is "somewhat hard." A rating of 15 is "hard." A rating of 17 is "very hard." A rating of 19 is "very, very hard."

71. d. Riding a stationary bike at 5.5 mph is approximately 3.5 METs. Descending a flight of stars is approximately 4 to 5 METs. Ironing is approximately 3.5 METs. Ambulating 5 to 6 mph is approximately 8.6 METs.

72. c. Patients with chronic obstructive airway disease are often given this set of instructions, which is known as the method of pursed-lip breathing. This method helps a patient regain control of his or her breathing rate and increase tidal volume and amount of oxygen absorbed.

73. a. The incentive spirometer provides visual feedback of maximal inspiratory efforts. The PTA is qualified to answer the patient's question. Incentive spirometry should only be used in acute episodes of chronic obstructive pulmonary disease. There is a risk for air trapping with long-term use.

74. d. Choice a increases the strength of the scalenes and sternocleidomas-toid. Choice b strengthens the latissimus dorsi. Choice c increases the strength of the upper trapezius. All of these are accessory inspiratory muscles. Choice d strengthens the abdominals, which are muscles of forceful expiration.

75. b. Training effects usually include increases in myocardial mass, stroke volume, ventilation, and respiratory muscular endurance.

76. d. As pregnancy advances, oxygen and carbon dioxide have more challenge transferring from the air to cells. Although there is increased cardiac output, there is also increased demand. Pregnant women compensate for this by breathing more deeply and with increased frequency.

77. a. Ultrasound was found to be an effective treatment approach for calcified tendons in the shoulder based on double-blind placebo studies.

78. a. Because this area has the largest girth of the choices, it will have the most edema. It also has the most volume loss as edema decreases. Edema control measures should be introduced immediately after the amputation.

79. a. Knee extensor strength should be maximized in this patient population because strong knee extension is essential for transferring from a seated to a standing position. It is also critical in using a prosthesis.

80. b. The frequency and direction of exercise are determined by the clinical status of the particular patient, but choice b is the best recommendation for initiation of weight training for patients with cancer.

81. b. There has been a false belief that children should not exercise intensely or participate in strength training. In fact it has been shown that children beginning at 8 years of age can safely exercise and strength train with sufficient supervision

82. d. High-resistance training exercise has been of significant benefit for sarcopenia. Strength training has been shown to improve insulin-stimulated glucose uptake in both healthy older adults and in individuals with diabetes. Aging muscle may be resistant to insulin-like growth factor (IGF)-I. Exercise may be able to help aging muscle that is resistant to IGF-I by reversing this effect. Increased strength leads to improved function and a decreased risk for falls, injuries, and fractures.

83. d. Joint proprioception, described as sensations generated to increase awareness of joint orientation at rest and in motion, declines with age, especially in the knee and ankle.

84. b. It has been shown that a limited amount of weight lifting improves strength in a child's muscle, but there is little gain in muscle mass. Strength increases result from improved coordination in neuromuscular recruitment.

85. d. Strength training has many benefits for the geriatric population. Choices a, b, and c are just a few of those benefits. However, strength training will not increase maximal oxygen uptake beyond normal. Endurance training will improve oxygen uptake.

86. c. Aerobic endurance training for fewer than 2 days per week at less than 50% maximal oxygen uptake and for less than 10 minutes is generally not a sufficient stimulus for developing and maintaining cardiovascular fitness in healthy adults.

87. c. Early in the course of intervention, the joint should be rested. This could be accomplished by splinting, traction, or casting. The splint should be removed periodically to perform simple range motion.

88. b. Given the potential complications of surgery and immobilization and the potential for tissue loss, a comprehensive rehabilitation program is necessary to maximize function. Active range-of-motion exercise is initiated early as soon as the infection begins to subside and treatment appears to be successful, which is often within 48 hours.

89. d. Choice a describes an expandable metal rod with prosthetic knee that is implanted into the bone, whereas choice b describes a tibia turn up. In a rotationplasty, the nerves, muscles, and blood supply are preserved. The posterior-facing ankle now functions as a weight-bearing knee joint in a specially fitted prosthesis.

90. b. For individuals diagnosed with osteoporosis or previous history of vertebral fractures, activities such as golfing, bowling, biking, rowing, sit-ups, or other exercise with a major component of spinal flexion, side bending, or spinal rotation should be avoided.

91. d. Immobilization is no longer advocated with this condition, although rest from the aggravating activity is necessary. Treatment should include exercises to address the mechanical inefficiencies of the extensor mechanism, stretching for any tight areas, and strengthening areas of weakness such as ankle dorsiflexion and pain-free quadriceps strengthening. When conservative care fails to resolve painful symptoms, full extension immobilization of the leg through a cast or splint may be prescribed for 6 to 8 weeks. This is only in chronic unresolved cases.

92. a. Stiffness of relatively short duration can occur after periods of inactivity, including sitting or sleeping. Morning stiffness usually only lasts 5 to 10 minutes after awakening. In rheumatoid arthritis, morning stiffness can last several hours.

93. b. Patients with long-standing osteoporosis almost always exhibit a forward posture when sitting and standing, making the anterior musculature chronically tight. The only anterior muscle listed is choice b.

94. c. Weight-bearing exercises are important to reduce bone demineralization. Swimming is not a weight-bearing exercise. Caution should be used in prescribing high-intensity exercise in a client with advanced osteoporosis.

95. c. Each of the choices is an impairment associated with osteoporosis, but choice c is the most important because of an associated risk for falls. Falls can fracture already brittle bones, leading to hospitalizations and more potential problems for the client.

96. c. An acute spinal compression fracture is very painful for this population. The other choices involve ways to mitigate pain, and resistive exercise should be avoided because it increases pain at this stage.

97. a. Spinal flexion should only be performed in conjunction with spinal extension, but the program of extension and resistive exercises only had the best outcome of reducing new spinal fractures.

98. d. Narrowing the base of support (or pulling the feet together in the anatomic position) only makes the person unstable. All the other choices make the person more stable.

99. c. To compensate for the extra weight of the backpack, the body leans forward to put the center of gravity more anterior. The other choices put the center of gravity more posterior.

100. d. Modifiable causes of poor posture include conditions that can be changed with therapy. This list would include tight or weak muscles or poor posture habits. Nonmodifiable causes would be bony or genetic changes that cannot be corrected.

101. a. All of the choices should be part of a comprehensive postural program, but biofeedback to correct poor posture habits should be considered first. Muscles can be at the appropriate strength and length, but if the patient falls back into poor posture habits, then any gains made with soft tissue will quickly revert to incorrect positions.

102. b. Low-load, long-duration stretching is best for chronically tight muscles. Serial casting may be correct in severe cases. Spring-loaded devices may provide this type of stretch.

103. d. Muscle power is defined as the rate of work, or amount of work per unit time. Strength is the ability of a muscle to exert a maximal force or torque at a specified or determined velocity.

104. c. The SAID principle is the systematic approach to progression of the load applied during exercise to optimize improvements in muscle performance and resultant functional ability.

105. d. Muscle type and number of fibers cannot be changed with any form of exercise.

106. a. The most cross-bridge sites are available between the actin and myosin filaments at normal resting length.

107. c. The question refers to a one-time muscle contraction; the other choices require time as an element in their definition.

108. c. Aerobic activities involve low load and long duration, whereas anaerobic activities are short, quick bursts of power.

109. d. Because a baseball pitch is an open-chain activity, the exercises to help the patient achieve that goal should be open chain as well. Choices a and b are closed chain. Although a biceps curl is open chain, it does not come close to the joint speed involved with a pitch or isokinetic strengthening.

110. c. Aggressive passive range of motion would only inflame the arthritis. Interventions should only decrease symptoms and increase strength.

111. b. Appropriate exercise increases strength and does not increase the number of joints affected by arthritis.

112. b. A good rule of thumb for rest is 8 to 10 hours of sleep per night and 30 to 60 minutes of rest per day.

113. b. Heat modalities should always be used before range-of-motion exercises. Heat does cause tissue extensibility. Using heat modalities after exercise would only increase inflammation.

114. c. Choice c is the only choice that involves joint rest. An aquatics program, changing patient's exercise program, and adding exercises would only increase the inflammation and warmth that is already present.

115. a. This patient's diagnosis of frozen shoulder will not improve without aggressive ROM exercises. Although strengthening, cryotherapy, and education will assist this patient, there should be a heavy emphasis on ROM exercises. Joint mobilization and ultrasound are also important, but ROM is easily the most important facet of this patient's program.

116. a. Compression forces along with movements that allow the natural process of self-lubrication of cartilage to occur are beneficial to a healthy joint. Range of motion without the compression of weight bearing does not provide enough nutrition to maintain cartilage integrity over time.

117. c. In grade 1 tendinopathy, minimal pain occurs only with activity. Grade 2 is characterized by minimal pain but does not interfere with the activity; grade 3 presents with pain that disappears between exercise sessions. Grade 4 tendinopathy is described in the question. In grade 5 tendinopathy, there is loss of function and maximum complaints of pain.

118. c. Tensor fascia lata tendonitis is usually caused by inadequate flexibility of the iliotibial band, gluteus medius weakness, and inappropriate

footwear or training surface. Strengthening the hip adductor muscles would only increase this patient's difficulties.

119. c. A characteristic Trendelenburg gait involves the patient's opposite hip dropping inferiorly upon weight bearing of the involved lower extremity. This is due to weakness of the hip abductor musculature on the involved lower extremity.

120. c. During an acute inflammatory stage of osteoarthritis, high-impact repetitive motions should be avoided. Any exercise that requires repetitive weight-bearing stress, such as running or treadmill walking, should be avoided. Low-impact exercises and gentle range-of-motion exercises should be emphasized.

121. a. Forward-flexion exercises tend to relieve pain associated with lumbar spinal stenosis. The spinal cord stretches with flexion, decreasing its cross-sectional area. This allows for less compression of the spinal cord in the thickened spinal canal.

122. a. Because most pregnancy lumbar pain is due to damage at the sacroiliac joint, the sacroiliac belt has the best chance of decreasing her symptoms. The posture of a pregnant female cannot be easily changed because of the anterior displacement associated with pregnancy. Lumbar exercises have not been shown to be effective in decreasing low back pain during pregnancy.

123. c. Patients with extension dysfunction have a loss of extension range of motion, poor posture with loss of movement, and some loss of function. End-range extension exercises should focus on stretching the patient into a more normal posture.

124. d. This patient is classified under the McKenzie classification syndrome as having a derangement 1 syndrome, which is usually first treated with repeated extension exercises to centralize the patient's pain. The patient should be given a home exercise program of extension exercises to move the pain away from the involved lower extremity.

125. d. The patient exhibits significant indicators of possible serious medical pathology. He should be immediately referred to a physician for more accurate testing and possible emergency medical intervention.

126. c. The straight leg raise test is used to evaluate for involvement of lumbar nerve roots. The patient is placed supine, and the involved lower extremity is kept straight as the hip is passively flexed. A positive test elicits a reproduction of the patient's symptoms.

127. c. The multifidus and transversus abdominis muscles work together to stabilize the spine before any upper extremity or lower extremity movement. Patients with chronic low back pain often exhibit weakness of either or both of these muscles. Therapists can teach patient techniques to master abdominal bracing with co-contraction of these specific muscles

128. c. Choices a and b involve some weight bearing to the ankle joint and are contraindicated according to the question. Choice d does not involve weight bearing, but also would not increase ankle range of motion.

129. a. Ballistic stretching involves quick repetitive bouncing movements that should only be used with athletic individuals. Care should be taken not to cause pain or soreness with this type of stretching, even in athletic individuals.

130. b. Elbow extension is difficult to regain after a total elbow arthroplasty because of the scarring and adhesions of the triceps musculature. Scarring of the triceps is due to the approach used in the surgery. Loss of extension is also consistent with the capsular pattern of damage to the elbow.

131. b. The subscapularis muscle is an internal rotator of the shoulder joint. Because this muscle is cut and repaired during surgery, active internal rotation of the shoulder is limited. External rotation is limited because of the stretching that would occur to the repaired subscapularis muscle.

132. d. Choice d is the only choice that does not push the femur posteriorly. Following the concave/convex rule, choices a, b, and c all stress the posterior capsule after a total hip replacement.

133. a. A typical Trendelenburg gait involves the contralateral side dropping during weight bearing of the involved side. This is due to a lack of strength of the involved hip abductors. The hip abductors of the involved lower extremity cannot hold the weight of the body during single-limb support during gait. Strengthening of the involved hip abductors (in this case the right) would alleviate this gait deviation.

134. c. Sixty-five degrees of knee flexion is required for normal gait, and 105 degrees is required for rising comfortably from a chair.

135. b. Because the normal gait pattern only requires 65 degrees of knee flexion, 95 degrees is more than adequate for normal gait. Patients are able to walk with 4/5 strength in the quadriceps and hip abductors. Full extension is required to maintain a stable knee during single-limb support. Furthermore, without full knee extension, the screw home mechanism would not stabilize the knee.

136. c. A functioning rotator cuff is the most important factor for a good outcome of a total shoulder replacement. The outcome is poor when the infraspinatus or subscapularis is involved.

137. d. It is generally accepted that a patient should be able to return to driving 4 to 6 weeks after a right total hip replacement. However, this is not up to the PTA to decide. The physician is the only one who should make this decision. Other factors to consider when returning to driving should be the use of narcotic pain medication, site of the surgery, and postsurgical precautions.

138. d. High-impact activities such as gymnastics, jogging, singles tennis, and soccer should be avoided after a total hip replacement. Low-impact activities such as swimming, walking, and stationary biking are allowed.

139. a. The greatest risk for dislocation of the prosthesis is in the first week after surgery. This is when the patient is least familiar with range-of-motion restrictions and when the surrounding hip tissues are the weakest. Most surgeons require that precautions be maintained for 12 weeks after surgery.

140. b. Because the patella moves inferiorly during knee flexion range of motion, the patella must have full inferior glide to maximize knee flexion range of motion.

141. c. Patella mobilization is important to limit adhesions in the suprapatellar pouch. Patella mobilizations would not affect the intracondylar notch. The lateral retinaculum and quadriceps tendon would be affected by patellar mobilizations, but this is not in the most common area for the adhesions to develop.

142. d. Deep squats should be avoided after total knee arthroplasty because the increased knee joint loading can damage the replaced surfaces, including the posterior portions of the patella.

143. d. Choices a, b, and c are too aggressive at this stage of rehabilitation. Passive and sometimes active ranges of motion are used for the first several weeks after total shoulder arthroplasty. Range of motion to the uninvolved joints such as the wrist and elbow should also be initiated at this stage.

144. a. In the supine position, gravity assists the rotator cuff in limiting humeral head migration superiorly. A weak rotator cuff and humeral head migration is thought to be the main cause of failure in total shoulder arthroplasty.

145. b. Appropriate mechanical stress of the involved ligament can lead to stimulation of collagen synthesis. This collagen synthesis causes the collagen fibers to orient in the direction of the force of the transmission from the muscle to the ligament attachment at the bone. This increases the structure of the ligament by increasing the amount of collagen in the ligament during healing.

146. b. Ice and compression are part of the PRICE (*protection, rest, ice, compression,* and *elevation*) regimen. All other choices could increase inflammation by being too aggressive with the joint. Any thermal modality is contraindicated at this stage of recovery.

147. d. High-intensity strength testing is often contraindicated in the initial postoperative period after surgery of the soft tissues. The other choices are all important aspects of an initial examination.

148. a. During the first several weeks after soft tissue repair surgery, the joint needs to be protected as much as possible. This is accomplished with assistive devices or possibly a splint or cast. As the rehabilitation and healing progress, exercises and weight bearing can be more aggressive.

149. d. This patient shows signs and symptoms of being in the final stages of rehabilitation. This phase is known as active strengthening/return to activity phase. The patient is ready for return to work and sport activities.

150. a. Patients with posterior horn tears appear to have less a favorable long-term outcome than those with any other type of meniscus tear.

151. d. Because the lateral retinaculum has been released, the patella should not be stretched medially. This would further stretch the retinaculum and possibly lead to poor tissue healing.

152. c. In choices a, b, and d, there are usually range-of-motion restrictions early in rehabilitation. Forced range of motion in these situations would cause abnormal tissue healing and damage the surgery. Knee extension after anterior cruciate ligament reconstruction should be a focus of physical therapy treatment.

153. a. The combination of wrist extension and subsequent passive finger flexion is referred to as a tenodesis grip. Some tightness in the long finger flexors should be preserved to allow this grip.

154. b. This position is considered a position of rest for the shoulders. Although passive range of motion should be performed on this patient several times per day, the shoulders should be placed in this position at rest.

155. c. If hamstring length is too short, it will pull the pelvis into a posterior tilt, which would lead to falling backward in a long sitting position. Hamstring lengths greater than 100 degrees would allow excessive anterior tilt.

156. a. Application of cold in hypertonic muscles will generally increase tone. Choices b, c, and d are all treatment options to decrease tone in vegetative patients.

157. c. The triceps will be responsible for the increases in elbow extension required to hold the body up to maintain the non–weight-bearing status. The latissimus dorsi muscle is responsible for the shoulder depression required to elevate the body.

158. c. Hip flexion contractures would manifest with anterior pelvic tilt rather than posterior pelvic tilt. The other choices would typically involve posterior pelvic tilt for compensation.

159. d. Weakness in the iliopsoas will cause inadequate hip flexion at initial contact through loading response.

160. a. Increased action of the knee extensor such as the quadriceps would cause extension throughout the gait cycle, including initial contact. All the other choices could possibly lead to excessive knee flexion at initial contact or anywhere in the gait cycle.

161. c. Weakness of the ankle dorsiflexors would allow rapid plantar flexion of the ankle at initial contact, leading to a foot slap. The other choices are possible causes of the forefoot making first contact at initial contact rather the heel.

162. c. This is a common gait deviation seen after a stroke. Inadequate hip flexion or knee flexion can also cause foot or toe drag during the swing phase of gait.

163. a. Patients often exhibit hip hiking or circumduction to compensate for a leg length discrepancy. A gluteus maximus lurch is characterized as a posterior trunk lean during the stance phase of gait to compensate for gluteus maximus weakness. Antalgic gait is a decrease in weight bearing on a limb because of pain during the gait cycle. A Trendelenburg gait is caused by weakness of the hip abductors.

164. c. A varus deformity at the knee would typically have a decreased base of support during double stance. All of the other changes would widen the base of support during double stance.

165. b. Scissoring gait is characterized by hip adduction and is often seen after central nervous system dysfunction. Ataxic gait is an uncoordinated pattern of gait and is seen as a symptom of brain dysfunction. A quadriceps avoidance pattern is a decrease in the typical amount of flexion seen during stance phase of gait to prevent excessive anterior tibial translation. This is usually in response to an anterior cruciate ligament injury.

166. a. Massage involves the systematic use of various manual strokes to produce certain physiologic, mechanical, and psychological effects. Myofascial release involves manual stretching of the layers of the fascia, which are the connective tissues that surround the muscle and other soft tissue in the body. Myofascial release techniques are reported to soften and reduce restrictions in muscles and fascia that are limiting normal movement.

167. c. Passive range of motion may be provided manually by the PTA or mechanically by the machine. When performing active assistive range of motion, the patient may be assisted either manually or mechanically if the prime muscle mover is weak. Pendulum exercises in which the patient is not receiving any support or resistance are an example of active free exercises. In active resisted exercises, an external force resists the movement.

168. c. Muscular strength is the maximal amount of tension that an individual can produce in one repetition. Muscle endurance is the ability to produce and sustain power over a prolonged period. Muscle power is the amount of work produced by the muscle in a given time.

169. b. If the goal of a program is to increase strength, the program will concentrate on low repetitions with heavy resistance. If the goal is to increase endurance, the program will concentrate on using low resistance for high repetitions. When the goal is to increase power, the exercise program will consist of a high-intensity muscle activity such as jumping.

170. c. Pushing against the wall is an example of isometric exercise, whereas flexing the elbow with a dumbbell in the hand in the standing position is an example of isotonic concentric exercise. The down phase of a push-up is an example of isotonic eccentric exercise for the triceps muscle.

171. d. In a closed kinetic chain exercise, movement at one joint affects movement in the other joints. Because the lower extremity typically functions with the foot on the ground, closed kinetic chain exercises are particularly important in rehabilitation of the lower extremity. Therefore, exercise involving the movements of the joint while the foot is on the ground facilitates movement that mimics function.

172. c. The superior pole is in most contact at about 90 degrees of knee flexion.

173. b. Because eccentric exercise makes the muscle work the hardest, this type of exercise will exacerbate DOMS. DOMS symptoms will alleviate in 2 to 3 days with stretching and ice application.

174. a. The popliteus, biceps femoris, and iliotibial band offer active restraint for the lateral side of the knee joint. The gastrocnemius assists in active restraint of the posterior side of the knee joint.

175. b. The anterior cruciate ligament is located within the articular cavity but outside the synovial lining. The anterior and posterior cruciate ligaments have their own synovial lining.

176. b. Plantar flexors have to contract in quiet standing. Other muscles are recruited with movement of the center of gravity.

177. b. Reduction indicates that the condyle is able to slide under the disk (reduce), causing a click.

178. c. The right side-lying position would create pressure on the right greater trochanter and right lateral malleolus. There is not pressure on the occiput or ischial tuberosity in the side-lying position.

179. c. Shortened hip flexors and lengthened anterior abdominals will contribute to an anterior tilt. Choices a and d would create a posterior pelvic tilt, and choice b would likely present with a more neutral position of the pelvis.

180. c. Patella cartilage. Every structure in the knee has pain nerve fibers except the articular cartilage.

181. b. Synovial fluid has been shown to inhibit healing of ligament tissues. This is demonstrated by the poor healing of intraarticular structures of all synovial joints.

182. d. Jumping (plyometrics) can generate up to 7 times body weight at the patella. Running is next most stressful at 3.5 times body weight.

183. a. Rotator cuff tear is rare before 40 years of age. It can occur from either side and is very common. Cadaver studies confirm that cuff tear is not usually symptomatic.

184. d. Traction from operative positioning, retractor placement, or lengthening of the leg leads to most cases of sciatic traction neurapraxia and foot drop.

185. a. Sever's apophysitis is a physeal stress injury. Tight Achilles tendons are uniformly seen, and frequently there is tendinitis.

186. b. Pes planus is common and usually painless. Hyperlaxity is a powerful risk factor for development of pes planus. In most cases, no treatment is necessary.

187. b. Flexion, biceps femoris. A hip flexion contracture increases flexor torque across the anterior hip. This increases muscle demand on the hip extensors. The biceps femoris is an extensor of the hip.

188. d. The axillary nerve is in close proximity to the surgical field in this patient. Range of motion is normal, so choice B is incorrect; poor compliance would lead to a multitude of problems rather than just deltoid weakness. The musculocutaneous nerve is not involved with this procedure, and it innervates muscles involved in elbow flexion.

189. d. The other choices will be important later in the rehabilitation of this diagnosis. Range of motion is important early to reduce abnormal scar tissue formation.

190. b. Children require more caloric intake (and hydration) than adults in athletics. Children have a greater surface area per body weight and a decreased ability to sweat compared with adults. This makes exercise in the heat a greater concern for the adolescent athlete. An adult weight-training program should be much more aggressive than a child's program. Children can cause many musculoskeletal dysfunctions with aggressive weight training.

191. c. Increased external rotation range of motion. Excessive femoral anteversion is related to increased internal rotation and decreased external rotation range of motion. It also results in a reduced hip abductor moment arm.

192. c. Trunk side-bending to the left. The superior gluteal nerve innervates the gluteus medius muscle. A lesion would result in a Trendelenburg stance, leading to left side-bending of the spine (to maintain an upright posture).

193. a. Right lumbar rotators. The single-leg stance would result in activation of all of the left-sided hip abductors and the right quadratus lumborum.

194. c. Coxa vara. Coxa valga would be a larger than normal angle of inclination at the hip. Anteversion is the angle made by the femoral neck and the femoral condyles (as measured from the coronal plane). Excessive medial rotation is anteversion, and excessive lateral rotation is retroversion.

195. d. Gluteus minimus, posterior fibers. Hip abductors and hip extensors do not limit hip extension. All the other choices may.

196. c. Normal. Genu valgum is an abnormal inward "bowing" of the knees (knock-kneed). Genu varus is an outward anatomic presence of the knee (bow-legged).

197. c. Medial tibia; sartorius, gracilis, semitendinosus. An interesting pneumonic to remember the pes anserine insertion is "Say Grace before SupperTime" (*S*artorius, *G*racilis, *SemiT*endinosus).

198. a. Increases, less stable. As the patella rides superiorly out of the trochlear groove, the joint becomes less stable because less of the patella is in contact with the trochlear groove.

199. b. Lateral, superior, and anterior. This is the normal anatomic presentation of the glenoid.

200. a. The scapula upwardly rotates 60 degrees, and the humerus abducts 120 degrees. The scapula upwardly rotates 1 degree for every 2 degrees of humeral abduction. Abnormalities of this relationship could signal deficiencies in the rotator cuff musculature.

201. b. Hill-Sachs lesion. Although many of these injuries are seen with shoulder dislocation, a Hill-Sachs lesion is by far the most common. A Hill-Sachs lesion to the humerus is caused when the smooth surface of the humerus hits the outer rim of the glenoid fossa.

202. d. Increased trochlear groove depth increases patellar instability. An internally rotated femur causes the patella to track laterally. A lateral patella is unstable. Weakness of the hip external rotators will lead to a more internally rotated femur. A superior patella (as in patella alta) will move the patella out of the trochlear groove. However, increased trochlear groove depth makes the patella MORE stable.

203. b. Travell and Simons report that myofascial pain syndrome of the quadratus lumborum muscle is the most common myofascial pain syndrome of the lower back.

204. b. The superior angle of the scapula commonly rests at the same level as vertebra T2. The spine of the scapula is approximately at T3. The inferior angle of the scapula and xiphoid process represent T7.

205. d. Choices a, b, and c would increase the functional length of the right lower extremity and possibly cause a circumduction during gait. Choice d would not change the functional leg length.

206. a. The briefcase should be carried in the right hand. Carrying the briefcase in the left hand would increase the amount of force that the right gluteus medius would have to exert to maintain a stable pelvis during gait.

207. d. Patellofemoral joint reaction forces increase as the angle of knee flexion and quadriceps muscle activity increase. Choice d involves the greatest knee flexion angle and quadriceps activity.

208. c. Leaning the trunk over the involved hip decreases joint reaction force and strain on the hip abductors. These factors together decrease pain in the involved hip.

209. b. Choice b is the correct answer. Choice a is a posterior pelvic tilt.

210. a. The lowest point in the gait cycle occurs when both lower extremities are in contact with the ground (double support).

211. a. Abdominal muscles attach to the lower border of the ribs and the superior surface of the pelvis. Strong abdominals prevent excessive anterior rotation of the pelvis during gait.

212. b. The fifth lumbar nerve root is impinged because it arises from the spinal column superior to the L4-5 lumbar disk.

213. b. This gait deviation is caused by the patient leaning back to decrease the flexion moment created at the hip at initial contact. The gluteus maximus is most responsible for counteracting this flexion moment.

214. c. The pelvis is dropping on the right side because the left gluteus medius is weak. The patient also may lean toward the left hip joint to move the center of gravity, making it easier to hold up the right side of the pelvis.

215. a. When the hindfoot is pronated, the forefoot (transverse tarsal joints) can compensate for uneven terrain. If the hindfoot is supinated, the forefoot also is likely to supinate and possibly cause damage to the lateral ankle ligaments.

216. a. A patient with severe knee flexion contractures has a line of gravity that is anterior to the hip, posterior to the knee, and anterior to the ankle. This causes a flexion moment at the hip, knee, and ankle.

217. b. To maintain balance, the lumbar spine must laterally flex toward the supporting lower extremity during single-limb support.

218. a. The tibialis anterior, extensor digitorum longus, and extensor hallucis longus contract concentrically to achieve a neutral ankle position before initial contact.

219. a. The hamstrings bring the knee to about 60 degrees of flexion during acceleration. The hip flexors, ankle dorsiflexors, and toe extensors are also active.

220. c. The geriatric population would have a longer period of double support in an attempt to maintain balance. They also would have a shorter step and stride length.

221. c. Cyriax's classic description describes the obvious cause of a springy end feel as being that of the torn part of a meniscus in the knee engaging between the bone ends blocking extension.

222. b. The power grasp often is used to control tools or other objects. The hook grasp is used when strength of grasp must be maintained to carry objects. Lateral pinch is used to exert power on or with a small object. Opposition of the thumb tip and the tip of the index finger, forming a circle, describes the tip pinch, which is used to get small objects.

223. d. The lateral triangle (composed of the radial head, olecranon process, and lateral epicondyle) is the most likely of the choices to exhibit joint edema. Joint edema is common after a surgical procedure.

224. b. All four muscles are hamstring muscles of the posterior thigh. All four muscles extend the hip. Only the hamstring portion of adductor magnus does not cross the knee. It inserts on the adductor tubercle of the femur. The other three muscles cross the knee posteriorly and therefore flex the knee.

225. c. Dupuytren's contracture is a progressive thickening of the palmar aponeurosis of the hand. The progression is gradual, and the interphalangeal joints are pulled into flexion.

226. d. The hip strategy is used to compensate for large movements in the center of mass, and the ankle strategy is used to compensate for small movements.

227. d. All of the listed muscles participate in mandibular elevation with the exception of the lateral pterygoid muscle. The lateral pterygoid muscle and the suprahyoid muscles participate in mandibular depression.

228. a. The anterior cruciate ligament prevents excessive posterior roll of the femoral condyles during flexion of the femur at the knee joint.

229. b. The extensor carpi radialis brevis absorbs most of the stress placed on the involved upper extremity in the position of wrist flexion, ulnar deviation, forearm pronation, and elbow extension (as with a backhand swing in tennis).

230. c. Swan-neck deformity involves hyperextension of the proximal interphalangeal (PIP) joint and flexion of the distal interphalangeal (DIP) joint. Splinting to avoid this deformity is the treatment of choice. Boutonnière deformity involves flexion of the PIP joint and DIP joint hyperextension. Dupuytren's contracture is contracture of the palmar aponeurosis. Claw hand is the result of laceration of the ulnar nerve.

231. b. The extensor carpi ulnaris is frequently subluxed after rupture of the triangular fibrocartilage complex. Subluxation leads to many mechanical changes in the wrist common in patients with rheumatoid arthritis.

232. d. A patient with hammertoes exhibits hyperextension of the distal interphalangeal joints and metatarsophalangeal joints and flexion of the proximal interphalangeal joints.

233. c. Race has no role in progression of scoliosis, idiopathic or congenital.

234. d. In clubfoot, the calcaneus is small, the hindfoot is in varus, and there is equinus of the ankle. There is typically no tibial involvement.

235. b. Although these diagnoses can occur in most joints, the hip is the most common.

236. d. Hip pain is common with this diagnosis, as is a traumatic history, although a slipped capital femoral epiphysis can have a chronic onset as well. Because a standard anterior or posterior view can miss the slip, the frog-leg radiograph will need to be viewed to determine the correct diagnosis.

237. d. Training errors are common if the correct techniques are not taught vigorously. Musculotendinous imbalances can occur if training emphasizes a certain muscle group over its antagonist. Malalignment of the lower extremities is seen with muscular imbalances over a period of time. Grass or turf has not been shown to increase risk for overuse injury.

238. d. Clicking that occurs during opening and closing. Reciprocal clicking is caused by the disk being displaced partially anteriorly. The condyle slides under the disk and clicks into its normal position during opening, then slips back out during closing.

239. b. The only possible correct answer is b. It is the typical pattern one sees with a Trendelenburg gait, in which because of gluteus medius weakness of the weight-bearing leg, the hip on the contralateral side lowers.

240. c. Tightness of the gastrocnemius–soleus muscle complex can cause a loss of dorsiflexion at the ankle. Having adequate ankle dorsiflexion throughout the stance phases of gait is important to the kinematics of tibial movement. When there is inadequate ankle dorsiflexion, which can result from gastrocnemius–soleus complex tightness, one common finding is knee hyperextension, or genu recurvatum.

241. d. Transferring from a sitting position to standing will pose the greatest challenge because of the need to generate force in the extensor muscles. Going from sitting to standing requires the recruitment of the hip and knee extensors.

242. c. Choice b describes a swan-neck deformity.

243. d. With a separation of this size, gentle abdominal strengthening should be utilized while binding the abdominal region.

244. a. Immobilizing the extremities would not allow for normal growth and development. Care must be taken for proper positioning and management of possible fractures, but immobilizing the extremities would not allow for motor milestones to be reached. Proper positioning will also promote muscle strengthening and bone mineralization.

245. d. Children with osteogenesis imperfecta should be allowed to mature at the same rate as other children. Social skill development may be compromised if the child is not allowed to participate in some activities. Keeping the extremities immobilized will not allow for a more normal growth and development.

246. d. Choice a may result in undue stress to the pubic symphysis or sacroiliac spine and can be dangerous because of changes in center of gravity. Hip extension in quadruped position may cause abnormal hyperextension of the lumbar spine, and bilateral straight leg raises could cause diastasis recti because of the additional stress to the abdominal muscle group.

247. a. Center of mass is at its highest point. The center of mass is at its highest during single-limb support.

248. c. Fractured sites should remain stable to promote healing and realignment of the bones. However, the PTA should encourage the movement of adjacent joints to assist in maintaining muscle strength and lengthening of tendons and muscles.

249. d. When grading shoulder flexion, the next step after achieving full shoulder flexion in side lying is to begin to work or perform activities against gravity to begin increasing strength. Shoulder flexion against gravity is achieved with the individual in the sitting or standing position.

250. a. A person with a hip fracture should avoid any activity, such as shoe tying, which could potentially cause hip flexion to 90 degrees or greater. Such a position could actually undo the benefits of the surgical procedure.

251. c. When ascending or descending stairs, the cane should move with the painful or weak leg. Specifically, when ascending the stairs, the leg without the cane should move first, allowing the weak leg and cane to bear the weight for only a short amount of time until the strong leg is able to provide the needed stability.

252. b. Discomfort and damage can occur if the scapula is not gliding with the humerus during movement. Passive range of motion can cause damage if the structures are not moving properly. An orthopedic specialist may be beneficial if therapy interventions have not been successful.

253. b. The term *soft end feel* is a spongy quality at end range of a joint contracture. It usually indicates that the joint has the potential to remodel. A low-load, long-duration stretch may yield the best results.

254. d. With the seat close to the pedals, the lumbopelvic region is flexed, separating the posterior facets and disk space at L5-S1. Adding a lumbar pillow supports the lumbar curve at the same time.

255. c. The pitcher is moving into D2 extension with the throwing motion. He is strengthening the muscles involved in shoulder internal rotation, adduction, and forearm pronation.

256. a. Isometric exercises in the shortest range of the extensor muscle are used to begin strengthening. In contrast, weak flexor muscles should be strengthened in the middle-to-lengthened range because they most often work near their end range.

257. d. This position places the least amount of stress on the lumbar spine in the sitting position.

258. c. Rhythmic stabilization involves a series of isometric contractions of the agonist, then the antagonist.

259. d. The patient with anterior cruciate ligament tear has a significant rotatory instability. Bracing may prevent some of this instability. Sports that are especially difficult on the knees (e.g., skiing, competitive tennis) are contraindicated.

260. b. Passive extension is the most important motion to gain after an anterior cruciate ligament reconstruction, regardless of the graft type. Active extension can be achieved after passive extension is full (or equal bilaterally).

261. a. Because of poor balance, geriatric patients should increase the treadmill grade rather than the speed. Use of machines allows better posture and low intensities and limits the exercise within the patient's safe range of motion.

262. d. Movements that stress the posterolateral hip joint capsule should be avoided. Sources vary on the exact amount of flexion that should be avoided. Passive hip abduction should be maintained after surgery with a wedge.

263. b. The patient has an extension lag, which may be due to any source that has inhibited the quadriceps and results in an inability to fully extend the knee actively.

264. d. The treatment techniques should be performed in the order of mobility, stability, controlled mobility, and skill.

265. a. Tennis elbow results from overuse of the wrist extensors. The shoulder external rotators should be used to power a backhand.

266. a. Lateral step-ups are probably too difficult for a patient who received an anterior ligament reconstruction with a patella tendon autograft 2 weeks ago.

267. c. The wrists should be in neutral position when the fingers are on the middle row of the keyboard.

268. d. Grade III injuries are complete ruptures of the ligament involved. Grade I injuries are considered minor, whereas grade II injuries will have associated edema, pain, and some loss of joint stability.

269. c. Tools with small handles require more grip strength. Tasks below shoulder height reduce the risk for impingement, and more force can be applied to tasks if they are kept below elbow height.

270. c. Upper trapezius strengthening will only exacerbate this dysfunction, and the elbow exercise is irrelevant to this type of biomechanical problem. The supraspinatus responds best to gravity resistance exercise early and a slow progression of resistance not to exceed 3 to 5 lb.

271. b. The arthrokinematics of the shoulder joint would lead one to believe that the posterior capsule is the most in need of mobilization.

272. b. The shoulder is still early in rehabilitation 6 days after surgery. Protection by the sling (along with ice for pain control) is a good suggestion. It is too early for aggressive exercise, and heat should never be used at this stage of recovery.

273. c. Anterior digastric trigger point refers to the incisors of the mandible.

274. a. Other symptoms may include pain and tenderness located at the joint, clicking, and crepitation. Although tinnitus, headache, and dizziness may be associated with a temporomandibular joint disorder, they are not caused by the disorder.

275. c. 38 mm is a reasonable opening range for function: eating, placing food in the mouth, brushing teeth, singing, and yawning.

276. a. Add stabilization exercises within the click free range. These patients may need anterior stabilization splinting if painful clicking and catching persists.

277. b. Plantar flexor spasticity. Spastic plantar flexors will produce excessive plantar flexion, and also knee extension throughout the stance phase, and prevent adequate passive knee flexion in preswing. The hamstrings are not responsible for knee flexion in preswing phase of gait. Plantar flexor weakness would cause tibial forward collapse and therefore excess knee flexion. Dorsiflexors are not responsible for knee flexion in preswing.

278. a. Adductor hypertonicity of the swing leg. The swing leg is adducting because of hypertonicity. The quadriceps does not play a key role during swing. The plantar flexors are not active in swing; weakness is not going to create a significant problem in this phase. Plantar flexor weakness affects terminal stance. A person with plantar flexor weakness would demonstrate excessive hip flexion in swing, not adduction. Gluteus medius hypertonicity would cause excess hip abduction, NOT adduction.

279. a. The PTA would use a PNF D1 diagonal to encourage the combined movements of hip flexion, adduction, and knee flexion. The diagonal

also encourages the combined movements of hip adduction and extension. This is the combination of muscle activity most needed for gait.

280. b. Patients with decreased executive functions should be taught time management techniques, and the client should be included in group activities. Patients with slowed information processing should have all environmental distractions removed. External aids and multiple approaches to improve retention of information should be used for patients with memory deficits

281. b. Moderate selective weakness characterizes stage II. The patient will have slight decreased independence in ADLs, such as difficulty climbing stairs, raising arms, and buttoning clothing. ALS is generally graded from stage I to stage VI, with stage VI being bedridden and completely dependent in all ADLs.

282. d. Exercises should be short and simple and be done in the same order each time. Patients with Alzheimer's disease respond to treatment sessions with decreased sensory input and increased repetition of exercises.

283. c. Children with Duchenne's muscular dystrophy are identified when the child has difficulty getting off of the floor, falls frequently, has difficulty climbing stairs, and starts to walk with a waddling gait pattern secondary to proximal muscle weakness. Another symptom of proximal muscle weakness is increased lumbar lordosis. Although a tight iliopsoas can contribute to lordosis, muscle weakness is more common in this population.

284. b. Choice a refers to an ASIA class A injury, and choice c is indicative of a class C injury. Choice d describes a class D injury. In ASIA class E, sensory and motor functions are normal.

285. c. According to ASIA, the level of motor innervation is determined by the most distal key muscle with a grade of 3 or better, with the segment above being a 5.

286. d. When the descending tracts are involved, immediate flaccidity is present, and reflexes are absent at and below the level of injury. This is followed by autonomic symptoms, including sweating and reflex incontinence of bladder and rectum.

287. a. Initially the sacrum, heel, and scapula are the most common sites of ulcer formation because of time spent in bed. As the individual begins to use a chair for mobility, the trochanter and ischium become common sites of pressure ulcers.

288. a. Normally, the asymmetrical tonic neck reflex is integrated by 6 to 8 months. In a child with quadriplegic cerebral palsy, this reflex could continue for several years, limiting function.

289. d. The abnormal pull of the spastic iliopsoas and adductor muscles is the initiating deforming force in hip dislocations.

290. a. Joint restrictions associated with cerebral palsy are a result of a decrease in the number of sarcomeres per muscle fiber. Muscles also demonstrate an increased variation in fiber size and type with both hypertrophy and atrophy present, possibly representing an ongoing dynamic process. Increases in fat and fibrous tissue and a decrease in blood flow have been identified. In this process, bone grows faster than muscle, resulting in a disadvantageous length–tension relationship of the muscle and an increased risk for subsequent contracture.

291. d. A child that sits with a wide base is compensating for poor trunk control. This decreases the ability to turn and rotate in and out of the sitting position.

292. a. Choices b, c, and d are all effects of hypertonia in a child with cerebral palsy.

293. c. Botox is injected directly into the muscle at the motor point and is used to block the neuromuscular junction by acting to reduce the release of acetylcholine. Muscle weakness and decrease in muscle spasm occur in 3 to 7 days and gradually reappear in 4 to 6 months.

294. a. The presence of primitive reflexes beyond age 2 years will lead to a poor ambulation potential. The absence of postural reactions beyond age 2 years also has a poor ambulation potential.

295. b. Programming based on cognitive outcomes has relatively stronger support than programming aimed at solely motor outcomes.

296. d. A significant number of children with a diagnosis of spastic cerebral palsy present with low muscle tone early in the first year of life and later develop spasticity.

297. b. In the case of postoperative casting, the PTA can instruct the family to wash and dry the skin at the edge of the cast frequently, inspecting often for signs of skin breakdown. Repositioning and ventilation under the cast with a cool-air blow-dryer can assist in preventing skin breakdown. A flashlight can be used daily to inspect beneath the cast. It is critical that an intensive therapy intervention program begin after surgery to assist with strengthening and improving functional performance.

298. c. Appropriate wheelchair positioning has been shown to encourage smoother and faster reach, decrease extensor tone, increase vital capacity, and improve functional cognitive testing.

299. d. Nonambulators and beginning standers require a solid ankle-foot orthosis neutral to +3 degrees of dorsiflexion. An ambulator with excessive pronation at the ankles would require a supramalleolar orthosis.

300. d. As a general rule, the thicker the myelin sheath, the faster the conduction velocity of a nerve. Proprioception has the fastest conduction velocity, and pain has the slowest.

301. c. Axonotmesis occurs when the axon has been damaged but connective tissue coverings that support and protect the nerve remain intact. Prolonged compression that produces an area of infarction and necrosis causes an axonotmesis.

302. b. Flattening of the hypothenar eminence along with abduction of the little finger coincides with weakness of the palmaris brevis and abductor digiti minimi. Paralysis of the flexor carpi ulnaris produces a radial deviation of the hand when wrist flexion is attempted. Impaired sensation may be expected along the fifth digit and the ulnar aspect of the ring finger.

303. a. Postural and breathing exercises and gentle stretching are the cornerstones of the initial conservative program. This is followed by strengthening exercises for the shoulder girdle musculature, especially the trapezius, levator scapulae, and rhomboids. PTAs are cautioned against forceful stretching to mobilize the first rib.

304. b. Partially denervated muscle does not have the physiologic capacity to respond to a conventional strengthening program. Instead, programs aimed at nonexhaustive exercise and general body conditioning are preferable. The client should never exercise to the point of fatigue. Caution the client to stop if pain or weakness persists.

305. a. Although individuals exhibit symptoms of areflexia, weakness is not common, and when it occurs, generally it is related to an inability to sustain the contractions secondary to impair proprioceptive feedback.

306. c. Initially the skin is hot and dry with increased hair and nail growth. As complex regional pain syndrome moves into the dystrophic phase, the skin becomes thin, glossy, cool, and sweaty. In the atrophic phase the skin is thin, shiny, cyanotic, and dry.

307. b. Damage to the peripheral nerves in the distal upper extremity will have little effect on postural control. Controlled posture comes from the trunk and lower extremity musculature.

308. b. The patient will require a period of adaptation secondary to loss of vestibular system. The somatosensory systems and the visual systems will allow the patient to return to normal activities. However, adaptation in the elderly population will be significantly delayed.

309. b. The Romberg test is similar to the test for drunken driving. The patient stands with the feet together and maintains balance with the eyes open, then closes the eyes. A loss of balance is a positive test. A positive test means there is impairment to the vestibular system. This patient is obviously using the visual system to compensate. She should always use the visual system; thus, keeping a light on at night is beneficial.

310. a. Choice a is the only answer that provides treatment while the patient is in the standing position. Choice b has little effect on balance, and choice c is in the sitting position.

311. d. The Brandt-Daroff exercises involve the patient in a sitting position and moving to the supine position. The head is also turned to 45 degrees as the patient lies down. This stimulates the vestibular system to return to normal function.

312. b. The motor system is responsible for selecting and adjusting muscle contractile patterns to maintain body control. The other choices are products of the sensory system.

313. a. The ankle strategy primarily controls body sway during stance. It begins with contractions of the dorsiflexor or plantar flexor muscles and could continue to the more superior hip and trunk musculature if necessary.

314. d. As we age, we are more likely to use the hip strategy than the ankle strategy during gait and quiet standing. Without a functioning ankle strategy, the amount and duration of sway during standing can also affect progression throughout the stance phase of gait. Special care should be taken to optimize ankle strategy in the older adult.

315. d. Brainstem lesions will most likely cause vertigo and incoordination, and basal ganglion lesions will cause slower involuntary movements. There are specific portions of the brain for visual field deficits and impaired spatial perception. The cerebellar lesions control movement, and lesions in this area are more likely to cause ataxia.

316. c. Single-leg stance to tandem stance to normal stance is the correct progression from small base of support to large base of support.

317. b. Choices a and d will most likely use the ankle strategy, and choice c will use the stepping strategy. Choice b is appropriate for initiating the hip strategy.

318. c. Even though all the other choices are good as goals for working with a fall prevention program, preventing injury from falls is the number one goal of any fall prevention and balance intervention program.

319. c. Each stage of motor development builds on the previous stage. Choice c lists these stages in the correct order.

320. b. Mobility is characterized by development of antigravity movement, and controlled mobility is defined as proximal movement on a fixed distal extremity. Skill combines mobility in a non–weight-bearing position.

321. d. Ninety percent of infants can sit without upper extremity support at about 8 months of age; 50% of infants can perform this activity at about 6 months of age.

322. d. Most infants can roll prone to supine with or without trunk rotation at about 9 months of age. About 50% of infants can perform this at 6 months of age.

323. c. Activity-focused intervention is repetition of functional actions. This could be transfers, activities of daily living, or as in this case, climbing stairs.

324. d. Impairment-focused interventions include neurodevelopmental treatment, strength training, electrical stimulation, biofeedback, and aerobic conditioning. Activity-focused interventions use adaptive equipment and sometimes therapeutic equipment.

325. c. All of the answer choices are examples of proprioceptive neuromuscular facilitation techniques. Alternating isometrics would be appropriate to gain stability in a joint. Slow reversal and agonistic reversals are appropriate for a patient attempting to gain controlled mobility and skill.

326. d. Because most functional tasks require a variety of movements, choice d is most appropriate. Feedback is given every other trial so that patients can reflect on their past performance and possibly solve their own problem with the task.

327. a. This upper extremity synergy is often paired with wrist and finger flexion. This is a common upper extremity synergy after traumatic brain injury or stroke.

328. a. Neurodevelopmental treatment involves reducing abnormal muscle tone and facilitating a normal movement pattern for the patient.

329. d. Choices a, b, and c are all core principles of PNF. PNF is designed to increase contraction or relaxation of various muscle groups. Tone does not need to be normalized before initiating PNF.

330. d. Intrinsic feedback includes any type of feedback that is naturally available to the individual such as somatosensory, proprioceptive, or visual input. The other three choices involve verbal or tactile cues, usually from the physical therapist.

331. b. A posterior pelvic tilt can be performed with similar hand placement, but the cues would be posterior rather than anterior. To use proprioceptive neuromuscular facilitation in this scenario, resistance would be applied through the anterior-superior iliac spine to promote anterior pelvic tilt in sitting.

332. b. Knee extension force has been correlated with increased sit-to-stand ability for a variety of diagnoses, including nonprogressive neurologic disorders.

333. a. A combination of these motions would facilitate rolling from side lying to prone. The PTA would most likely use rhythmic initiation, slow reversals, or agonistic reversals in this situation.

334. b. Patients with Parkinson's disease exhibit rigidity, impaired balance, and poor postural control.

335. a. Because the pathology of Parkinson's disease is a degeneration of neurons that produce dopamine in the brain, physical therapy will not alter the disease process.

336. c. Studies have shown that excessive heat can actually increase the symptoms of multiple sclerosis. Excessive fatigue will also increase symptoms. It is appropriate with this patient to reduce exercise intensity and possibly introduce energy conservation techniques.

337. b. Choices a, c, and d usually manifest as spasticity in muscles without the additional passive stretch. There is rigidity or tremor in the muscles associated with Parkinson's disease.

338. a. There is a possibility of overwork damage or overuse fatigue with aerobic conditioning for patients with amyotrophic lateral sclerosis. The therapist should keep track of symptoms of overuse during conditioning.

339. b. Balance training should begin with all of these diagnoses, but Parkinson's disease is the most important. Parkinson's disease will often cause a forward trunk lean and rigidity during gait. These symptoms are usually seen early in the disease process, so balance training should begin immediately.

340. b. Frenkel's exercises are a series of exercises emphasizing normal daily activities. They increase in difficulty and are performed in lying, sitting, standing, and walking. Although the patient can begin at any point during the exercises, it is general practice to begin with lying and progress through walking.

341. d. With a thorough knowledge of the typical return of sensation, the therapist can guide the intervention appropriately. When there is complete nerve transection, a therapist may want to move straight toward protective sensation rather than beginning with discriminative touch.

342. b. Nerve gliding techniques are usually performed by the physical therapist. Constant reexamination of the patient is necessary to make sure no damage is being done to the nerve involved. Application of electrical stimulation to the denervated muscle may cause damage to the nerve, and choice d might be necessary, depending on the particular nerve involved. Choice b is the most applicable during this scenario.

343. d. Because of the distal weakness associated with Charcot-Marie-Tooth disease, patients will often present with foot drop and a steppage gait. This could be corrected with an ankle-foot orthosis.

344. c. Frequent tripping is often the result of dorsiflexor weakness. These patients also complain of difficulty walking on uneven surfaces. All the other choices are indicative of proximal muscle weakness.

345. c. Because of the distal weakness associated with Charcot-Marie-Tooth, pes cavus and hammertoes are common.

346. b. Because delayed-onset muscle soreness has lasted more than 24 hours, this patient's exercise intensity should be lowered. Eccentric exercise will increase muscle damage and soreness. Eccentric exercise and increasing the patient's intensity should be avoided.

347. a. Glossopharyngeal breathing uses the upper inspiratory accessory muscles to expand the oral cavity and draw air into the mouth. This creates negative pressure to facilitate inspiration. Air is then pushed into the lungs by pulling the chin and tongue back toward the neck, creating a positive pressure in the mouth. Although this is not an energy method of respiration, it can be used as an emergency procedure if mechanical ventilation fails.

348. d. Patients with neuropathic ulcers sometimes require aerobic exercises or strengthening exercises. This is best performed with a non–weight-bearing intervention such as a bicycle. The other choices would possibly cause the ulcer to become worse.

349. c. Off-loading is the redistribution of foot pressures to eliminate areas of high peak pressure during weight bearing. This would decrease stress at the wound site.

350. c. Carpal tunnel syndrome is often associated with menopause, hysterectomy, pregnancy, obesity, physical inactivity, and decreased physical fitness. Increased pressure in the carpal tunnel results in ischemia of the median nerve, which impairs nerve conduction and causes pain and paresthesia.

351. b. If the motor component of the visual-ocular system is damaged, visual and vestibular controlled eye movements are abnormal. If the sensory component is damaged, visually controlled eye movements are usually normal, but vestibular dependent eye movements are abnormal.

352. d. The posterior canal is placed in the vertical position if the body is supine and the head is extended beyond neutral and rotated 45 degrees to the same side.

353. b. Once medical and orthopedic clearance is obtained, vigorous functional training can begin. This could occur in the acute stage of the patient's recovery, or later when the patient is admitted to other physical therapy units.

354. d. Developed by Dr. Kabat, a neurologist associated with the physical therapists Margaret Knott and Dorothy Voss, proprioceptive neuromuscular facilitation emphasizes specific patterns of movement in the retraining process. From his observations of normal human movement, he emphasized that most human activities require multidimensional movements; that is, various muscles at various joints complement and enhance one another's activities.

355. b. Locomotor training with the body supported is the technique that focuses on facilitating automatic walking patterns using intensive tasks specific training. The patient dons a harness that goes around the trunk with straps attached to an overhead suspension system. Training can be performed on a treadmill, with the therapist facilitating automatic walking pattern.

356. c. Observations of generations of children tells us that walking is initiated at about 10 to 13 months, yet some infants take their first steps as early as 8 months or as late as 18 months.

357. c. Pediatric therapists play a crucial role in determining the absence of movement components that may impede the accomplishment of developmental milestones or functional goals for a child.

358. c. Studies have shown that electrical stimulation had no effect on prevention of idiopathic curve progression; therefore, its use in a clinical practice is not supported.

359. c. In the dynamical systems theory, the internal components of the patient and the external context of the task are equally important and contribute to functional movement. This theory emphasizes the process of moving rather than the product of the movement.

360. b. Through the use of a motivating environment with the child's active participation, therapists use manual facilitation and inhibition techniques to present the child with a normal sensory experience and thereby encourage facilitation of a more functional motor response.

361. a. Infants accomplish this task between about 5 and 10 months of age. The response in choice a would prevent the parent from excessive unnecessary worry. Sources vary widely about the exact month when developmental milestones are reached, but choice a is the correct answer in this scenario.

362. c. Increasing motor ability is not independent of motor learning. A therapist must facilitate motor learning with proper sensory cues and by promoting appropriate motor activity. Answer d is true because infants begin spontaneous movement, which later develops into more deliberate movement. Answer a is true because reflex movement can be used to develop more deliberate movement.

363. a. Isometric control develops before isotonic control.

364. a. This result is typical in normal development because as the child begins to acclimate to the upright position, the neck will gain control to allow the child appropriate interaction with the environment.

365. a. Ballistic movements are high-velocity movements requiring antagonist muscle groups to contract. Coactivation would not produce movement, and visual guidance is not needed for random, ballistic movements. Proprioception is not an issue.

366. d. Because the head is large (compared with the body) at this stage of development, weight must be shifted to the thighs and lower abdomen to raise the head in prone.

367. c. In normal development, gaining postural control will allow for more rapid change of positions. This change will allow more normal movement patterns. An infant may not be able to understand feedback, and a single way of performing the skill is not advisable.

368. b. Four-year-olds typically can manage buttons, and 3-year-olds still show dysmetria with block stacking. Infants just beginning the skill of walking are unafraid of falling.

369. a. It is known that flickering lights or repetitive noises can trigger epileptic episodes. Although anticonvulsants are quite effective, it is recommended to avoid such aversive stimuli in these patients.

370. a. A shuffling gait and difficulty with initiating gait are typical signs of Parkinson's disease. This population would also present with a small base of support.

371. b. The obturator nerve innervates the adductor brevis, adductor longus, adductor magnus, obturator externus, and gracilis muscles. Choice a has no motor function. Choice c innervates the sartorius, pectineus, iliacus, and quadriceps femoris. The ilioinguinal nerve innervates the obliquus internus abdominis and transversus abdominis.

372. c. No activity = 0. Slight contraction = 1+. Normal response = 2+. Exaggerated response = 3+. Severely exaggerated = 4+.

373. d. Choices a, b, and c all receive innervation from that branch of the brachial plexus. The triceps brachii is innervated by C7-C8.

374. d. Left torticollis and resultant plagiocephaly would cause flattening of the left frontal and right occipital regions with bulging of the opposite areas.

375. a. The danger in using a hot tub for a person with multiple sclerosis is that it may cause extreme fatigue. There is no need to avoid the other activities listed.

376. c. Choice c is the most appropriate. Some of the other choices may be mastered, but c is the most necessary. Choice b is achieved at about 3 months of age, and choice d at about 9 months of age.

377. c. The deltoid is innervated by the axillary nerve arising from vertebral level C5-6. Shoulder flexion would be the most limited in this case.

378. c. The most consistent area of L5 sensation loss is between the first and second toes. The ankle jerk tests the S1 level. The nerve that comes out of L5-S1 interspace is S1. Sensation loss on the bottom of the foot could result from S1 or S2 involvement. Weakness in the calf incriminates S1.

379. c. To reach as described in the question, the patient must shift weight to the right buttock and elongate the right side of the trunk. With the same circumstances given in the question, but to the left side, the patient would shift weight to the left buttock and elongate the left side of the trunk.

380. d. The skill of holding and drinking from a bottle typically emerges at about 6 months of age.

381. a. The asymmetrical tonic neck reflex (ATNR) is present in utero until 6 to 8 months of age while the child is awake and until up to 42 months of age while the child is sleeping. Because of the ATNR reflex, the child's head turns toward the extended arm and leg, and the opposite arm and leg bend. This reflex may help in the birthing process, assist in the development of visual-motor integration, and protect the airway while the child is in the prone position.

382. a. The prone position is the best for facilitating neck and trunk extension whether on a ball, bolster, or wedge.

383. d. The most common and effective position to place a child in is sitting, with attention given to the head and neck control, visual regard, and visual tracking. Although the child can be placed in the supine and side-lying positions, sitting is the most commonly used position.

384. b. Amyotrophic lateral sclerosis is a degenerative disease without a cure that results in death. Stage 3 is characterized by moderate dependence in self-care and independent activities of daily living along with severe weakness of the arms and legs. At this stage of the disease, conserving energy and maintaining quality of life are paramount.

385. a. Hand-propelled tricycle models are available for children who do not have the ability to pedal with their legs. These can provide mobility outdoors, in hallways, and in corridors.

386. c. Patients with Alzheimer's disease often have difficulty with change. The family members can contribute information about what items are valuable and should be retained and can also assist the client in gradually changing in the environment to reduce stress and allow time to adjust.

387. b. D2 flexion patterns support upper trunk extension, which is important for patients with Parkinson's disease who tend to develop excessive kyphosis.

388. a. An electric wheelchair definitely uses less energy but does not require the physical effort needed by this patient to maintain functional mobility. Ambulation with a knee-ankle-foot orthosis is probably possible but requires much more energy than locomotion with a manual wheelchair. Ankle-foot orthoses alone do not provide enough support for the patient to attempt ambulation.

389. d. To assist a patient in developing a tenodesis grip, the therapist should allow the patient's finger flexors to tighten. This grip functions with active extension of the wrist, which allows flexion of the fingers because of shortened flexor tendons.

390. d. Choice d is the correct answer because in the supine position, the abdominal contents are located more superiorly than in the other positions. This places the diaphragm in a more elevated resting position, which allows greater excursion of the diaphragm. Semi-Fowler's position resembles a reclining position, with the knees bent and the upper trunk slightly elevated. Semi-Fowler's position, without an abdominal binder, allows gravity to pull the abdominal contents downward, which does not put the diaphragm in an optimal resting position. Semi-Fowler's position is, however, the position of choice for patients with uncompromised innervation of the diaphragm who have chronic respiratory difficulty. The standing and sitting positions present the same problem, but to a greater extent, as semi-Fowler's position.

391. d. The pressure applied by the PTA should be applied as the patient coughs to assist in a forceful exhalation. Placing the heel of one hand about 1 inch above the umbilicus applies pressure immediately inferior to the diaphragm.

392. a. As perception improves, objects should be moved into the area of the deficit (the right side in this case), but initially they should be placed in plain view of the patient (the left side in this case).

393. a. Prone and side-lying positions would encourage flexion of the extremities with this patient. In this population, prone positioning allows more efficient cardiovascular function. Lying on the right or left side does not make any difference in this situation.

394. c. A prolonged stretch assists in decreasing tone.

395. a. Avoiding the interossei helps to inhibit tone. Direct pressure to any hand musculature may increase tone. Hyperextension of the meta-carpophalangeal joints also may cause an increase in tone.

396. a. Bottle feeding or breastfeeding is rarely performed successfully before 34 weeks of gestational age. Side-lying position allows the infant to move the hands toward the mouth. The prone position encourages flexion. Full contact with the hand is more comforting to the infant.

397. d. Although vibration often elicits a muscle contraction, a therapist should first choose stimuli that are more likely to occur naturally.

398. c. When an exaggerated symmetrical tonic labyrinthine reflex is present, supine positioning increases extensor tone and prone positioning increases flexor tone. Side lying also provides an opportunity for the PTA to stimulate flexion. Right or left side lying makes no difference in this case.

399. b. Tarsal tunnel syndrome is caused by compression of the posterior tibial nerve as it travels through the tarsal tunnel. The tarsal tunnel is formed by the medial malleolus, medial collateral ligament, talus, and calcaneus.

400. b. Flexed postures should be avoided with this patient population. Positions of shoulder adduction, internal rotation, and wrist flexion are contraindicated, as are wrist, finger, thumb flexion, and finger thumb adduction.

401. d. Cervical flexion opens up the cervical intervertebral joint spaces. Any extension or lateral flexion toward the impingement will result in nerve root compression.

402. c. Maintain finger flexion to protect extrinsic finger flexors. Tenodesis is passive insufficiency of the extrinsic finger flexors. After spinal cord injury lesion at C6, people can use preserved wrist extension combined with passive finger flexion to grip objects. Preserving extrinsic finger flexor tightness is essential to maintaining passive insufficiency.

403. c. A brachial plexus injury is a lower motor neuron injury and therefore does not cause spasticity, an upper motor neuron sign.

404. a. Activities that unduly increase body temperature are not recommended for patients with multiple sclerosis. Keep in mind that spasticity is a significant complication of multiple sclerosis and can adversely affect gait parameters. If the patient is presenting with poor balance and decreased strength, hill training and plyometric training may be too aggressive for this particular patient. At this age, improving balance, strength, and coordination is paramount to preventing falls and future injury.

405. c. Treatment of acute cutaneous skin injuries is generally symptomatic. Antiperspirants and talcum powder should be avoided in the radiation field. Active and passive ranges of motion exercises are important for retention of mobility and reduction of contractures, especially in the axillary region.

406. c. The patient is experiencing Raynaud's phenomenon. Closure of the muscular digital arteries, precapillary arterioles, and arteriovenous shunts of the skin causes the hand to become numb and white and then bluish in color as blood flow remains blocked. About 10 to 15 minutes later, blood flow will return, and the fingers (or toes) will become red and warm. This is often the first sign of scleroderma.

407. d. Rubbing or massaging the area can cause further tissue damage and should be avoided. Weight bearing should be avoided until the patient has been evaluated further.

408. b. Because this patient has intact latissimus dorsi and triceps, he is able to perform the push-up technique from a sitting position. This is the preferred method for pressure relief.

409. d. This is correct advice to decrease the chance of pressure ulcers. The skin should be kept clean and dry, and the patient should have adequate nutrition. Proper positioning in the wheelchair is also critical to decrease the chance of developing pressure ulcers.

410. d. Although correct wheelchair positioning will also help temporarily normalize tone and reflexes, it will not increase strength. All other choices are goals of a positioning protocol program.

411. c. The interventions mentioned in the question should be part of any treatment plan to care for or prevent pressure ulcers. These interventions could be provided by any person assisting the patient with the wound.

412. b. Generally 30 to 40 mm Hg of pressure at the ankle is the recommended level of compression to assist with venous insufficiency. Usually the therapist should ask the patient, "What is the strongest compression that you can be compliant with?"

413. c. Because the venous system is compromised and cannot return blood to the heart, compression intervention is necessary. The other choices are sometimes necessary, but compression therapy is the most important of the choices given.

414. b. The question describes a venous ulcer. Arterial ulcers have necrotic wound bed with regular and distinct margins. Edema is only present in arterial insufficiency if a venous component is present as well.

415. c. This patient's wound could be infected. Infections are difficult to determine in arterial ulcers because of the lack of blood flow to the area. The body does not produce a normal inflammatory response to these ulcers.

416. b. Nonadherent dressings are less likely to remove viable tissue when removed from the wound. Adherent dressings could possibly tear the viable tissue away from the wound. All wounds heal better in a moist, clean environment.

417. a. Choices b, c, and d should all be performed by a trained professional. The patient should be instructed in daily inspection of the foot, with emphasis on skin protection.

418. b. Because of the severity of the burn injury in this question, there is muscle catabolism. It is thought that the body uses protein from muscle as fuel secondary to the increased energy it needs to heal the burn.

419. d. This position puts the anterior and inferior portions of the shoulder capsule at a stretch position. If the shoulder was moved into adduction, there could possibly be frozen shoulder after an axillary burn of this type.

420. a. It is imperative for any patient with a possible contracture after a burn injury to receive splinting as soon as possible. This would alleviate the need for painful physical therapy as the patient begins more aggressive rehabilitation.

421. c. During remodeling, scar tissue is deposited in a disorganized fashion without specific alignment. Range of motion in this phase and during the proliferation phase will allow scar to be deposited in a more organized fashion.

422. b. If the patient begins ambulation and has excess lower extremity edema, care must be taken to increase the compression of the lower extremities bandages. Edema should not be excessive in the lower extremities when the patient begins ambulation after a burn injury.

423. a. Superficial burns are usually classified as sunburn and should be treated with a moisturizing skin lotion as soon as possible. Other burns should be treated with an antimicrobial ointment and appropriate dressing. Deep partial-thickness and full-thickness burns should be treated with an antimicrobial agent before possible surgical intervention.

424. d. A skin graft must not be disturbed by movement or pressure until it becomes vascularized and adheres to the tissue bed. This generally takes at least 48 hours. However, the surgeon should be consulted before intervention is initiated.

425. a. This type of end feel is normal for abrupt end range of motion such as knee or elbow extension. Regardless of the diagnosis, bone-to-bone end feels of knee flexion are abnormal.

426. d. The garments should only be removed for bathing of the patient and washing of the garments. They should be worn at all other times to minimize scarring.

427. c. Depending on the circumstances, the maturation phase may also be the phase when work hardening and work conditioning exercises are energetically pursued. The PTA can generally be more aggressive with manipulation of the wound site during this phase.

428. b. Other areas at risk for pressure ulcer development in a seated position are elbows, spinous processes, sacrum, coccyx, greater trochanters, and heels. The occiput and scapulae are associated with pressure ulcer development in the supine position, and the side-lying position promotes pressure ulcer development at the malleoli.

429. a. Arterial wounds and neuropathic ulcers should be cleansed when dressings are changed. Dressings that maintain or increase moisture at the wound site should be used because of the lack of exudate from the wound.

430. c. Venous wounds should be managed by wound care and compression of the affected extremity. Compression of the extremity helps reduce swelling and venous hypertension in the limb.

431. d. Anticontracture positions are positions of extension at each affected joint region, such as elbow extension with supination or a neutral ankle position with no flexion of the toes. Splints may be used as static positioning devices to hold the joint in a certain position.

432. c. Turning schedules should be established and followed for patients in danger of developing pressure ulcers. In a typical turning schedule, the patient is turned every 2 hours with equal time spent supine, prone, lying on the right side, and lying on the left side.

433. d. The relative weakness of the musculature of a child will allow scar tissue to contract the palmar aponeurosis. Careful splinting of this area should be considered.

434. b. The shrinker should be removed only for bathing. Because the surgical scars are healed, the stump can be immersed in water.

435. c. Transverse (perpendicular to the scar) or circular massage assists in mobilization of scar tissue.

436. c. This answer is correct because the most common deformities after a severe burn such as this are related to hip flexion, hip adduction, knee flexion, and ankle plantar flexion.

437. b. Choices a, c, and d are key to early ambulation after a burn. Bandages should not be loosened unless they are painful. Loose bandages might cause edema.

438. d. Burn patients lose heat more rapidly than other individuals. It is advisable to keep room temperatures at a higher than normal level.

439. d. A resting heart rate of more than 130 beats/minute or less than 40 beats/minute would stop any exercise session, as would an oxygen saturation of less than 90%. An acute infection or a temperature greater than 100° F would also stop any exercise session. A rise in systolic blood pressure to more than 250 mm Hg or diastolic blood pressure to more than 115 mm Hg also could stop a session.

440. c. Surgical revascularization to restore perfusion is preferred when possible. The vessel segments to be treated are identified by angiography. The involved artery is then bypassed with a vein harvested from elsewhere in the body or a synthetic graft.

441. a. When pulmonary medications are used through a metered dose inhaler 15 to 20 minutes before exercise, their effects should improve the individual's ability to exercise and more effectively obtain the benefits of training.

442. a. Activities that require short bursts of energy do not frequently bring on an episode of exercise-induced asthma. Sports that involve endurance exercise such as soccer, basketball, distance running, or biking will often trigger an attack.

443. d. If a patient's oxygen saturation decreases during gait, then respirations increase. Choices a, b, and c are all indicators of decreased oxygen saturation during gait.

444. a. During the course of training, resting blood pressure will decrease over time. Physical exertion would always increase blood pressure immediately.

445. a. Oxygen saturation values of 95% to 100% are generally considered normal. Values less than 90% could be a red flag to deterioration of status, and values below 70% are considered life threatening.

446. c. Walking is the easiest form of exercise for this patient population. It requires no equipment, and patients are able to stop when they feel tired. Walking can also be supported with assistive devices early on in rehabilitation.

447. d. Heart rate can be easily monitored by the therapist during an intervention. However, the therapist should be aware of any medications that the patient is taking that would affect heart rate. Certain medications will not allow heart rate to increase during intense exercise.

448. d. Sitting at rest is considered 1 MET. Adding any activity to sitting at rest would increase the MET range for the activity.

449. c. A rating of 10 to 12 on the scale is considered light exertion. This is an appropriate level for patients just beginning a deconditioning program.

450. b. The heart rate reserve is calculated by subtracting the resting heart rate from the maximum heart rate, in this case $170 - 80 = 90$ beats/minute.

451. c. Circuit weight training is proposed to add an aerobic component to traditional weight training. For this reason the intensity of exercise is decreased in order to increase the repetitions of exercise.

452. b. Before initiating a program to increase patients' endurance, they have to be ready to change their behavior. The program needs to be maintained over a long period of time. The therapist should be careful to tailor the exercise program to patients' specific needs and background.

453. c. This patient is considered overweight by the body mass index scale. Strenuous activities would be contraindicated for this patient at this point. They should begin with low-level activities and increase as tolerated.

454. c. This exercise strengthens the muscles that open the upper esophageal sphincter, the "gate" that allows food or drink to slide down the esophagus to the stomach. This exercise works best for people with a weak or ineffective esophageal sphincter.

455. d. As part of the stomach herniates through a weakness in the diaphragm, regurgitation and motor impairment will cause the major clinical manifestations associated with this type of hernia. Anything that weakens the diaphragm or alters the hiatus and increases intraabdominal pressure can predispose a person to hiatal hernia.

456. c. For nocturnal reflux, encourage the individual to sleep on the left side with a pillow in place to maintain this position. Right side lying makes it easier for acid to flow into the esophagus because of the effect of gravity on the esophagus (the lower esophagus bends to the left and this straightens out with left side lying).

457. a. The semi-Fowler position (head of the bed raised 6 to 12 inches with the knees slightly flexed) facilitates breathing and drainage after any type of gastrectomy.

458. d. Gluteus medius, hamstrings, and psoas muscles are affected first and most severely, resulting in gait impairments, difficulty rising from low seats, or difficulty accomplishing functional activities such as getting in and out of a bathtub.

459. b. Individuals with chronic renal disease benefit from stationary bicycle exercise protocols requiring exercise three times per week at intensities of 40% to 70% of target heart rate. Clients with renal disease will often have lower MET levels than their age-matched counterparts. Exercise can be performed on dialysis days or nondialysis days; this decision is usually left to the client.

460. a. Restoring normal pelvic floor strength and bladder control is essential before performing vigorous physical activity. The physical PTA is instrumental in teaching contraction of the appropriate muscles without contraction in the anal area or of the gluteal muscles, with complete relaxation of the pelvic muscles between contractions.

461. c. Because chronic pelvic pain syndrome has periods of exacerbation and remission, pelvic floor strengthening could be indicated for this patient population.

462. c. Bicycle seats can aggravate prostatitis; thus, a recumbent bicycle is recommended because it puts less pressure on the groin.

CHAPTER 4

Nonsystem Topics

Questions

1. A patient presents to physical therapy requiring bracing secondary to scoliosis. What are some of the common precautions given to patients using this type of orthotic?
   a. Wear a thick protective layer under the brace.
   b. Monitor the skin under the brace for redness.
   c. Direct heat improves the integrity of brace materials.
   d. Braces should fit tightly.

2. All prosthetic feet do which of the following?
   a. Compress at heel contact
   b. Permit the wearer to tiptoe
   c. Accommodate shoes of various heel heights
   d. Store energy during late stance

3. The distal end of the heel in a solid ankle cushion heel (SACH) foot does which of the following?
   a. Permits midfoot inversion
   b. Is the site of forefoot hyperextension
   c. Absorbs shock
   d. Releases substantial stored energy

4. A resilient socket liner makes it easier for the client to do which of the following?
   a. Make adjustments to accommodate volume changes
   b. Wear snugly fitting trousers
   c. Eliminate wearing a sock
   d. Perspire less when wearing the prosthesis

5. Compared with a cuff, supracondylar brim suspension provides more of which of the following?
   a. Distal weight bearing
   b. Resistance to knee hyperextension
   c. Adjustability
   d. Mediolateral stability

6. Compared with a transfemoral exoskeletal shank, an endoskeletal shank is more of which of the following?
   a. Easy to adjust
   b. Durable
   c. Unrealistic in appearance
   d. Heavy

7. Which of the following is TRUE about hydraulic swing phase control knee units?
   a. Are unsuitable for polycentric axis systems
   b. Increase resistance when the client walks faster
   c. Decrease stance stability when the client walks faster
   d. Exaggerate knee flexion in early swing phase

8. A transfemoral prosthesis has a knee unit with a manual lock. Which of the following is TRUE about this prosthesis?
   a. Provides stability during early stance
   b. Requires the client to remain sitting with an extended knee
   c. Should be slightly longer than the contralateral intact extremity
   d. Is more difficult to don than a prosthetic without a manual lock

9. Compared with a totally rigid socket, a transfemoral socket, which includes flexible plastic, is more of which of the following?
   a. Durable
   b. Comfortable
   c. Warm
   d. Difficult to adjust

10. What is a common gait deviation after a transmetatarsal amputation?
    a. Decreased midswing
    b. Decreased knee extension at heel contact
    c. Decreased time at late stance
    d. Increased hip flexion throughout the gait cycle

11. Which of the following is more commonly known as Chopart's disarticulation?
    a. Phalangeal amputation
    b. Transmetatarsal amputation
    c. Midtarsal disarticulation
    d. Ray resection

12. What portion of the foot remains after a Syme's amputation?
    a. Metatarsal heads
    b. Cuboid bone
    c. Navicular bone
    d. Calcaneal fat pad

13. A patient has recently undergone a transtibial amputation. The PTA is beginning to teach the patient about proper positioning after the surgery. Which of the following is correct advice for this patient?
    a. Place pillows under the knee at all times.
    b. Maintain knee extension and hip extension by lying prone.
    c. Place pillows under the lumbar spine.
    d. Place pillows under the thigh while in supine.

14. Which of the following areas on the residual lower limb after a transtibial amputation tolerates pressure best from the prosthetic socket?
    a. Patella ligament
    b. Tibial tuberosity
    c. Tibial crest
    d. Fibular head

15. What is a disadvantage of the pelvic band suspension system in a transfemoral prosthesis?
    a. Better control of hip abduction
    b. Better control of hip adduction
    c. Better control of hip rotation
    d. Weight of the suspension system

16. A patient is beginning rehabilitation after receiving a preparatory prosthesis for a transtibial amputation. How long should the prosthesis be worn before the patient removes it to check the skin for breakdown?
    a. 2 hours
    b. 15 minutes
    c. 1 hour
    d. 6 hours

17. The patient is just beginning ambulation after receiving a transtibial prosthesis. The patient shows excessive knee flexion or "buckling" of the knee at early stance. Which of the following are possible causes of this gait deviation?
    a. Low shoe heel
    b. Excessive plantar flexion
    c. Socket too far posterior
    d. Stiff heel cushion

18. What is the lightest terminal device for a prosthesis for the upper extremity after a transhumeral amputation?
    a. Myoelectric hand
    b. Hook
    c. Battery-powered hand
    d. Cable-controlled hand

19. Which of the following would be an advantage of an ankle-foot orthosis used by a patient with polyneuropathy?
    a. Improve muscle tone
    b. Improve sensation
    c. Reduce the risk for falls
    d. Assist with regeneration of the involved nerves

20. Paul is trying to learn to go up a curb in his wheelchair. To perform this skill successfully, it is critical that he do which of the following?
    a. Have good timing and good command of the wheelie skill
    b. Have exceptional upper extremity strength and normal upper extremity motor control
    c. Be able to use his preserved lower extremity function enough to at least assist during the technique with pelvic and lower extremity control
    d. Have a specially modified wheelchair designed to assist with this type of mobility

21. In a clinical setting, which are the most common types of exercise equipment used during assessment of aerobic capacity?
    a. Treadmill and stationary bicycle
    b. Stationary bicycle and rowing ergometer
    c. Treadmill and self-paced walking
    d. Treadmill and manual muscle testing

22. Which of the following is NOT recommended for compression intervention in patients with a venous ulcer?
    a. Short-stretch elastic wraps
    b. Custom-fit stockings
    c. Removable orthotic devices
    d. Long stretch elastic wraps (ACE bandages)

23. Which of the following is incorrect for the assessment of proper shoe fit of a patient with diabetes?
    a. The widest part of the shoe should be at the first metatarsophalangeal joint
    b. There should be approximately ½ inch of space between the end of the longest toe and the end of the shoe with the patient standing
    c. The collar or back portion of the shoe should slide up and down on the heel
    d. There should be no areas of stitching over the forefoot of the shoe

24. Which of the following is NOT true regarding the use of total contact casting for treatment of neuropathic ulcers?
    a. Cast should be replaced every 5 days in ulcers with a Wagner grade 4
    b. Fragile skin is a relative contraindication and should be monitored closely

   c. Cast should usually be used with a Wagner grade 2 plantar ulcer with loss of protective sensation

   d. The ankle and knee should be positioned at 90 degrees

25. The most common assistive device for mobility is which of the following?
   a. Forearm crutch
   b. Underarm crutch
   c. Cane
   d. Pickup walker

26. Which part of the home interferes least with use of assistive devices for mobility?
   a. Floor surface
   b. Doorways
   c. Stairs
   d. Bed height

27. Which of the following is NOT a purpose of assistive devices for ambulation?
   a. Improve balance
   b. Assist propulsion
   c. Reduce load on a lower extremity
   d. Minimize sensory input

28. A long cane is most useful to the person with visual impairment because of which of the following?
   a. Alerts passersby not to impede the patient
   b. Increases load on the lower extremities
   c. Increases the user's comfort
   d. Protects the skin

29. The underarm crutch should terminate proximally at which of the following?
   a. Axilla
   b. Elbow
   c. Lateral chest
   d. Mid-forearm

30. A properly fitted cane places the elbow at approximately what angle?
   a. 30 degrees of flexion
   b. 45 degrees of flexion
   c. 15 degrees of flexion
   d. Full extension

31. Wheelchair use can improve all of the following EXCEPT which?
   a. Respiration
   b. Lower extremity strength

    c. Communication

    d. Swallowing

32. Which muscles are most important for propelling a manual wheelchair?
    a. Triceps
    b. Biceps
    c. Latissimus dorsi
    d. Pectoralis major

33. The most common way to control a powered wheelchair is with which of the following?
    a. Sip-and-puff mechanism
    b. Joystick mechanism
    c. Head control mechanism
    d. Eye control mechanism

34. A wheelchair intended for a patient with lower extremity amputation should have which of the following?
    a. An extended backrest
    b. Large anterior wheels
    c. Rear wheels located farther posteriorly
    d. Solid tires

35. The patient who has edematous legs should have a wheelchair that includes which of the following?
    a. Elevating leg rests
    b. Pneumatic tires
    c. Desk-type armrests
    d. A titanium frame

36. A wheelchair seat that is too narrow is most likely to do which of the following?
    a. Facilitate transfer into and out of the wheelchair
    b. Irritate the skin over the greater trochanters
    c. Interfere with propulsion
    d. Reduce pressure on the ischial tuberosities

37. A wheelchair with a high backrest will do which of the following?
    a. Increase the stability of the wheelchair
    b. Protect the patient from tipping forward
    c. Make the patient vulnerable to kyphosis
    d. Impede shoulder girdle mobility

38. Which of the following would make a manual wheelchair easier to propel with the upper extremities?
    a. Moving the seat closer to the rear wheels
    b. Pneumatic wheels inflated to 50 psi

c. Large-diameter casters

d. Tall armrests

39. Which of the following is the best way to determine whether a wheelchair cushion is performing adequately?

a. Asking for the patient's subjective complaints of ischial tuberosity pain

b. Contacting the wheelchair manufacturer for their specific specifications

c. Placing the PTA's hand between the cushion and seat of the wheelchair for palpable bony prominences

d. Observing the ischial tuberosities after 5 minutes of sitting in the wheelchair

40. If a patient's walker is adjusted too high, which of the following would the PTA likely observe?

a. Limited front wheel rotation of the walker

b. Patient ambulating with the walker too far forward from the trunk

c. Forward bending of the trunk

d. Limited hip extension during the stance phase of gait

41. Which of the following is considered the proper fit for triceps crutches?

a. Upper cuff middle third of the upper arm, lower cuff 6 cm below the olecranon process

b. Upper cuff distal third of the upper arm, lower cuff 1 to 4 cm below the olecranon process

c. Upper cuff proximal third of the upper arm, lower cuff 6 cm below the olecranon process

d. Upper cuff proximal third of the upper arm, lower cuff 1 to 4 cm below the olecranon process

42. Which of the following is a purpose for tennis balls or other glide mechanisms on the rear uprights of rolling walkers?

a. Reduce friction

b. Aid in stair gait

c. Allow the patient to put more weight on the rear uprights of the walker during ambulation

d. Allow for easier turning of the walker

43. A 65-year-old man has recently suffered a motor vehicle collision. The orders from the physician are to begin gait training immediately. The orders also state that the patient is to be non–weight bearing on the left lower extremity and right wrist. Which of the following would be the best assistive device choice for this patient?

a. Forearm crutches

b. Triceps crutches

c. Rolling walker with right platform attachment

d. Four-wheel rolling walker with brakes and seat attachment

44. Assuming the patient is in normal erect stance, where should the tip of a cane be located on the ground in relation to the foot?
    a. 8 inches out from the toes at a 90-degree angle
    b. 2 inches out from the toes at a 45-degree angle
    c. 6 inches out from the toes at a 90-degree angle
    d. 6 inches out from the toes at a 45-degree angle

45. A 19-year-old woman has recently suffered a motor vehicle collision. She has sustained multiple fractures to the bilateral lower extremities, and will remain non–weight bearing for several months. She will continue to attend college while she rehabilitates her injuries. What is the most appropriate assistive device for this patient?
    a. Forearm crutches
    b. Rolling walker
    c. Wheelchair
    d. Axillary crutches

46. Which of the following would the PTA observe if a patient's wheelchair was built so that the seat was too deep within the wheelchair frame?
    a. Increased pressure on the ischial tuberosities
    b. Excessive hip abduction during sitting
    c. Excessive hip external rotation during sitting
    d. Excessive posterior pelvic tilt with kyphotic posture

47. An ankle-foot orthosis (AFO) worn with a shoe that has a heel higher than that for which the orthosis was made will cause the wearer to have which of the following?
    a. Experience laterally directed force at the knee at midstance
    b. Maintain the knee extended during stance phase
    c. Experience medially directed force at the ankle at midstance
    d. Flex the knee excessively in early stance

48. Which of the following cervical orthosis most restricts neck motion?
    a. Four-post
    b. Rigid collar
    c. Three-post
    d. Two-post

49. The orthosis that is secured directly to the skeleton is which of the following?
    a. Minerva
    b. Milwaukee
    c. Taylor
    d. Halo

50. The best candidate for a scoliosis orthosis has which of the following?
    a. Immature spine with a moderate curve
    b. Immature spine with a severe curve
    c. Mature spine with a severe curve
    d. Mature spine with a moderate curve

51. Orthotics are NOT used for which of the following purposes?
    a. To assist motion
    b. To prevent motion
    c. To speed the healing process
    d. To protect a body part

52. Orthoses are often helpful for which of the following dysfunctions?
    a. Poor balance
    b. Decreased sensation
    c. Weakness
    d. Poor endurance

53. What is the difference between a splint and an orthosis?
    a. A splint is a temporary orthosis.
    b. Splints and orthoses are used on different parts of the body.
    c. A splint is made of flexible material, and an orthosis is always made of hard material.
    d. An orthosis should be worn 23 hours per day, and a splint can be removed several times per day.

54. Orthotics are NOT designed to provide which of the following functions?
    a. Support musculoskeletal deviations
    b. Correct musculoskeletal deviations
    c. Improve the function of moveable parts of the body
    d. Improve sensation

55. Which of the following is TRUE regarding the comfort of an orthosis?
    a. The area covered by the orthosis should be minimized to decrease pressure.
    b. An orthosis could be lengthened to provide comfort.
    c. A functional orthosis would be used by the patient even if it is uncomfortable.
    d. The straps that attach the orthosis should be as tight as possible.

56. A PTA has decided to use a knee-ankle-foot orthosis to control genu valgum of the knee. Where must the force be applied to control this deformity?
    a. Superior force medially, knee force medially, ankle force medially
    b. Superior force laterally, knee force laterally, ankle force laterally

    c. Superior force laterally, knee force medially, ankle force laterally

    d. Superior force medially, knee force laterally, ankle force medially

57. A child with an ankle-foot orthosis breaks his orthosis about every 2 to 3 months. What material property is the most likely cause of this orthosis failure?
    a. Compressive stress
    b. Tensile stress
    c. Fatigue resistance
    d. Shear stress

58. Which of the following orthosis materials is most easily adapted to fit a patient's limb?
    a. Thermoplastic
    b. Thermosetting plastic
    c. Metal
    d. Steel

59. What portion of a shoe should be modified if the shoe is to be used with an ankle-foot orthosis that has an insert at its distal attachment?
    a. Toe box
    b. Sole
    c. Heel
    d. Upper

60. Which of the following types of orthosis is molded into the sole of a shoe to transfer force posteriorly from metatarsal heads?
    a. Ankle-foot orthosis
    b. Metatarsal pad
    c. Metatarsal bar
    d. Medial heel wedge

61. Which of the following types of ankle-foot orthosis (AFO) contributes least to frontal and transverse plane control?
    a. Spiral AFO
    b. Solid ankle AFO
    c. Hinged AFO
    d. Posterior leaf spring AFO

62. Which of the following is FALSE regarding wearing an ankle-foot orthosis after a stroke?
    a. There is more dorsiflexion range of motion in the early stance.
    b. It is associated with decreased overall rehabilitation time.
    c. There is longer single stance time on the involved lower extremity.
    d. There is greater quadriceps activity.

63. What is the most common type of knee control used in a knee-ankle-foot orthosis?
    a. Pawl lock
    b. Drop ring lock
    c. Carbon fiber lock
    d. Stance phase knee lock

64. What is the primary effect of a lumbar corset?
    a. Decrease abdominal musculature activity
    b. Decrease erector spinae muscle activity
    c. Compress the abdomen to increase intraabdominal pressure
    d. Reduce pain

65. What type of upper extremity splint is most commonly prescribed for repetitive motion injuries such as carpal tunnel syndrome?
    a. Long opponens splint
    b. Short opponens splint
    c. Cockup splint
    d. Prehension orthosis

66. What is the purpose of most shoulder orthoses?
    a. To decrease rotator cuff involvement
    b. To reduce pain
    c. To prevent shoulder subluxation
    d. To reduce anterior deltoid involvement in shoulder flexion

67. Which of the following is an example of an assistive device?
    a. Bedside commode
    b. Raised toilet seat
    c. Grab bar secured to the wall in the bathroom
    d. Cane

68. The PTA is treating a patient who received an above-elbow amputation 2 years ago. The prosthesis has a split cable that controls the elbow and the terminal device. With this type of prosthesis, the patient must first lock the elbow to allow the cable to activate the terminal device. This is accomplished with what movements?
    a. Extending the humerus and elevating the scapula
    b. Extending the humerus and retracting the scapula
    c. Extending the humerus and protracting the scapula
    d. Extending the humerus and depressing the scapula

69. The PTA is crutch-training a 26-year-old man who underwent right knee arthroscopy 10 hours ago. The patient's weight-bearing status is toe-touch weight bearing on the right lower extremity. If the patient is going up steps, which of the following is the correct sequence of verbal instructions?
    a. Have someone stand below you while going up, bring the left leg up first, then the crutches and the right leg.
    b. Have someone stand above you while going up, bring the left leg up first, then the crutches and the right leg.
    c. Have someone stand below you while going up, bring the right leg up first, then the crutches and the left leg.
    d. Have someone stand above you while going up, bring the right leg up first, then the crutches and the right leg.

70. A patient is receiving crutch training 1 day after a right knee arthroscopic surgery. The patient's weight-bearing status is toe-touch weight bearing on the right lower extremity. The PTA first chooses to instruct the patient how to perform a correct sit to stand transfer. Which of the following is the most correct set of instructions?
    a. (1) Slide forward to the edge of the chair; (2) put both the crutches in front of you and hold both grips together with the right hand; (3) press on the left armrest with the left hand and the grips with the right hand; (4) lean forward; (5) stand up, placing your weight on the left lower extremity; (6) place one crutch slowly under the left arm, then under the right arm.
    b. (1) Slide forward; (2) put one crutch in each hand, holding the grips; (3) place crutches in a vertical position; (4) press down on the grips; (5) stand up, placing more weight on the left lower extremity.
    c. (1) Slide forward to the edge of the chair; (2) put both the crutches in front of you and hold both grips together with the left hand; (3) press on the right arm rest with the right hand and the grips with the left hand; (4) lean forward; (5) stand up, placing your weight on the left lower extremity; (6) place one crutch slowly under the right arm, then under the left arm.
    d. (1) Place crutches in close proximity; (2) slide forward; (3) place hands on the armrests; (4) press down and stand up; (5) place weight on the left lower extremity; (6) reach slowly for the crutches and place under the axilla.

71. Which of the following is NOT a physiologic benefit associated with the use of continuous passive motion?
    a. Prevent muscle atrophy by simulating a normal concentric contraction
    b. Prevent adhesions by orienting collagen fibers as they heal
    c. Reduce edema by facilitating the movement of fluid in an out of the joint
    d. Reduce pain via the stimulation of joint mechanoreceptors

72. The PTA makes recommendations to a patient after hip replacement surgery for positioning in a wheelchair. Which set of instructions would adhere to safety precautions?
    a. Keep legs abducted with abductor pillow and affected leg in neutral.
    b. Keep legs together by using an adductor strap to prevent external rotation of legs.
    c. Sit in a regular wheelchair with feet supported on foot rest.
    d. Sit in regular wheelchair with affected leg in full extension.

73. The PTA is ambulating a patient with an above-knee amputation. The new prosthesis causes the heel on the involved foot to move laterally at toe-off. Which of the following is the most likely cause of this deviation?
    a. Too much internal rotation of the prosthetic knee
    b. Too much external rotation of the prosthetic knee
    c. Too much outset of prosthetic foot
    d. The prosthetic foot is set in excessive dorsiflexion

74. The use of compression stockings on the feet and ankles is contraindicated in which patient population?
    a. Chronic venous disease
    b. Recent total knee replacement
    c. Burn patients
    d. Chronic arterial disease

75. The PTA is ambulating a 42-year-old man who has just received an above-knee prosthesis for the left leg. The PTA notices pistoning of the prosthesis as the patient ambulates. Which of the following is the most probable cause of this deviation?
    a. The socket is too small.
    b. The socket is too large.
    c. The foot bumper is too soft.
    d. The foot bumper is too hard.

76. While examining a patient who has just received a new left below-knee prosthesis, the PTA notes that the toe of the prosthesis stays off the floor after heel strike. Which of the following is an unlikely cause of this deviation?
    a. The prosthetic foot is set too far anterior.
    b. The prosthetic foot is set in too much dorsiflexion.
    c. The heel wedge is too stiff.
    d. The prosthetic foot is outset too much.

77. Which of the following is the most appropriate orthotic for a patient with excessive foot pronation during static standing?
    a. Scaphoid pad
    b. Metatarsal pad

    c. Metatarsal bar

    d. Rocker bar

78. A PTA is instructing a patient in the use of a wrist-driven prehension orthotic. What must be done to achieve opening of the involved hand?
    a. Actively extend the wrist
    b. Passively extend the wrist
    c. Actively flex the wrist
    d. Passively flex the wrist

79. The PTA has just given the patient a custom wheelchair. The patient has a long-standing history of hamstring contractures resulting in fixation of the knees into 60 degrees of flexion. The patient is also prone to develop decubitus ulcers. Which of the following is incorrect advice for the PTA to give the family and patient?
    a. Keep the patient's buttocks clean and dry.
    b. Make sure that the wheelchair cushion is always in the wheelchair seat.
    c. Keep the leg rests of the wheelchair fully elevated.
    d. Never transfer using a sliding board from one surface to another.

80. A PTA is ordered to provide gait training for an 18-year-old girl who received a partial medial meniscectomy of the right knee 1 day earlier. The patient was independent in ambulation without an assistive device before surgery and has no cognitive deficits. The patient's weight-bearing status is currently partial weight bearing on the involved lower extremity. Which of the following is the most appropriate assistive device and gait pattern?
    a. Crutches, three-point gait pattern
    b. Standard walker, three-point gait pattern
    c. Standard walker, four-point gait pattern
    d. Crutches, swing-to gait pattern

81. A PTA is ordered to provide gait training to a 78-year-old man who received a right cemented total knee replacement 24 hours earlier. The patient also had a traumatic amputation of the left upper extremity 3 inches above the elbow 40 years ago. If the patient lives at home alone, which of the following is an appropriate assistive device?
    a. Rolling walker
    b. Standard walker
    c. Hemi-walker
    d. Wheelchair for 2 weeks

82. Which of the following is a FALSE statement about below-knee amputations?
    a. Gel socket inserts should be left in the prosthesis overnight.
    b. The PTA should puncture any blisters that appear on the stump.

c. Areas of skin irritation on the stump can be covered with a dressing, then a nylon sock before donning the prosthesis.
d. When not in use, the prosthesis should be placed on its side on the floor.

83. A PTA is assisting a patient with pregait activities who has been fitted with a hip disarticulation prosthesis. To ambulate with the most correct gait pattern, what must be mastered first?
a. Forward weight shift on to the prosthesis
b. Swing-through of the prosthesis
c. Maintenance of stability while in single-limb support on the prosthesis
d. Posterior pelvic tilt to advance the prosthesis

84. A 68-year-old man is being treated by a PTA after a right below-knee amputation. The patient is beginning ambulation with a preparatory prosthesis. In the early stance phase of the involved lower extremity, the PTA notes an increase in knee flexion. Which of the following is a possible cause of this gait deviation?
a. The heel is too stiff.
b. The foot is set too far anterior in relation to the knee.
c. The foot is set in too much plantar flexion.
d. The heel is too soft.

85. A patient begins ambulation with axillary crutches for the first time. The gait required will be non–weight bearing for the right foot. What is the best advice to give the patient in regard to crutch placement during static standing?
a. Stand with the crutches and weight bearing foot in a parallel line.
b. Stand with both crutches under the right arm.
c. Stand with both crutches under the left arm.
d. Stand with both crutches about 4 inches to the front and side of the shoulders.

86. Of the walkers listed below, which is the least stable?
a. Folding walker
b. Reciprocal walker
c. Rolling walker
d. Nonfolding standard walker

87. The PTA is providing intervention for a patient with a recent stroke. Gait training with a new ankle-foot orthosis (AFO) will begin today. What is the most important aspect of the fit of the AFO?
a. The ankle should be flexed to 90 degrees.
b. The top of the AFO should be 4 inches below the knee joint.
c. Any complaints of pain or discomfort should be addressed.
d. The bottom of the AFO should stop at the metatarsal heads.

88. A physician orders gait training for a 16-year-old boy with recent open-reduction internal fixation of the left femur. The patient is non–weight bearing on the affected leg. Which of the following assistive device is most appropriate for this patient?
    a. Forearm crutches
    b. Front-wheel walker
    c. Axillary crutches
    d. Quad cane

89. Postoperative knee braces have been associated with all the following complications EXCEPT which?
    a. Deep vein thrombosis
    b. Peroneal nerve injury
    c. Avascular necrosis
    d. Ankle edema

90. Which of the following is indicated for treatment directly over a tumor?
    a. Ultrasound
    b. Diathermy
    c. Ice pack
    d. Hot pack

91. What modality should NOT be used to increase tissue extensibility before a stretching session?
    a. Short-wave diathermy
    b. Ice packs
    c. Hot packs
    d. Ultrasound

92. A patient presents to outpatient physical therapy today to begin rehabilitation following a grade 1 ankle sprain. Treatment today consists of ankle range of motion (ROM), weight-bearing exercises, resisted ankle exercises, and cryotherapy. When would the cryotherapy be MOST appropriately used for this patient?
    a. Before treatment begins
    b. After the weight-bearing exercises
    c. After ROM exercises
    d. At the conclusion of treatment

93. A PTA wishes to use a superficial heating modality to a patient's lumbar extensors before today's treatment. Which of the following modalities would NOT be appropriate to use to produce a superficial heat intervention?
    a. Ultrasound
    b. Diathermy
    c. Electrical stimulation
    d. Hot packs

94. Which of the following electrical stimulation parameters are appropriate for reduction of edema?
    a. Polyphasic pulsed current with a pulse rate of 120 pulses per second, and the cathode at the site of inflammation
    b. Monophasic pulsed current with a pulse rate of 240 pulses per second, and the anode at the site of inflammation
    c. Polyphasic pulsed current with a pulse rate of 240 pulses per second, and the cathode at the site of inflammation
    d. Monophasic pulsed current with a pulse rate of 120 pulses per second, and the cathode at the site of inflammation

95. Which of the following is the primary modality to relieve pain at a fracture site?
    a. Monophasic pulsed electrical current
    b. Transcutaneous electrical nerve stimulation
    c. Ultrasound
    d. Neuromuscular electrical stimulation

96. Which of the following is NOT a proposed mechanism for the effectiveness of low-intensity pulsed ultrasound on the healing of a delayed or nonunion fracture?
    a. Increased blood vessel formation
    b. Increased synthesis or cartilage matrix
    c. Local vasoconstriction
    d. Increased cartilage formation at the fractured callus

97. Which of the following modalities would be contraindicated over a recent cemented total hip arthroplasty?
    a. Ultrasound
    b. Transcutaneous electrical nerve stimulation unit
    c. Ice pack
    d. Neuromuscular electrical stimulation

98. Which of the following is appropriate to use after surgical repair of the ulnar nerve?
    a. Heating pads
    b. Cold application
    c. Continuous ultrasound
    d. Diathermy

99. Transcutaneous electrical nerve stimulation may help control neuropathic pain by which of the following mechanisms?
    a. Stimulating A-beta sensory fibers
    b. Stimulating nerve growth
    c. Stimulating C fibers
    d. Stimulating muscle fibers

100. The PTA decides to use deep heat on a patient's calf secondary to complaints of pain. The patient has a diagnosis of advanced diabetic neuropathy. Of the choices given, what is the best deep-heating agent to use for this situation?
   a. Pulsed ultrasound
   b. Continuous ultrasound
   c. Moist heat
   d. Heating agents are contraindicated

101. The PTA decides to use pneumatic compression pumping for patient's edematous lower extremity. How much pressure should the compression pump exert for this particular patient?
   a. 15 mm Hg
   b. 45 mm Hg
   c. 60 mm Hg
   d. 90 mm Hg

102. A stage IV sacral ulcer has a large amount of necrotic tissue and a minimal to moderate amount of exudate on the old dressings. The patient has no fever, chills, or other signs of systemic infection. The most appropriate adjunct modality to facilitate wound healing at this point would be which of the following?
   a. Electrical stimulation
   b. Ultraviolet C
   c. Vacuum-assisted closure
   d. Pulsed lavage with suction

103. Which of the following mechanisms is NOT a way in which vacuum-assisted closure (VAC) facilitates wound healing?
   a. Reducing the bacterial load
   b. Effectively managing exudates and thereby preventing further periwound skin damage
   c. Increasing the amount of granulation tissue in the wound bed
   d. Removing necrotic tissue

104. Which of the following is a false statement regarding the application of superficial heat to a client's lumbar area?
   a. It will decrease blood flow.
   b. It will increase metabolism.
   c. It will decrease pain.
   d. It will decrease stiffness.

105. Short-wave diathermy is an example of what type of physical agent used in physical therapy?
   a. Superficial heat
   b. Deep heat
   c. Cold
   d. Electrical stimulation

106. What heating agent uses corncobs finely chopped into a sawdust-type substance?
    a. Paraffin treatment
    b. Fluidotherapy
    c. Hot packs
    d. Short-wave diathermy

107. Which of the following is NOT a normal clinical indication for the use of electrical stimulation on a client?
    a. Pain
    b. Inflammation
    c. Joint stiffness
    d. Wounds

108. The terms below refer to properties of water that make hydrotherapy valuable to a variety of patient populations. Match the following terms with the statement that best relates to each term.
    1. Viscosity
    2. Buoyancy
    3. Relative density
    4. Hydrostatic pressure
    A. This property can assist in prevention of blood pooling in the lower extremities of a patient in the pool above waist level.
    B. This property makes it harder to walk faster through water.
    C. A person with a higher amount of body fat can float more easily than a lean person because of this property.
    D. This property makes it easier to move a body part to the surface of the water and harder to move a part away from the surface.
    a. 1-B, 2-C, 3-D, 4-A
    b. 1-B, 2-D, 3-C, 4-A
    c. 1-C, 2-B, 3-A, 4-D
    d. 1-A, 2-C, 3-B, 4-D

109. A PTA begins to treat a patient using iontophoresis. The order indicates that the purpose of the treatment is to attempt to dissolve a calcium deposit in the area of the Achilles' tendon. When preparing the patient for treatment, the PTA connects the medicated electrode to the negative pole. Which of the following medications is the PTA most likely preparing to administer?
    a. Dexamethasone
    b. Magnesium sulfate
    c. Hydrocortisone
    d. Acetic acid

110. A PTA is performing ultrasound over the lumbar paraspinals of a patient. Which of the following conditions would cause the PTA to use a lower intensity and shorter dosage of treatment?
    a. Diabetes
    b. Hypertension
    c. Hypothyroidism
    d. Parkinson's disease

111. A PTA is instructed to provide electrical stimulation to a patient with a venous stasis ulcer on the right lower extremity. What is the correct type of electrical stimulation to promote wound healing?
    a. Biphasic pulsed current
    b. Direct current
    c. Interferential current
    d. Transcutaneous electrical stimulation

112. Which of the following is a contraindication to ultrasound at 1.5 watts/cm^2 with a 1-MHz sound head?
    a. Over a recent fracture site
    b. Over noncemented metal implant
    c. Over a recently surgically repaired tendon
    d. Over the quadriceps muscle belly

113. The PTA routinely places ice on the ankle of a patient with an acute ankle sprain. Ice application has many therapeutic benefits. Which of the following is the body's first response to application of ice?
    a. Vasoconstriction of local vessels
    b. Decreased nerve condition velocity
    c. Decreased local sensitivity
    d. Complaints of pain

114. Which of the following theories supports the use of a transcutaneous electrical nerve stimulation unit for sensory-level pain control?
    a. Gate control theory
    b. Sensory interaction theory
    c. Central summation theory
    d. Sensory integration theory

115. Which of the following tissues absorbs the least amount of an ultrasound beam at 1 MHz?
    a. Bone
    b. Skin
    c. Muscle
    d. Blood

116. The PTA decides to use electrical stimulation to increase a patient's quadriceps strength. Which of the following is the best protocol?
    a. Electrodes placed over the superior/lateral quadriceps and the vastus medialis obliquus—stimulation on for 15 seconds, then off for 15 seconds
    b. Electrodes over the femoral nerve in the proximal quadriceps and the vastus medialis obliquus—stimulation on for 50 seconds, then off for 10 seconds
    c. Electrodes over the vastus medialis obliquus and superior/lateral quadriceps—stimulation frequency set between 50 and 80 Hz, pps
    d. Electrodes over the femoral nerve in the proximal quadriceps and the vastus medialis obliquus—stimulation frequency set between 50 and 80 Hz, pps

117. A PTA should consider using a form of treatment other than moist heat application on the posterior lumbar region of all of the following patients EXCEPT which?
    a. Patient with a history of hemophilia
    b. Patient with a history of malignant cancer under the site of heat application
    c. Patient with a history of Raynaud's phenomenon
    d. Patient with a history including many years of steroid therapy

118. A PTA chose to work with a patient using fluidotherapy rather than paraffin wax. The patient has lack of range of motion and also needs to decrease hypersensitivity. There are no open wounds on the hand to be treated. Which of the following would NOT be an advantage of using fluidotherapy versus paraffin wax in the above scenario?
    a. The PTA can assist range of motion manually while the hand is in the fluidotherapy and not while in the paraffin wax.
    b. The fluidotherapy can be used to assist in desensitization by adjusting air intensity.
    c. The fluidotherapy can be provided at the same time as dynamic splinting, and this cannot be done while in paraffin wax.
    d. The fingers can be bound, to assist gaining finger flexion, with tape while in fluidotherapy and not in paraffin wax.

119. A PTA is treating a 35-year-old man who has suffered loss of motor control in the right lower extremity due to peripheral neuropathy. The PTA applies biofeedback electrodes to the right quadriceps in an effort to increase control and strength of this muscle group. The biofeedback can help achieve this goal in all of the following ways EXCEPT which?
    a. Providing visual input for the patient to know how hard he is contracting the right quadriceps
    b. Assisting the patient in recruitment of more motor units in the right quadriceps

    c. Providing a measure of torque in the right quadriceps

    d. Providing the PTA input on the patient's ability and effort in contracting the right quadriceps

120. A patient is receiving electrical stimulation for muscle strengthening of the left quadriceps. One electrode from one lead wire, 4 × 4 inches in size, is placed on the anterior proximal portion of the left quadriceps. The two other electrodes from one lead wire are each 2 × 2 inches in size. One of the electrodes is placed on the inferior medial side of the left quadriceps and one on the inferior lateral side of the left quadriceps. This is an example of what type of electrode configuration?

    a. Monopolar

    b. Bipolar

    c. Tripolar

    d. Quadripolar

121. In comparing the use of cold pack and hot pack treatments, which of the following statements is FALSE?

    a. Cold packs penetrate more deeply than hot packs.

    b. Cold increases the viscosity of fluid, and heat decreases the viscosity of fluid.

    c. Cold decreases spasm by decreasing sensitivity to muscle spindles, and heat decreases spasm by decreasing nerve conduction velocity.

    d. Cold decreases the rate of oxygen uptake, and heat increases the rate of oxygen uptake.

122. A patient is being treated with iontophoresis, driving dexamethasone, for inflammation around the lateral epicondyle of the left elbow. The PTA is careful when setting the parameters and with cleaning the site of electrode application to prevent a possible blister. This possibility is not as strong with some other forms of electrical stimulation, but precautions must be taken to ensure that the patient does not receive a mild burn or blister during the treatment session with iontophoresis using which form of stimulation?

    a. Alternating current

    b. Direct current

    c. Pulsed current

    d. Transcutaneous electrical nerve stimulation

123. A physician has ordered a specific type of electrical stimulation that uses a frequency of 2500 Hz with a base frequency at 50 Hz and with a 50% duty cycle to achieve fused tetany. What type of electrical stimulation has the physician ordered?

    a. Iontophoresis

    b. Transcutaneous electrical nerve stimulation

    c. Intermittent flow configuration

    d. Russian stimulation

124. A PTA who is pregnant has been studying the use of transcutaneous electrical nerve stimulation during labor and birth to decrease pain perception. Which of the following is the most effective technique in this situation?
    a. Place the electrodes over the upper abdominals during the first stages of labor and over the lower abdominals during the later stages.
    b. Place the electrodes over the paraspinals at the L5 level and S1 level throughout labor and delivery.
    c. Place the electrodes in a V pattern above the pubic region during labor and delivery.
    d. Place electrodes over the paraspinals at the L1 and S1 levels initially during labor, and over the pubic region during the latter stages.

125. A patient with chronic back pain is referred to physical therapy for application of a transcutaneous electrical nerve stimulation unit. The parameters chosen by the PTA are set to provide a noxious stimulus described as an acupuncture type of stimulus. Which of the following lists of parameters produces this type of stimulation?
    a. Low intensity, duration of 60 μsec, and a frequency of 50 Hz
    b. High intensity, duration of 150 μsec, and a frequency of 100 Hz
    c. Low intensity, duration of 150 μsec, and a frequency of 100 Hz
    d. High intensity, duration of 150 μsec, and a frequency of 2 Hz

126. Use of functional electrical stimulation in patients with longstanding spinal cord injury does NOT improve which of the following?
    a. Aerobic capacity
    b. Muscle strength
    c. Osteopenia
    d. Muscle mass

127. A PTA is using a cold pack to decrease inflammation after a therapeutic exercise session. Which of the following areas needs to be monitored most closely during the ice pack application?
    a. Lateral knee
    b. Lumbar area
    c. Quadriceps area
    d. Acromioclavicular joint

128. In which of the following patient conditions would it be safe to apply spinal traction to help decompress a spinal nerve root?
    a. Acute rheumatoid arthritis
    b. Degenerative joint disease
    c. Osteoporosis
    d. Spinal tumor

129. Which of the following best describes the patient's position when administering positional traction?
    a. Hanging upside down on an inversion table (or with inversion boots)
    b. Hanging by the hands (right side up) from an overhead bar
    c. Side lying with a pillow placed under one side of the lumbar spine
    d. Sitting with head in a halter that is attached to an over-the-door traction system

130. You plan to administer lumbar traction as directed by the plan of care to a patient who has back pain and nerve root impingement. You determine from the history provided in the initial evaluation that this patient has no contraindications to the use of traction. What other piece of information do you need to obtain from this patient in order to determine the appropriate intensity for your traction treatment?
    a. Age
    b. Body weight
    c. Medications currently taken
    d. Pain rating

131. You administer cervical traction to a patient in your clinic to help stretch the tight soft tissues along the posterior aspect of her neck. She responds well to the initial treatment, so you arrange for her to lease a home cervical traction unit to continue this treatment on a daily basis. In what position would you instruct her to place the traction unit to produce the optimal effect?
    a. At a downward angle that pulls her neck into slight extension
    b. At an upward angle that slightly flexes her neck
    c. At an upward angle that fully flexes her neck
    d. Lying flat with no angle (no extension or flexion)

132. When the goal of a lumbar traction treatment is to cause distraction of the vertebrae, the magnitude of the traction force should approximate what percentage of the patient's body weight?
    a. 10
    b. 25
    c. 50
    d. 75

133. A patient with venous insufficiency in his lower extremities is referred for instruction on the use of a pneumatic compression pump at home. What inflation pressure and treatment time will you use to initiate this compression treatment?
    a. Continuous pressure equal to the patient's diastolic blood pressure for 20 to 30 minutes
    b. Continuous pressure between 30 and 50 mm Hg for 20 to 30 minutes
    c. Intermittent pressure no higher than 30 mm Hg for 1 hour
    d. Intermittent pressure between 40 and 80 mm Hg for 2 hours

134. Which of the following conditions would contraindicate the use of an intermittent pneumatic compression pump?
    a. Congestive heart failure
    b. Lymphedema
    c. Recent joint arthroplasty
    d. Venous stasis ulcers

135. If you are using iontophoresis to deliver dexamethasone (−) to an inflamed tissue, which of the following would be the most appropriate treatment parameters?
    a. (+) Active electrode; intensity = 1.5 mA; treatment time = 30 minutes
    b. (−) Active electrode; intensity = 2 mA; treatment time = 20 minutes
    c. (+) Active electrode; intensity = 4 mA; treatment time = 10 minutes
    d. (−) Active electrode; intensity = 8 mA; treatment time = 5 minutes

136. If you want move ions into the tissue, as in the application of iontophoresis, what type of electrical current will you need to use?
    a. Continuous biphasic
    b. Continuous monophasic
    c. Pulsed biphasic
    d. Pulsed monophasic

137. You are treating a patient who is recovering from a muscle strain, and you want to help increase the blood flow to that muscle as well as enhance its extensibility. Which thermal agent is most likely to produce these effects in muscle tissue?
    a. Hot pack
    b. Infrared radiation
    c. Pulsed ultrasound
    d. Short-wave diathermy

138. You are treating an athlete who strained his hamstring muscle. Which of the following modalities would be contraindicated if this patient had a cardiac pacemaker?
    a. Ice massage
    b. Hydrotherapy
    c. Short-wave diathermy
    d. Ultrasound

139. You are directed by the physical therapist to use sensory-level (i.e., conventional) transcutaneous electrical nerve stimulation (TENS) to provide some relief for incisional pain in your patient who recently underwent knee surgery. The physiologic mechanism by which this form of TENS is thought to provide immediate pain relief is known as what?
    a. Autogenic inhibition
    b. Descending inhibition

    c. Presynaptic inhibition

    d. Reciprocal inhibition

140. When you apply cryotherapy to a patient, in what way can you expect it to affect that patient's sensory and motor nerve conduction velocity?
   a. Decrease
   b. Increase
   c. Initially increase, then decrease
   d. Not change

141. You have a patient with subacute rheumatoid arthritis in her hands who also has a history of Raynaud's disease. Which of the following modalities would be contraindicated for this patient?
   a. Cold pack
   b. Fluidotherapy
   c. Paraffin wax bath
   d. Ultraviolet light

142. You plan to administer a combination of ultrasound and electrical stimulation to a patient who is experiencing muscle spasm in her upper trapezius and posterior neck muscles following a recent whiplash injury. To perform this type of treatment, what type of electrode set-up would you use?
   a. Bipolar technique using a dispersive pad that is equal to the size of the soundhead
   b. Monopolar technique using a dispersive pad that is much larger than the soundhead
   c. Monopolar technique using a dispersive pad that is much smaller than the soundhead
   d. Quadripolar technique using two soundheads and two equal-sized dispersive pads

143. You are treating a 12-year-old patient with Osgood-Schlatter disease and want to apply a modality treatment over his tibial tuberosity to help relieve his pain. Which of the following modalities should you probably avoid using in a patient this age?
   a. Ice massage
   b. Iontophoresis
   c. Transcutaneous electrical nerve stimulation
   d. Ultrasound

144. You have an older patient with balance problems who you think would benefit from walking in a therapeutic pool. However, this patient also has some lower extremity edema associated with venous insufficiency. What effect might the pool therapy have on her edema?
   a. The hydrostatic pressure exerted by the water should reduce her edema.
   b. The relaxing effect of the water is likely to slow her circulation and diminish her edema.

c. Her edema will probably worsen because therapeutic pools are usually heated to at least 100° F.

d. It should have no effect on her edema because walking in water is not that strenuous.

145. You are treating a patient with adhesive capsulitis of the glenohumeral joint. You decide to administer some ultrasound in order to increase the extensibility of the patient's joint capsule before your joint mobilization procedures. Which ultrasound parameters are most likely to produce the desired results in this particular tissue?

a. 1 MHz continuous ultrasound

b. 1 MHz pulsed ultrasound

c. 3 MHZ continuous ultrasound

d. 3 MHz pulsed ultrasound

146. Which of the following patient conditions would contraindicate the use of most thermal, mechanical, and electrical modalities?

a. Diabetic neuropathy

b. Hypertension

c. Metastatic cancer

d. Urinary incontinence

147. Which of the following patients would NOT be an appropriate candidate for electromyography biofeedback training?

a. Individual with tension headaches

b. Older adult with Alzheimer's dementia

c. Post-stroke patient who needs balance training

d. Quadriplegic patient who has had a recent tendon transfer

148. Which of the following physiologic changes would NOT be associated with the application of superficial heat?

a. Decreased interstitial fluid

b. Decreased pain perception

c. Increased extensibility of collagen tissue

d. Increased metabolic activity

149. Which of the following modalities produces its thermal effects through evaporation?

a. Hot pack

b. Ice massage

c. Paraffin wax

d. Vapocoolant spray

150. If you apply a cold pack or ice massage over a patient's biceps muscle for 5 minutes before a session of resistive exercise, what change would you expect to see in that muscle?
    a. An immediate increase in isometric strength
    b. An immediate decrease in muscle tone and tendon reflex
    c. Elimination of any exercise-induced muscle soreness
    d. Faster recruitment of type II muscle fibers

151. Heat modalities are generally contraindicated in the presence of an infectious lesion because they may do which of the following?
    a. Increase circulation, which can spread the organism to other parts of the body
    b. Increase the rate of cellular mitosis and cause the organism to mutate
    c. Mask the pain associated with the lesion, which may cause further tissue damage
    d. Reduce the effectiveness of the body's immune system

152. In most cases, it is considered safe to apply ultrasound over or near which of the following?
    a. Cemented and plastic implants
    b. Metal screws, plates, implants
    c. A pacemaker
    d. Reproductive organs

153. You are administering ultrasound to a localized area around a patient's patellar tendon when she begins to complain of intense pain over her tibial tuberosity. What is the most likely cause of this response?
    a. You have the ultrasound intensity too low.
    b. There is a very low attenuation of ultrasound in bony tissue.
    c. You are using an ultrasound unit with a high beam nonuniformity ratio and/or are moving it too slowly.
    d. The crystal in the soundhead has been damaged.

154. You plan to give a short-wave diathermy treatment to a 42-year-old female patient who has low back pain. Which of the following questions would NOT be necessary or appropriate to ask this patient before giving her this treatment?
    a. Are you currently menstruating?
    b. Could you possibly be pregnant?
    c. Do you know if you might have a urinary infection or a pelvic tumor?
    d. Do you take birth control pills?

155. Why must a patient's skin be cleaned and débrided before applying electrodes?
    a. To avoid contaminating your electrodes
    b. To determine whether the patient's sensation is intact

c. To help decrease skin resistance

d. To reduce current density at the electrode–tissue interface

156. For which of the following patient conditions would electrotherapy be an inappropriate treatment modality?
    a. An infected wound
    b. Prior history of seizures
    c. Muscle spasticity
    d. Urinary incontinence

157. A high-frequency sinusoidal (i.e., biphasic) waveform that is typically delivered in bursts of about 50 per second and used for muscle strengthening is usually referred to as what?
    a. High-volt galvanic stimulation
    b. Interferential current
    c. Microcurrent
    d. Russian current

158. Why do most neuromuscular electrical stimulation protocols recommend frequency settings between 30 and 50 pulses per second?
    a. Frequencies lower than this range cannot produce a muscle contraction.
    b. Higher frequencies usually stimulate the nociceptors and make the patient uncomfortable.
    c. It produces a smooth, tetanic muscle contraction without excessive fatigue.
    d. Most muscle stimulators cannot produce frequencies above or below this range.

159. In which of the following situations would it be appropriate to use a low frequency (i.e., 1–5 Hz) to stimulate a muscle?
    a. When the muscle is only partially innervated and very weak
    b. When stimulating the intrinsic muscles of the hand or foot
    c. When you are trying to relax a muscle that is in spasm
    d. When you are trying to stretch a joint contracture

160. When using neuromuscular electrical stimulation, when would you want to use a long rise/ramp time (i.e., 2–3 seconds)?
    a. When stimulating a completely denervated muscle
    b. When stimulating a hypotonic (i.e., flaccid) muscle
    c. When stimulating a hypertonic (i.e., spastic) muscle
    d. When stimulating the antagonist of a hypertonic (i.e., spastic) muscle

161. Which muscles would you stimulate if you were using neuromuscular electrical stimulation to help correct a subluxed glenohumeral joint in a patient who has had a stroke?
    a. Anterior and posterior deltoid
    b. Rhomboids and serratus anterior

    c. Supraspinatus and latissimus dorsi/teres major
    d. Supraspinatus and posterior deltoid

162. If you are using electrical stimulation to limit edema formation in an acutely injured joint, the amplitude should be adjusted to produce what?
    a. Mild muscle contraction (tapping)
    b. Strong muscle contraction (beating)
    c. Sensory response only
    d. Subsensory response

163. Why is a modulated current recommended when using conventional transcutaneous electrical nerve stimulation (TENS) for pain control?
    a. It provides combined effects of sensory and motor level TENS.
    b. It helps prevent sensory adaptation/habituation.
    c. It reduces the placebo effect of TENS.
    d. It selectively activates A-beta fibers.

164. Nerves cannot achieve a continuous state of excitation because of what period?
    a. Threshold
    b. Depolarization period
    c. Repolarization period
    d. Refractory period

165. When utilizing electrical stimulation, what is the pulse frequency range for tetany?
    a. 25 to 50 pps
    b. 0 to 10 pps
    c. 10 to 20 pps
    d. 75 to 100 pps

166. What is the duty cycle for an electrical stimulation program with 6 seconds on time and 18 seconds off time?
    a. 25%
    b. 15%
    c. 33%
    d. 50%

167. When stimulating the wrist extensors, which is the best current type and electrode configuration?
    a. Symmetric biphasic and monopolar
    b. Symmetric biphasic and bipolar
    c. Asymmetrical biphasic and monopolar
    d. Asymmetrical biphasic and bipolar

168. A 29-year-old woman fractured her right mid-tibia in a skiing accident 3 months ago. After cast removal, a severe foot drop was noted. The patient desires to try electrical stimulation orthotic substitution. You would set up the functional electrical stimulation to contract the appropriate muscles during what phase?
    a. Toe-off
    b. Push-off
    c. Foot flat
    d. Swing phase

169. You are applying pulsed current to the quadriceps to improve patellar tracking during knee extension. Your patient complains that the current is uncomfortable. To make the current more tolerable to the patient, yet maintain a good therapeutic effect, you should consider adjusting which of the following?
    a. Current intensity
    b. Pulse rate
    c. Pulse duration
    d. Current polarity

170. Exposure to which of the following bodily fluids presents the highest risk for HIV transmission?
    a. Tears
    b. Sweat
    c. Saliva
    d. Semen

171. Influenza is commonly spread by which mode of transmission?
    a. Contact transmission
    b. Airborne transmission
    c. Droplet transmission
    d. Vehicle transmission

172. According to the Centers for Disease Control and Prevention, when is it *essential* to wash hands with soap and water?
    a. Before putting on latex gloves
    b. After removing latex gloves
    c. After the hands are visibly soiled with body fluid
    d. After routine contact with a patient

173. A PTA has contracted varicella-zoster (shingles) virus. When should the PTA be allowed to return to patient contact?
    a. After fever has subsided
    b. In 14 days
    c. After all lesions are dry and crusted
    d. After all lesions have healed completely

174. Which of the following is an absolute contraindication to airway clearance techniques?
    a. Open wounds over the chest
    b. Pulmonary edema
    c. Hypotension
    d. Large pleural effusion

175. Which of the following describes the transmission mode of tuberculosis?
    a. Exchange of body fluids
    b. Skin-to-skin contact
    c. Inhalation of infected airborne particles
    d. Through fecal material

176. Which of the following complications after a fracture is considered a medical emergency?
    a. Fat embolism
    b. Refracture
    c. Delayed union
    d. Malunion

177. The PTA is beginning treatment for a client with traumatic brain injury in the intensive care unit. The patient has a chest tube secondary to hemothorax. Which of the following is a correct statement regarding management of the chest tube during treatment?
    a. The drainage tube should be kept below the level of the chest at all times.
    b. The drainage tube should be kept at the level of the chest at all times.
    c. The drainage tube should be kept above the level of the chest at all times.
    d. Patients with a chest tube should not receive intervention from the PTA.

178. What is the primary hemodynamic dysfunction in autonomic dysreflexia?
    a. Hypotension and vasodilation
    b. Hypertension and vasoconstriction
    c. Hypotension and vasoconstriction
    d. Hypertension and vasodilation

179. Which of the following interventions should be avoided if a patient has a positive vertebral artery test?
    a. Cervical traction
    b. Upper extremity range of motion
    c. Upper extremity strengthening
    d. Lumbar stabilization exercises

180. A patient who sustained a humerus fracture 3 weeks ago can participate in all of the following exercises for cardiovascular fitness EXCEPT which?
    a. Elliptical trainer
    b. Stationary bicycle
    c. Treadmill walking
    d. Upper body ergometer

181. What is the primary health risk for a patient following a total knee replacement?
    a. Lack of range of motion
    b. Lack of strength
    c. Pain
    d. Deep vein thrombosis formation

182. A patient who has undergone a total joint replacement of the hip complains of increased leg swelling, calf pain, and shortness of breath. You suspect which of the following?
    a. Pneumonia
    b. Prosthetic loosening
    c. Deep vein thrombosis
    d. Decreased aerobic capacity and postoperative pain

183. A patient presents to outpatient physical therapy for treatment after a lateral ankle ligament repair surgery. Which of the following would NOT be a red flag to contact the physician for further medical evaluation?
    a. Decreased superficial skin sensation over the area of edema after the surgery
    b. Yellow drainage from the patient's wound
    c. 103° F body temperature
    d. Significant edema and redness in the calf area

184. A patient diagnosed with multiple sclerosis is beginning aquatic exercises. The PTA lowers the pool temperature to 85° F. Why did the PTA lower the pool temperature for this patient?
    a. Cooler pool temperatures stimulate increases in strength.
    b. Water is easier to exercise in when it is cooler.
    c. Patients with multiple sclerosis will have an adverse reaction to higher temperatures.
    d. Water is more buoyant at cooler temperatures.

185. In which of the following patients is the PTA most concerned about bruising and fractures of the long bones of the extremities?
    a. Patients with Parkinson's disease
    b. Patients with Huntington's disease
    c. Patients with amyotrophic lateral sclerosis
    d. Patients with multiple sclerosis

186. Which of the following tests is contraindicated if it is believed that the patient could have an unstable cervical spine?
    a. Oculovestibular reflex test
    b. Oculocephalic reflex test
    c. Pupillary reflex test
    d. Corneal reflex test

187. The physician has requested that the PTA take temperature readings before a patient's exercise session. This particular patient has tuberculosis. What type of thermometer should be used to assess this patient's temperature?
    a. Electronic thermometer
    b. Disposable thermometer
    c. Tympanic thermometer
    d. Mercury-in-glass thermometer

188. In which of the following circumstances would you terminate an exercise session with a patient with heart failure?
    a. Dyspnea index rating of 3/4
    b. Borg Scale of Perceived Exertion rating of 12
    c. Angina scale rating of 1
    d. Increase of 15 beats/minute over resting heart rate

189. Which of the following groups of people will most likely present with head, neck, and facial injuries after an episode of domestic violence?
    a. Children
    b. Intimate partner violence victims
    c. Elder abuse victims
    d. Alcoholic abuse victims

190. Which of the following heat illnesses is a medical emergency?
    a. Heat syncope
    b. Heat cramps
    c. Heat stroke
    d. Heat exhaustion

191. A PTA is providing intervention for a client in the intensive care unit of a hospital. The patient has recently undergone surgical excision of a brain neoplasm. The PTA notes an intracranial pressure of 20 mm Hg. What should the PTA do upon learning this information?
    a. Increase level of intervention
    b. Decrease level of intervention
    c. Continue at the same level of intervention
    d. Contact the nurse or physician

192. Which of the following is considered a medical emergency?
    a. Tonic-clonic seizures
    b. Status epilepticus

    c. Myoclonic seizures

    d. Atonic seizures

193. Which of the following is a FALSE statement regarding epilepsy?
    a. You should restrain someone during a seizure.
    b. It is impossible to swallow your tongue during a seizure.
    c. Status epilepticus can cause death.
    d. People with epilepsy hold jobs with a high degree of responsibility.

194. Which of the following conditions is a medical emergency?
    a. Benign prostatic hyperplasia
    b. Orchitis
    c. Epididymitis
    d. Testicular torsion

195. When should physical therapy intervention begin and drains be removed from the surgical site after mastectomy?
    a. 2 hours postoperatively
    b. 1 day postoperatively
    c. 3 days postoperatively
    d. 5 days postoperatively

196. A patient with type 1 diabetes presents to the outpatient physical therapy clinic. The client informs the PTA that she has not eaten all day and is feeling lightheaded. A blood glucose level of 54 mg/dL is found with handheld glucometer testing. What should the PTA do first?
    a. Contact the supervising physical therapist
    b. Call 911
    c. Contact the referring physician
    d. Administer fruit juice for the patient

197. A patient starting to use antihypertensive medications must be observed when getting up or leaving a warm therapeutic pool in order to avoid an episode of which of the following?
    a. Bradycardia
    b. Orthostatic hypotension
    c. Dysrhythmias
    d. Skeletal muscle weakness

198. What is the single most important measure to prevent the spread of infectious diseases?
    a. Handwashing
    b. Proper cooking
    c. Canning
    d. Pasteurization

199. A 30-year-old female patient presents with right calf pain and may have a deep vein thrombosis (DVT). What would be the MOST appropriate initial course of action?
    a. Prescribe rest and inactivity until symptoms subside
    b. Treat with RICE protocols until symptoms subside
    c. Treat with massage, muscle stripping, and stretching procedures
    d. Refer for medical evaluation

200. The most important step to take upon involvement in an emergency is which of the following?
    a. Let the patient know that you have arrived
    b. Assess the scene and environment
    c. Make sure that you have plenty of gloves
    d. Immediately care for the patient

201. What is the BEST method for controlling bleeding and should be attempted first?
    a. Elevation
    b. Direct pressure
    c. Trauma dressing
    d. Tourniquet

202. When caring for a fractured, dislocated, or sprained extremity, when is it important to check for pulses, sensation, and motor function?
    a. After the splint has been removed at the hospital
    b. Before applying a splint
    c. Before and after applying a splint
    d. During the detailed physical examination of the patient, usually en route to the hospital

203. A patient at an outpatient facility experiences the onset of a grand mal seizure. Which of the following is the most appropriate course of action by the PTA?
    a. Assist patient to a lying position, move away close furniture, loosen tight clothes, and prop the patient's mouth open.
    b. Assist patient to a lying position, move away close furniture, and loosen tight clothes.
    c. Assist the patient to a seated position, move away close furniture, and loosen tight clothes.
    d. Assist the patient to a seated position, move away close furniture, loosen tight clothing, and prop the patient's mouth open.

204. A PTA is setting up a portable whirlpool unit in the room of a severely immobile patient. What is the most important task of the PTA before the patient is placed in the whirlpool?
    a. Check for a ground fault circuit interruption outlet.
    b. Check to make sure the water temperature is below 110° F.

c. Make sure the whirlpool agitator is immersed in the water.

d. Obtain the appropriate assistance to perform a transfer.

205. A 37-year-old man fell and struck his left temple area on the corner of a mat table. He begins to bleed profusely but remains conscious and alert. Attempts to stop blood flow with direct pressure to the area of the injury are unsuccessful. Of the following, which is an additional area to which pressure should be applied to stop bleeding?

a. Left parietal bone 1 inch posterior to the ear

b. Left temporal bone just anterior to the ear

c. Zygomatic arch of the frontal bone

d. Zygomatic arch superior to the mastoid process

206. A PTA is scheduled to provide intervention for the shoulder of a patient with hepatitis B. The PTA notices no open wounds or abrasions and also notices that the patient has good hygiene. The physical therapist has ordered passive range of motion to the right shoulder because of adhesive capsulitis. Which of the following precautions is absolutely necessary to prevent the PTA from being infected?

a. The PTA must wear a gown.

b. The PTA must wear a mask.

c. The PTA must wear gloves.

d. There is no need for any personal protective equipment.

207. A contraindicated activity for a child with osteogenesis imperfecta would be which of the following?

a. Spontaneous active extremity movement

b. Pull-to-sit maneuver

c. Prone scooter activity

d. Light weights attached close to joints

208. The best recommendation for strength training in prepubescent children is which of the following?

a. No strength training is recommended.

b. Strength training programs should be the same as adolescents.

c. Strength training should be done only for the lower extremities.

d. Strength training should be closely supervised, correctly taught, and involve low load/high repetition tasks.

209. You are working with a 2-year-old child who has a tumor in the posterior fossa. She demonstrates a significant right torticollis. Which intervention is most likely contraindicated?

a. Facilitated active range of motion

b. Gentle anterior-posterior glides in the upper cervical region

c. Home positioning program

d. Upper trapezius strengthening

210. A physical therapist has determined that hamstring stretching should be incorporated in the intervention of 75-year-old woman with complaints of low back pain. Which of the below is a contraindication to stretching of the hamstring muscle group by the PTA?
    a. Soreness lasting 2 to 3 hours after therapy
    b. Hemophilia
    c. Patient's age
    d. Minimal complaints of pain in the lumbar area

211. A PTA is about to begin intervention for a patient with recent total hip replacement using an anterior approach. Which of the following is a contraindicated motion of the hip during early rehabilitation?
    a. Hip flexion above 90 degrees
    b. Hip hyperextension
    c. Hip adduction past neutral
    d. Hip internal rotation

212. Which of the following is proper placement of a catheter bag?
    a. In the patient's lap while in a wheelchair
    b. On the patient's stomach while in the supine on a hospital bed
    c. Hooked onto the PTA's pocket during ambulation
    d. Below the waist of the patient

213. A physical therapist decides to use cervical traction for a patient with complaints of cervical pain. The PTA is consulted for intervention. Which of the following conditions is a contraindication for cervical traction?
    a. Hyperthyroidism
    b. Hypertension
    c. Diabetes
    d. Down syndrome

214. Which of the following positions should be avoided in postpartum patients?
    a. Left side lying
    b. Right side lying
    c. Supine with a pillow under the knees
    d. Prone with the knees pulled to the chest

215. What motions should NOT be stretched early in rehabilitation after an open rotator cuff repair?
    a. Horizontal abduction, extension, and internal rotation
    b. Horizontal adduction, extension, and internal rotation
    c. Horizontal abduction, flexion, and internal rotation
    d. Horizontal abduction, extension, and external rotation

216. Which of the following vital sign issues should cause concern?
    a. The systolic blood pressure falls during exercise.
    b. The pulse rate increased by 15 beats/minute with activity and recovered within 2 minutes.
    c. The patient reported the activity was rated a 13 on the Borg Scale of Perceived Exertion.
    d. The 6-year-old child had a resting pulse rate of 90 beats/minute.

217. Deep vein thrombosis (DVT) can be described as which of the following?
    a. Can break off and cause a pulmonary embolism
    b. Usually occurs in people who are highly mobile
    c. Is usually prevented by daily administration of a thrombolytic
    d. Is a clot that develops in a superficial vein

218. PTAs should be immunized against many diseases. Which of the following diseases requires an immunization injection each year?
    a. Hepatitis B
    b. Influenza
    c. Measles
    d. Tetanus

219. A patient reports to the PTA that she has pain at night that awakens her from sleep. What should the PTA do with this information?
    a. Increase intensity of current rehabilitation
    b. Decrease intensity of current rehabilitation
    c. Continue at the current intensity of rehabilitation and monitor the patient closely
    d. Contact the referring physician or supervising physical therapist

220. Physiatrists are described as which of the following?
    a. Physical therapists who specialize in spinal cord–injured patients
    b. PTAs who specialize in spinal cord–injured patients
    c. Physicians who specialize in physical medicine and rehabilitation
    d. Specially trained physical therapists who manage rehabilitation units in a hospital

221. What portion of patient management by the PTA includes interventions and goals for the patient?
    a. Examination
    b. Evaluation
    c. Diagnosis
    d. Prognosis

222. PTAs provide what portion of patient management?
    a. Interventions
    b. Examination

    c. Prognosis

    d. Diagnosis

223. A patient with a diagnosis of pneumonia is receiving inpatient rehabilitation. Before today's intervention, the nurse informs the PTA that the most recent oral temperature is 101.5° F. What is the appropriate action by the PTA?

    a. Contact the physician.

    b. Proceed with intervention as planned.

    c. Cancel the intervention.

    d. Contact the supervising physical therapist.

224. What is the name of the document produced by the American Physical Therapy Association that describes the approach of the PTA to patient care?

    a. Guide to Physical Therapist Practice

    b. Model Definition of Physical Therapy for State Practice Acts

    c. Physical Therapist Scope of Practice

    d. Guide to State Practice Acts

225. What part of the physical therapy patient management model includes establishing a diagnosis and prognosis that includes a plan of care?

    a. Examination

    b. Evaluation

    c. Intervention

    d. Research

226. For a PTA education program to be accredited, what type of degree should students attain upon graduation?

    a. Baccalaureate

    b. Associate of Applied Science

    c. Postbaccalaureate

    d. Doctorate

227. Which of the following is the most appropriate reason for periodic reassessment of a client receiving a structured physical therapy program?

    a. To ensure program effectiveness

    b. To maintain a billable relationship with the client

    c. To provide the physician with updates

    d. To provide the insurance company with updates

228. Which of the following is a comprehensive evaluation that would be performed by a physical therapist before a client's initiation into a work-hardening or work-conditioning program?

    a. Work training evaluation

    b. Functional work evaluation

    c. Work conditioning evaluation

    d. Functional capacity evaluation

229. In what part of the client management model would a physical therapist obtain a recent medical history?
    a. Examination
    b. Evaluation
    c. Diagnosis
    d. Prognosis

230. What is usually the final component of the examination performed by a physical therapist?
    a. History
    b. Systems review
    c. Tests and measures
    d. Prognosis

231. At what point in the client management model would a physical therapist design a plan of care?
    a. Examination
    b. Evaluation
    c. Diagnosis
    d. Prognosis

232. Which of the following is NOT a part of the plan of care in the client management model?
    a. Short-term and long-term goals
    b. Insurance information
    c. Outcomes
    d. Interventions

233. What part of the traditional SOAP note includes the client's history?
    a. Subjective
    b. Objective
    c. Assessment
    d. Plan

234. What part of the traditional SOAP note would include clinical judgment based on observations made by the PTA during the treatment session?
    a. Subjective
    b. Objective
    c. Assessment
    d. Plan

235. At what point in a client's rehabilitation would a PTA become substantially involved in the client's care?
    a. Examination
    b. Evaluation
    c. Diagnosis
    d. Procedural intervention

236. What should a PTA do if there are questions about a patient's plan of care after reviewing the initial examination and evaluation of a particular client?
    a. Proceed with the interventions carefully.
    b. Contact the referring physician.
    c. Contact the supervising physical therapist.
    d. Refuse treatment for this patient for today's session.

237. What document controls the day-to-day relationship of the physical therapist (PT) and the PTA?
    a. Balanced Budget Act of 1997
    b. Medicare and Medicaid Legislation of 1965
    c. A PTA position statement on PT and PTA communication
    d. State practice acts

238. Which of the following is outside the scope of care of a PTA?
    a. Performing manual muscle testing
    b. Developing a plan of care
    c. Performing hydrotherapy
    d. Performing range-of-motion measurements with a goniometer

239. Oversight of documentation for services rendered to each client at each physical therapy session is the responsibility of what clinician?
    a. The physical therapist
    b. The referring physician
    c. The PTA in contact with the client
    d. The clinical coordinator of the rehabilitation facility

240. According to the American Physical Therapy Association document, "Direction and Supervision of the Physical Therapist Assistant," when should a supervisory visit by the physical therapist occur?
    a. In response to a change in the client's medical status
    b. After a request by the referring physician
    c. Once every 2 weeks
    d. On every third physical therapy visit

241. Which of the following is NOT generally included in the supervisory visit?
    a. An onsite reexamination of the client
    b. Onsite review of the plan of care with appropriate revision or termination
    c. Evaluation of need and recommendation for use of outside resources
    d. Written communication by the referring physician that the supervisory visit is necessary

242. According to the American Physical Therapy Association, at what level of physical therapist supervision of the PTA is it appropriate to communicate by telephone?
    a. General supervision
    b. Direct supervision
    c. Direct personal supervision
    d. Direct onsite supervision

243. What is the Medicare supervision requirement for a PTA currently working in a home health agency?
    a. Direct onsite supervision
    b. Direct personal supervision
    c. Direct supervision
    d. General supervision

244. According to the American Physical Therapy Association, which of the following tasks should be performed by a PTA, NOT a technician?
    a. Performing ultrasound to a patient's lumbar spine
    b. Transporting a patient to treatment areas
    c. Assisting patients on and off equipment
    d. Cleaning equipment

245. What two specific physical therapy interventions are beyond the scope of a PTA's training according to the American Physical Therapy Association (APTA)?
    a. Selective sharp débridement and hydrotherapy
    b. Spinal joint mobilizations and hydrotherapy
    c. Selective sharp débridement and spinal mobilizations
    d. Hydrotherapy and electrical stimulation

246. What is the common term for coursework designed to maintain a PTA's licensure?
    a. Continued licensure coursework
    b. After-hours coursework
    c. Continuing education units
    d. Continuing education credits

247. Which of the following components of the American Physical Therapy Association (APTA) is considered to be at the national level?
    a. Membership
    b. Districts
    c. Chapters
    d. Sections

248. To become a member of the American Physical Therapy Association (APTA), which document must a PTA sign and pledge indicating compliance with throughout their career?
    a. Code of Ethics
    b. Mission statement of the APTA
    c. Standard of Ethical Conduct for the Physical Therapist Assistant
    d. APTA Vision Statement for Physical Therapy 2020

249. What organization is responsible for developing, maintaining, and administering the national licensure examination for physical therapists and PTAs?
    a. American Academy of Physical Therapy
    b. Federation of State Boards of Physical Therapy
    c. American Physical Therapy Association
    d. Foundation for Physical Therapy

250. Which federal statute requires that all health care providers who transmit patient information electronically adhere to federal guidelines on the type of information they disclose to protect patient confidentiality?
    a. Americans with Disabilities Act
    b. Health Insurance Portability and Accountability Act
    c. Social Security Amendments of 1965
    d. Individuals with Disabilities Education Act

251. What is the single most important statute regarding physical therapy in each state?
    a. Physical Therapy Practice Act
    b. Americans with Disabilities Act
    c. Physical Therapy Act
    d. Social Security Amendments of 1965

252. Which of the following is NOT generally found in a state practice act?
    a. Definition of physical therapy practice
    b. Reimbursement schedules
    c. Identification of providers who legally provide therapy services
    d. Supervisory requirements

253. What is the penalty for violating a particular states practice act?
    a. Censure by the American Physical Therapy Association
    b. Prosecution in a state court
    c. Prosecution in a federal court
    d. It varies state to state.

254. Which of the following creates a scope of practice, authorizes the individual to practice in a given state, and legally protects the use of a professional title?
   a. Licensure
   b. Certification
   c. Registration
   d. Nomination

255. What part of Medicare covers outpatient physical therapy services?
   a. Part A
   b. Part B
   c. Part C
   d. Part D

256. Which of the following is outside the scope of a state physical therapy regulatory board?
   a. Advise the legislature to clarify the scope of practice
   b. Change the state's practice act
   c. Assist in administering state licenses
   d. Act as consultants by prosecutors in professional misconduct cases

257. Which of the following examples could be considered malpractice?
   a. A patient falls on a slippery floor.
   b. A plinth breaks and a patient falls.
   c. A patient is injured from overly aggressive hamstring stretching.
   d. An exercise bike breaks causing a patient injury.

258. What is durable medical equipment?
   a. Gloves and gowns used for the professional's protection
   b. Insurance documents
   c. Complex machines such as magnetic resonance imaging scanners
   d. Personal medical equipment such as wheelchairs or hospital beds

259. Which of the following is TRUE of health care providers in a managed care organization?
   a. Can charge whatever they would like
   b. Must charge according to the Medicare Fee Schedule
   c. Must bill the patient directly
   d. Agrees on a fixed payment schedule

260. When working with individuals from a culture different than your own, which of the following should you do?
   a. Study the culture extensively.
   b. Stereotype the culture so that you can study it further.
   c. Avoid stereotyping based on ethnic and cultural expectations.
   d. Go to the patient's home and observe the family for cultural expectations.

261. The patient's preferred learning style is generally obtained during what portion of the SOAP note process?
    a. Subjective
    b. Objective
    c. Assessment
    d. Plan

262. A patient's lawyer calls the therapy clinic requesting his client's clinical records. The lawyer states that he or she needs the records to pay the patient's bill. What is the best course of action by the PTA?
    a. Tell the lawyer either to have the patient request a copy of the records or to have the patient sign a medical release.
    b. Fax the needed chart to the lawyer.
    c. Mail a copy of the chart to the patient.
    d. Call the patient and tell him or her of the recent development.

263. During a home health visit, the PTA observed several items that require modification in the home of an elderly patient. In terms of priority, which environmental hazard needs the most immediate attention?
    a. The cracked toilet seat
    b. A malfunctioning thermostat
    c. A throw rug
    d. A cluttered kitchen

264. Which is the BEST example of a statement that would be documented in the assessment portion of a subjective, objective, assessment, and plan (SOAP) note?
    a. Client and spouse participated in a discussion about planning activities of interest for the patient.
    b. Client complains of difficulty donning night-time splint and requests that the splint be reevaluated by the PTA.
    c. Family was referred to Social Services for consideration of alternative placement.
    d. Client demonstrates good understanding of the home program but requires supervision to perform independently.

265. Which statement would be the MOST appropriate for the PTA to document in the plan section of the SOAP note?
    a. Client was given educational materials to practice correcting posture and trunk balance during daily routine.
    b. Client is able to respond to verbal instructions and questions with correct responses three out of three times.
    c. Client indicates that the long-term goal is to return to work on a full-time basis.
    d. Client was assessed for use of compensatory techniques while cooking in the clinic kitchen.

266. After talking to nursing staff, the inpatient rehabilitation PTA treated the patient in the room for instruction in safety and adaptive equipment for toileting, along with dressing and grooming activities. The patient was motivated and worked hard throughout the treatment session. Which is the BEST choice for the subjective portion of the daily SOAP note?
    a. Patient was cooperative and engaged in social conversation throughout the treatment session.
    b. Patient reports feeling good today.
    c. Patient is unable to move the right upper extremity as well today as yesterday, although it doesn't really hurt but feels "tight."
    d. Nursing staff reports that patient is unsafe to toilet independently.

267. After a stroke, a patient had difficulty picking up pills from the table, difficulty buttoning, and difficulty completing jigsaw puzzles, which was a favorite leisure activity. During part of the treatment session, the patient worked on putting in and removing pieces from a jigsaw puzzle, and practiced manipulating different-sized coins from a flat table surface. When documenting the treatment, which is the BEST choice for an objective statement?
    a. Patient worked for 15 minutes placing and removing jigsaw puzzle pieces.
    b. Patient worked on tripod grasp using various coins and jigsaw puzzle pieces.
    c. Patient worked for 15 minutes on tripod grasp in order to be able to grasp objects used for leisure activities and activities of daily living.
    d. Patient worked on tripod grasp to be able to perform leisure activities and activities of daily living.

268. A PTA walks into a patient's room and finds the patient lying on the floor next to the bed. The PTA had been previously reprimanded for forgetting to put the bed rails up after treatment. After checking to be sure the patient has no broken bones and is not in severe pain, the PTA helps the patient back into bed, then leaves the room without reporting the incident. Which terms best describe the PTA's conduct?
    a. Legal and ethical
    b. Legal but unethical
    c. Ethical but illegal
    d. Illegal and unethical

269. To facilitate effective communication between a physical therapy supervisor and employee, the supervisor should do what?
    a. Communicate what is expected of the employee
    b. Express disappointment regarding the employee's behavior
    c. Offer criticism to stimulate discussion
    d. Meet with the employee away from the workplace to facilitate a conversation

270. The term that refers to the process of providing information to individuals to assist them in the decision-making process about their own health care is which of the following?
a. Beneficence
b. Fidelity
c. Autonomy
d. Informed consent

271. A patient tells the PTA how much the services provided have helped in coping with his depression. The patient then offers a gift of appreciation to the PTA. Which is the PTA's best response?
a. I love the gift, but I need to report it to my administrator in order to follow regulations.
b. Thank you, that's great. What is it?
c. Just knowing that you appreciate my helped is reward enough. I appreciate the gesture, but I cannot accept the gift.
d. Please mail it to my house. I cannot accept the gift on the hospital premises.

272. A 12-year-old boy has been referred to physical therapy after recently being involved in a car crash. The patient's mother has signed all the necessary paperwork for admission to the clinic, including a form allowing release of her son's records to the parties listed. The patient's mother included herself, doctors involved in the patient's care, and their attorney on the list. The patient's stepfather comes to the clinic after the patient is discharged and requests a copy of the stepson's record. Which of the following would be the correct response from the office staff?
a. Give the stepfather a copy of the records.
b. Give the stepfather a copy of the records after he has signed a release form.
c. Inform the patient's stepfather that he is not on the list that authorizes the records to be released to him.
d. Call the patient's mother and get verbal permission to release the records to the stepfather.

273. The home health PTA arrives late at the home of a patient for a treatment session just as the occupational therapist has finished. The patient is angry because the sessions are so close together. The patient becomes verbally abusive toward the PTA. What is the most appropriate response to the patient?
a. I'm sorry I'm late, but you must try to understand that I am extremely busy.
b. I know you are aggravated. It is inconvenient when someone does not show up when expected. Let's just do our best this session and I will make an effort to see that we do not have physical therapy and occupational therapy scheduled so close together from now on.

c. You have to expect visits at any time of the day with home health.

d. The occupational therapist and I did not purposefully arrive so close together. I apologize, please let's now begin therapy.

274. A PTA is performing a chart review and discovers that lab results reveal that the patient has malignant cancer. When examining the patient, the PTA is asked by the patient, "Did my lab results come back and is the cancer malignant?" What is the appropriate response of the PTA?

a. Tell the patient the truth and contact the social worker to assist in consultation of the family.

b. "It is inappropriate for me to comment on your diagnosis before the doctor has assessed the lab results and spoken to you first."

c. "The results are positive for malignant cancer, but I do not have the training to determine your prognosis."

d. Tell the patient the results are in but that PTAs are not allowed to speak on this matter.

275. Which of the following acts forced all federally supported facilities to increase corridor width to a minimum of 54 inches to accommodate wheelchairs?

a. Americans with Disabilities Act

b. National Healthcare and Resource Development Act

c. Civil Rights Act

d. Older Americans Act (Title III)

276. During documentation after an intervention, a mistake is made in the note. Which of the below is NOT an appropriate step to make in correcting the mistake?

a. Strike one line through the error so that it is still legible.

b. Write your initials in the margin near the mistake.

c. Write "mistaken entry" or "error" near the mistake.

d. Use liquid correction fluid or an eraser over the mistake.

277. When disrobing and draping a patient to prepare for intervention, which of the following is the most important advice?

a. Avoid wrinkles in the draping garment.

b. Do not use the patient's clothing for draping.

c. Obtain the patient's consent before disrobing.

d. Ask for appropriate assistance in situations in which gender of the patient could be concern.

278. According to the American Physical Therapy Association Guide for Physical Therapist Practice, what is the correct order of process of the following elements of patient management during an initial session?

a. Examination, assessment, impairment, treatment

b. Evaluation, treatment, documentation, assessment

    c. Examination, evaluation, diagnosis, prognosis

    d. Interview, evaluation, tests and measures, diagnosis

279. Which of the following pieces of legislation guarantees patients the right to make autonomous decisions about their health care?
    a. Americans with Disabilities Act
    b. Emergency Medical Treatment and Active Labor Act
    c. Health Insurance Portability and Accountability Act
    d. Patient Self-Determination Act

280. Which bioethical principle addresses a PTA's duty to provide honest information to his or her patients?
    a. Beneficence
    b. Fidelity
    c. Justice
    d. Veracity

281. You are treating an older adult who recently fell at home. The patient sustained no major injuries from the fall; however, the physical therapist's evaluation indicates that she is at high risk for falling again, and the cognitive screening suggests that she probably has mild dementia. The patient lives alone and desperately wants to stay in her own home. However, you and the physical therapist do not believe that she can live safely in this environment by herself and think it is in her best interests to investigate an alternative living arrangement. What ethical duty does this exemplify?
    a. Autonomy
    b. Beneficence
    c. Disclosure
    d. Nonmaleficence

282. You are ambulating a postoperative patient in the hospital corridor using a gait belt and appropriate guarding techniques. Suddenly the patient slips on an unnoticed wet spot on the floor and falls down. Although not seriously injured, the patient is in a lot of pain, has to spend extra days in the hospital, and requires additional rehab services. The patient's family sues the hospital and receives a financial settlement to cover the costs of additional hospitalization and home care. What is this settlement is an example of?
    a. Comparative justice
    b. Compensatory justice
    c. Distributive justice
    d. Fiduciary justice

283. You are treating a patient who recently underwent total hip arthroplasty when she tells you that she urgently needs to use the bathroom. You immediately take her to the bathroom and, observing

all positional precautions, assist her on and off the toilet using her walker, a gait belt, and a raised toilet seat. However, as the patient sits back down in her wheelchair, she states that she felt a "funny sensation" in her hip. You check out her hip position and movements but don't find anything unusual. Before returning to her room, the patient is transported to radiology for a previously scheduled radiograph. The next day one of the nurses informs you that the patient is back in surgery because she "dislocated her hip the previous day in physical therapy." You do not believe you were responsible for this patient's injury. What is your best defense against liability in this situation?

a. The patient was confused and did not follow instructions well.
b. You followed standard protocol and safety precautions during your treatment session.
c. One of your transporters reported that the radiology techs frequently mishandle patients.
d. It was an emergency situation, so you are protected from liability by Good Samaritan laws.

284. A male PTA is performing an initial prosthetic check-out on a female patient with a transfemoral amputation. She is complaining of pinching from her prosthesis when she bears weight on it or sits down. To determine whether or not the socket is too tight, the PTA takes the patient into a private treatment room and asks her to undress so that he can better palpate the tissues in her groin region. The patient doesn't say anything at that time, but later files a complaint against the PTA for sexual misconduct. What other action could this PTA have taken to protect him from this type of accusation?

a. Ask the patient to sign a specific written consent form for palpation procedures.
b. Distract the patient with some casual conversation to make her feel more comfortable.
c. Request the presence of a female chaperone during the patient's examination.
d. Wear gloves while performing the examination.

285. According to the Americans with Disabilities Act (ADA), what circumstances would legally preclude an employer from having to hire, or provide accommodations for, a disabled worker?

a. If the employer suspects that the worker's disability is not legitimate
b. If the employer has to spend more than $500 on accommodations
c. If the worker is not qualified to perform the essential job functions
d. If the employment setting is privately owned and employs less than 100 people

286. A PTA has been asked to determine whether a ramp to enter a local shopping mall meets the minimum accessibility standards required by law. The maximum grade for wheelchair ramps is best identified as how many inches of length for every inch of rise?
    a. 3
    b. 6
    c. 9
    d. 12

287. During a treatment session with a new patient on the psychiatric unit, the patient asks the PTA if he should divorce his spouse. What would be the best response?
    a. That's not a decision that I can make. I don't know what it is like to be in your situation, but we can talk about it and see if it helps you to make a good decision for yourself.
    b. Why don't you ask your doctor?
    c. Yes. Your spouse seems to be no good from what you have told me. Go ahead and divorce.
    d. If it were me, I'd dump your spouse.

288. In an attempt to establish a home exercise program, the PTA gives a patient written exercises. After 1 week, the patient returns and has not performed any of the exercises. After further questioning, the PTA determines that the patient is illiterate. What is an inappropriate course of action?
    a. Go over the exercises in a one-on-one review session.
    b. Give the patient a picture of the exercises.
    c. Give a copy of the exercises to a literate family member.
    d. Contact the physician for a social services consult.

289. A supervisor in a physical therapy clinic observes a new graduate performing incorrect exercises on a patient. The exercises are not life threatening but are incorrect. What is the best way to handle this situation?
    a. The supervisor should immediately tell the new therapist to stop exercising the patient and instruct the patient and therapist in the correct procedure.
    b. The supervisor should tactfully tell the new therapist to come into the supervisor's office and discuss the situation in private.
    c. The supervisor should put a note on the new therapist's desk to meet with the supervisor after work.
    d. The supervisor should give the new therapist research articles about the correct options.

290. The PTA has just returned from an inservice offering new treatment techniques in wound care. The PTA would like to share the information with interested members of the hospital staff. What is the best way to share this information?
    a. Prepare a handout on the new treatment techniques and give it to the members of the hospital staff.
    b. Schedule a mandatory inservice during lunch for all the hospital staff members who participate in some form of wound care.
    c. Post bulletins in view of all hospital staff and send memos to the department heads inviting everyone to attend an inservice during lunch.
    d. Call each department head and invite the heads and their staff to an inservice during lunch.

291. A patient is scheduled to undergo extremely risky heart surgery. The patient seems really worried. During the treatment session, the patient and family look to the PTA for comfort. Which of the following is an appropriate response from the PTA to the patient?
    a. Don't worry, everything will be okay.
    b. Your physician is the best, and he will take care of you.
    c. I know it must be upsetting to face such a difficult situation. Your family and friends are here to support you.
    d. Try not to worry. Worrying increases your blood pressure and heart rate, which are two factors that need to be stabilized before surgery.

292. What is the BEST strategy for communicating with a patient diagnosed with Wernicke's aphasia?
    a. Use writing board for communication
    b. Attend to nonverbal behaviors and emotional content of message
    c. Correct patient errors frequently to assist in his learning strategies
    d. Use easier who, what, and when questions

293. Evidence-based practice requires that clinicians NOT be guided by which of the following?
    a. Relevant clinical research data
    b. Pathophysiology of the patient's condition
    c. Success of interventions in the past based on the clinician's personal experience
    d. Individual patients' values and preferences

294. Which of the following is NOT a primary component of evidence-based practice?
    a. Patient preferences
    b. Clinician's expertise
    c. Research evidence
    d. Latest intervention techniques

295. What is the simplest study design?
    a. Single-subject research study
    b. Case report
    c. Large-group research study
    d. Randomized controlled trial

296. Which group of subjects would provide the best results in a controlled study for a physical therapy intervention?
    a. Animals
    b. Humans without the pathology being studied
    c. Humans with the pathology being studied
    d. In vitro subjects

297. What criterion must a study meet to be considered double blind?
    a. The clinician must be blind to the true intervention and placebo.
    b. The patient must be blind to the true intervention and placebo.
    c. The patient and clinician must be blind to the true intervention and placebo.
    d. The intervention and placebo must be blind to the tester.

298. Which of the following is the consistency or reproducibility of data from a particular test?
    a. Validity
    b. Reliability
    c. Probability
    d. Correlation

299. What type of test measures accurately what it intends to measure?
    a. Valid
    b. Reliable
    c. Probable
    d. Correlative

300. Which of the following is considered to be a quantitative review?
    a. Systematic report
    b. Meta-analysis
    c. Randomized clinical trail
    d. Double-blind randomized clinical trial

301. Which of the following type of studies has the potential for author bias?
    a. Meta-analysis
    b. Systematic review
    c. Randomized clinical trial
    d. Narrative report

302. A test that is proved to have a high probability of a positive result in individuals with the pathology in question is considered to have a high degree of which of the following?
a. Specificity
b. Sensitivity
c. Correlation
d. The p value

303. Which of the following is TRUE regarding efficacy and effectiveness?
a. Effectiveness is more relevant to the clinical setting.
b. Effectiveness is easier to evaluate in research trials.
c. Efficacy is the benefit of the intervention in a clinical setting.
d. Efficacy is more important because it takes into the account the variability of patients and clinicians.

304. Range-of-motion and strength measurements are what type of measurement?
a. Qualitative
b. Random
c. Included in the "S" portion of the SOAP note
d. Quantitative

305. Evidence-based practice is the determination of intervention strategies based on which of the following?
a. Extant research findings
b. Research findings, the physical therapist's and PTA's own experiences, and family priorities
c. A physical therapist's and PTA's expert opinion
d. Other disciplines' practice

306. A PTA is preparing a poster that will clarify some of the data in an inservice presentation. The poster reflects the mode, median, and mean of a set of data. The data consist of the numbers 2, 2, 4, 9, and 13. If presented in the above order (mode, median, mean), which of the following is the correct list of answers calculated from the data?
a. 4, 2, 6
b. 2, 4, 6
c. 6, 2, 4
d. 6, 4, 2

307. Which of the following clinical measures exemplifies an ordinal level of measurement?
a. Gait speed
b. Heart rate
c. Joint range of motion
d. Visual Analogue Scale pain rating

308. To meet the definition of "reliable," a test must be both consistent and what?
  a. Cost effective
  b. Efficient to use in a clinical setting
  c. Free from error
  d. Highly specific

309. If you wanted to graphically illustrate the relationship of two variables, which type of graph would you select?
  a. Bar graph
  b. Line graph
  c. Pie chart
  d. Scatterplot

310. A PTA conducted a study to compare the effects of real versus placebo laser radiation on the joint pain and mobility of patients with arthritic knee joints. Subjects' pain and mobility were measured before and after 2 weeks of daily laser treatments. What was the dependent variable in this study?
  a. Laser intensity
  b. Pain and functional ratings
  c. Treatment duration (2 weeks)
  d. Type of laser treatment received (real versus placebo)

311. One threat to internal validity may occur in a research study in which subjects know they are being studied, so they perform differently than usual, producing biased results. What is this phenomenon is known as?
  a. Hawthorne effect
  b. Maturation
  c. Placebo
  d. Selection

Answers

1. b. Skin under the brace should return to normal color and smooth-
ness within 10 minutes of removing the brace. The brace should fit
snugly with a finger's thickness of space. It should not fit tightly or
be kept in direct heat.

2. a. All prosthetic feet compress slightly at heel contact to accept the
weight of the wearer. A prosthetic foot does not allow varying heel
heights, nor is the patient able to tiptoe. Prosthetic feet do store
energy during the early stance phase of gait.

3. b. The distal end of the keel in a SACH foot bends to mimic forefoot
hyperextension. It does not permit inversion because the keel is
generally stiff along this area.

4. a. Patients with amputations generally have changes in the residual
limb. These changes could be from a variety of factors, including
salt and fluid intake. The resilient socket liner allows for adjustments
to accommodate these changes.

5. d. The supracondylar suspension features a brim extending over the
medial and lateral femoral condyles, making it very stable. The
socket also covers the patella and is recommended for patients with
a short residual limb.

6. a. In addition to being easier to adjust, the endoskeletal shank is more
cosmetic and is lighter in weight than an exoskeletal shank.

7. b. The hydraulic swing phase control knee units increase resistance when
the client walks faster to give it a more natural appearance. Oil or air
provides the friction in the cylinders of these fluid friction knees.

8. a. A prosthetic knee unit with a manual lock is not only more stable
during early stance but also more stable throughout the entire gait
cycle. With this type of device, the wearer walks with a stiff knee
but must unlock the device when sitting.

9. b. The flexible plastic socket is much more comfortable because it con-
forms to the contour of the chair when a person sits. The thin plastic
also transmits heat better, so the prosthesis is cooler.

10. c. Late stance is altered by the loss of metatarsophalangeal hyperextension. During swing phase, the shortened foot could also slip
from the shoe.

11. c. Chopart's disarticulation involves amputation between the talus and navicular on the medial side of the foot and between the calcaneus and cuboid on the lateral side of the foot.

12. d. The calcaneal fat pad is preserved after a Syme's amputation for weight-bearing purposes on the residual limb. This patient will require a prosthetic for long-distance ambulation and to equalize leg length.

13. b. One of the goals in early rehabilitation after this type of amputation is to avoid hip flexion and knee flexion contractures. The PTA should make every effort during this time to educate the patient to maintain knee and hip extension.

14. a. The patella ligament, triceps surae belly, and pes anserinus tolerate pressure the best. Areas that do not tolerate pressure well are the tibial tuberosity, tibial crest, tibial condyles, fibular head, hamstring tendons, and distal ends of the tibia and fibula.

15. d. Although the pelvic band provides better control of the hip musculature, it is bulkier and more apt to irritate the low back when the wearer sits.

16. b. Initially, the patient should check the residual limb every 5 to 15 minutes for skin tears. During this time the skin, is most vulnerable for blisters or other skin malformations.

17. d. Choices a, b, and c could be causes of insufficient knee flexion at early stance. If the patient's heel cushion is too stiff, it is not allowing for sufficient knee extension at early stance.

18. b. Choices a, c, and d require sometimes heavy batteries and motors for correct operation. Although the hook is the least cosmetically pleasing, it is the lightest and most popular option.

19. c. The ankle-foot orthosis used by people with polyneuropathies can prevent plantar flexion contractures and assist in gait. Polyneuropathies in the ankle usually cause dorsiflexor weakness.

20. a. Because this maneuver is a result of practice and skill, exceptional upper extremity strength is not required. Normal upper extremity strength is required for forward motivation and the wheelie skill. Ascending a curb is performed better when the patient can balance in the wheelchair using trunk control rather than relying on exceptional upper extremity strength.

21. a. The stationary bicycle and treadmill are usually used to test aerobic capacity because they are easy for patients to understand and easy

for the PTA to adjust during the test. Choices b and c would have excessive body movement during testing.

22. d. ACE bandages are not recommended for patients with venous ulcers because they apply high resting pressure when the patient is not moving, and they stretch too much when the calf muscle contracts and thus provide low compression when the patient walks.

23. c. When the shoe slides on the heel, it creates an area for possible blister formation. The shoe should fit snugly enough that it does not slide up and down on the heel. The other choices are all appropriate for proper footwear fit.

24. a. Total contact casting is absolutely contraindicated on a neuropathic ulcer with a Wagner grade of 3 to 5. It is also absolutely contraindicated for active infection or gangrene.

25. c. More than 4 million Americans use canes, and more than 1.5 million use walkers to improve their mobility.

26. d. Functional obstacles such as curbs, steps, and doorway thresholds are most likely to interfere with assistive devices. Although bed height may interfere with a sit-to-stand transfer, it will not interfere with the use of the assistive device.

27. d. Although an assistive device can help to perform choices a, b, and c, it will not change sensory input. Assistive devices also can decrease the risk for falls.

28. a. The typical long cane of a person with visual impairment is white with a red tip. This alerts passersby that the patient is visually impaired. The cane can also be used to find functional obstacles such as walls and chairs.

29. c. The underarm crutch should not come into contact with the axilla. Prolonged contact with the axilla can cause skin irritation, impingement to superficial nerves, and damage to local blood vessels.

30. a. This allows the triceps optimum position to accept body weight during mobility with a cane. This can quickly be assessed by having the patient stand in a normal posture. The cane should be adjusted so that it falls at the patient's wrist. After this adjustment is made, the PTA can assess whether the elbow is at the optimum 30-degree angle.

31. b. Although a wheelchair can improve upper extremity strength with prolonged use, lower extremity strength will decrease ultimately with use of the wheelchair.

32. d. Because shoulder flexion is primarily used to propel the wheel-chair, the pectoralis major muscle group will be responsible for this motion. The anterior deltoid is also pivotal in wheelchair forward mobility.

33. b. Most patients have good hand function and dexterity to control a joystick for the power wheelchair. For those with limited manual dexterity, the chair could be equipped with one of the other choices.

34. c. The rear wheels located farther back in the wheelchair frame allow increased stability, particularly when ascending ramps. Because of the lack of lower extremities, the patient's base of support is shifted posteriorly.

35. a. Elevating leg rests will allow this patient to perform the elevation component of PRICE (protection, rest, ice, compression, elevation). Although this patient's wheelchair could have any of the choices mentioned, choice a is the most important.

36. b. Because the greater trochanters could come into contact with the side armrest of the wheelchair, it is important that the wheelchair be wide enough to accommodate the patient.

37. d. A high backrest could be indicated for a patient with poor neck control. A high backrest could limit shoulder girdle mobility if the scapulae are in constant contact with the backrest.

38. a. Pneumatic tires should be inflated to 100 psi. Large-diameter casters make the wheelchair ride smoother, whereas small-diameter casters provide for ease of maneuverability and mobility. Armrests that are too high would not allow the patient adequate range of motion to propel the wheelchair forward.

39. c. Although the other methods could be used for proper pressure relief, the best method is for the PTA to attempt to palpate the ischial tuber-osities while the patient is sitting in the wheelchair.

40. b. If the walker handles are too high, the patient could push the walker farther forward from the trunk during ambulation. The other choices would be likely if the walker handles were adjusted too low. Patients may push hard onto the walker because of low handles and hinder wheel rotation. Forward bending of the trunk can also inhibit hip extension during the stance phase of gait.

41. d. The upper cuff should contact the proximal third of the upper arm about 5 cm below the anterior fold of the axilla. The lower cuff

should lie 1 to 4 cm below the olecranon process, avoiding bony contact but providing adequate stability.

42. a. Tennis balls or other glide mechanisms on the rear uprights reduce friction during ambulation and may decrease the amount of work required for ambulation.

43. c. This assistive device allows for the lower extremity and upper extremity both to be non–weight bearing. The patient's right upper extremity weight would be borne through the elbow and not the wrist.

44. d. This is the optimal location for a cane during stance. The elbow should be slightly flexed at an angle of less than 30 degrees.

45. c. Because the patient will remain non–weight bearing bilaterally for several months, the wheelchair is the most appropriate choice for this patient. She will remain on a college campus throughout the rehabilitation of her injury. It would be correct for the PTA to assume that the patient would have long-distance mobility challenges each day. The wheelchair will allow the patient to carry her books and other articles to and from class. The other choices would be appropriate for short-distance ambulation.

46. d. Increased pressure on the ischial tuberosities with hip abduction and external rotation would be seen with a shallow wheelchair seat. An excessively deep seat would cause pressure on the popliteal fossa. Patients compensate for this by tilting the pelvis posteriorly and adopting a kyphotic posture to prevent sliding forward.

47. d. A higher than normal heel will cause excessive plantar flexion during early stance. The response to increased plantar flexion will be excessive knee flexion in early stance.

48. a. The four-post cervical brace is commonly referred to as a halo vest. The halo vest is a circular band of metal that is fixed to the skull by four screws, and then four posts connect to the halo to the halo vest. This particular orthosis allows no cervical motion.

49. d. The halo attaches to the skull by four screws. All of the other choices are applied with Velcro or leather straps.

50. a. A mature spine will not respond to the correction of a scoliosis orthosis. An immature spine with a severe curve will also resist the forces applied by the orthosis.

51. c. Although an orthosis could aid in healing by protecting the body part or preventing motion, it will not speed the healing process. The body's response to injury cannot be changed with an orthosis.

52. c. Orthoses are often used to help single joint weakness such as dorsiflexion weakness associated with strokes. Orthoses will not help with balance, sensation, or endurance issues.

53. a. Both splints and orthoses could be made of hard or soft material. A splint is usually thought of as a temporary orthosis for a short-term dysfunction. An orthosis is used for large musculoskeletal deficits that could last for years.

54. d. Although orthotics serve to protect and support musculoskeletal dysfunctions, they cannot improve balance. Orthotics would also not help a decrease in endurance or poor sensation.

55. b. An uncomfortable orthosis will probably not be worn by the patient, even if it is completely functional. A major element in ensuring comfort is minimizing pressure by maximizing the area covered by the orthosis. Another way to improve comfort is to make the orthosis longer to provide greater leverage for the longitudinal segments of the orthosis to apply force.

56. c. A genu valgum deformity is commonly defined as knock-knee deformity. The orthosis should gently push the patient's knees medially. This is accomplished by a lateral force superior and inferior to the knee, with a medial force at the knee joint.

57. c. Fatigue resistance is the ability of the material to withstand cyclic loading. An active child who is prone to frequent falls or rough behavior may cause the material to fail because of constant damage. Compressive stress occurs when a force squeezes the material, and tensile stress involves pulling of the material. Shear occurs when the material slides over another surface.

58. a. Thermoplastics require relatively low temperature to make the material malleable. Usually, thermoplastics are warmed with hot water and molded directly to the patient. Thermosetting plastics such as polyester cannot be reshaped after they are molded. Metal and steel are difficult to mold to a patient's limb.

59. d. The upper is the portion of the shoe over the dorsum of the foot. If it is to be used with an ankle-foot orthosis, the upper should extend to the proximal portion of the dorsum of the foot to secure the orthosis high onto the foot. The upper should have a separation at the distal

margin of the lace stay to allow the foot to easily enter the shoe and for adjustability of fit.

60. c. Metatarsal bar is a flat strip of leather or other firm material placed onto or in the sole posterior to the metatarsal heads. At late stance, the bar transfers stress from the metatarsophalangeal joints to the metatarsal shafts. A metatarsal pad accomplishes this same task but is not molded into the sole of the shoe. A metatarsal pad is usually incorporated into the design of an insert or a separate component that is glued to the sole of the shoe.

61. d. A posterior leaf spring AFO has a single posterior upright and does not contribute to medial and lateral ankle stability. The spiral AFO contributes somewhat to medial and lateral stability, but does not eliminate the motion in all planes. Solid ankle AFOs and hinged AFOs have rigid sides to restrict motion in all planes.

62. b. Although the ankle-foot orthosis performs the other choices listed, there is no evidence to suggest that the patient's overall rehabilitation time is decreased. There is, however, a decreased risk for falls.

63. b. When the patient stands with the knee fully extended, the ring drops, preventing the uprights from bending. Both medial and lateral joints of the brace should be locked for maximum stability. The Pawl lock would lock both uprights simultaneously, but this type of lock is bulky and may release unexpectedly if the wearer bumps against a rigid object. The stance phase knee lock would lock in the late swing phase and unlock at the beginning of the next swing, but this could be dangerous to the uncoordinated patient.

64. c. Greater intraabdominal pressure increases spinal stability and reduces stress on posterior spinal musculature. Long-term reliance on a corset is contraindicated because it can promote muscle atrophy and contracture.

65. c. This orthosis prevents the wrist from dropping into palmar flexion, thereby assisting the median nerve enervated muscles by placing them in a more functional position. The other splints are designed to keep the thumb pad under the palmar surface of the index and middle fingers to help the patient achieve palmar prehension. Prehension orthoses are examples of substitutive appliances. These orthoses help the wearer to hold an object.

66. c. Most shoulder orthosis are intended to protect the glenohumeral joint from subluxation caused by flaccid hemiplegia or injury to the shoulder joint capsule. The simplest and most widely used shoulder orthosis is a sling.

67. d. Adaptive equipment allows an individual to perform a functional task with increased ease or independence. Choices a, b, and c are all examples of adaptive equipment. An assistive device is one that provides the individual with assistance during periods of mobility.

68. d. To lock the elbow with this type of prosthesis, the patient must extend the humerus and depress the scapula.

69. a. Choice a is the correct gait sequence for ascending stairs in the given scenario. A caregiver should stand below the patient because the patient is most likely to fall down the stairs. This same rule holds true for descending stairs.

70. a. The method used in choice a is the safest. The method used in choice c is too unstable.

71. a. Because this is passive movement only, continuous passive motion does not cause a muscle contraction, nor can it prevent atrophy.

72. a. Following hip precautions, it is essential to avoid hyperextension or flexion of the hip past 90 degrees. In a wheelchair, a cushion or pillow should be placed in the seat to reduce the angle of the hip while seated, and the legs should be positioned in neutral to prevent internal or external rotation with the use of an abductor pillow.

73. a. This deviation is commonly referred to as a lateral heel whip. Excessive internal rotation of the prosthetic knee is one of the causes of this deviation. Excessive external rotation of the knee causes a medial heel whip.

74. d. Compression stockings (e.g., Jobst, TED hose) are used in patients with poor venous return. A patient with chronic arterial disease already has difficulty getting blood to the lower extremities; there is no need to further inhibit the flow.

75. b. A socket that is too large may cause the prosthetic limb to "drop" during ambulation.

76. d. If the foot is outset too much, it is likely to cause the prosthetic knee to bow inward during standing.

77. a. Metatarsal pads, metatarsal bars, and rocker bars transfer weight onto the metatarsal shaft. A scaphoid pad is for patients with excessive pronation.

78. d. This type of orthotic uses tenodesis to achieve opening and closing of the hand. To close the hand, the patient actively extends the wrist. To open the hand, the patient passively flexes the wrist.

79. c. Fully elevating the leg rests of the patient's chair increases hip flex-ion. The already tight hamstrings (secondary to contracture) would tilt the pelvis posterior. This maneuver would increase weight on the ischial tuberosity, risking a decubitus ulcer. Choice d is correct advice because sliding board transfers can lead to abrasions. Choices a and b are also correct measures to decrease the chance of developing ulcers.

80. a. A patient of this age usually can begin with crutches instead of a standard walker. If the patient has no cognitive deficits and was independent in ambulation without an assistive device before surgery, she most likely will have the balance and coordination necessary to ambulate with crutches. A three-point gait pattern is necessary because of the current partial weight-bearing status. A swing-to pattern also can be used, but a three-point pattern assists more quickly in returning a more normal gait pattern.

81. c. Although the patient will have to use the hemi-walker with the right upper extremity, choice c is still the best answer for this patient. Choices a and b are unsafe with one upper extremity. Choice d does not encourage weight bearing and is not the most functional choice. A person with a cemented prosthesis can bear weight as tolerated on the involved lower extremity in early rehabilitation.

82. b. Blisters should be allowed to subside naturally. Gel inserts lose their shape if not left in the prosthesis overnight. The prosthesis should be propped up in a corner or laid on the floor to prevent it from falling and cracking.

83. d. All of the choices are important skills for a patient with a hip dis-articulation prosthesis to master, but posterior pelvic tilt should be mastered first to advance the prosthesis.

84. a. A heel that is too stiff causes excessive knee flexion. Choices b and c cause excessive knee extension during this stage of the gait cycle.

85. d. Choice a provides a very small base of support, whereas choice d widens the base of support. Crutches should never be placed under the same arm.

86. b. The reciprocal walker has hinges that allow each side of the walker to move with the lower extremity being advanced. This walker is unsafe. The order of most to least stable is: nonfolding standard, folding, rolling, and reciprocal.

87. c. Any complaints should be investigated immediately. Pain could be a sign of possible pressure areas or a compartment syndrome. The fit of the brace should be examined after there are no complaints.

88. c. Axillary crutches are the most appropriate device based on the patient's age and diagnosis.

89. c. Braces can cause many problems from direct pressure or constriction. Avascular necrosis has not been found with bracing.

90. c. All heating modalities are contraindicated directly over a tumor. An ice pack can be used for pain relief but must be monitored by the PTA.

91. b. Any modality that increases tissue temperature should be used before stretching. Cold modalities are appropriate after a stretch to mediate pain caused by the procedure.

92. d. Cryotherapy is used in this setting to control any localized inflammation that would occur because of the treatment. The natural vasoconstriction response to cryotherapy helps control edema. Ice application has also been shown to reduce pain after physical therapy intervention.

93. c. Ultrasound and diathermy are both considered to be heating modalities. Hot packs heat the superficial structures that are less than 1 cm deep. Electrical stimulation is not a thermal modality.

94. d. Choice d has the appropriate parameters for reduction of edema with electrical stimulation. The current amplitudes should be sufficient to produce a strong sensation, and the treatment duration is usually 20 to 90 minutes.

95. b. Choice b is the only choice that involves pain control. Monophasic pulsed current has been shown to control edema, and neuromuscular electrical stimulation has been shown to increase strength in muscles. Ultrasound is not a pain control modality for fractures.

96. c. Low-intensity pulsed ultrasound does not cause vasoconstriction at the intended site. It does, however, promote all of the other choices. It also increases blood flow at the fracture site during and shortly after the ultrasound treatment.

97. a. Ultrasound may rapidly heat the plastic or cement in a cemented total joint. All of the other choices are possible modalities to be used after a total hip replacement.

98. b. Like any other surgical procedure, there will be edema and inflammation after a surgical nerve repair. Cold application should be used to decrease this. Any heat application is contraindicated. Pulsed ultrasound may be used, but not continuous ultrasound.

99. a. A transcutaneous electrical nerve stimulation unit will stimulate A-beta sensory fibers while avoiding stimulation of C and A-Delta fibers. This is more effective in patients with nerve pain but intact sensation of touch.

100. d. Because patients with advanced diabetic neuropathy normally have sensation loss, deep-heating agents are contraindicated. There is a risk for burn if a patient is unable to distinguish temperature sensations.

101. c. Upper extremity pressures should be 45 mm Hg, with 60 mm Hg for the lower extremities. The recommended treatment includes 30 seconds of compression followed by a 5-second rest period for the upper extremity or a 10-second rest period for the lower extremity.

102. d. Because of the large amount of necrotic tissue with a wound and exudates on the old dressings, pulsed lavage would be the intervention of choice in this scenario. The necrotic tissue and drainage need to be removed before any of the other choices are recommended.

103. d. VAC therapy is contraindicated for wounds with more than 30% necrotic tissue. VAC-assisted wound healing promotes generation of healthy tissue, but does not remove tissue that is already necrotic.

104. a. The application of superficial heat or deep heat will increase blood flow to the area. Application of cold will decrease blood flow to the area.

105. b. Ultrasound and short-wave diathermy are the most common types of deep-heating agents used in physical therapy.

106. b. Fluidotherapy is the use of a self-contained unit filled with corncobs finely chopped into a sawdust-type substance. The particles are heated to the desired temperature and circulated by air pressure around the involved body part. In addition to receiving the effects of heating, the patient can exercise while the treatment is in progress.

107. c. Usually, superficial or deep heat is used for complaints of joint stiffness. Pain, inflammation, wounds, muscle weakness and imbalance, and nerve regeneration are all clinical indications for the use of electrical stimulation.

108. b. Viscosity is the friction of fluids. Buoyancy is the property that pushes up on the part immersed with a pressure that is equal to the weight of the amount of water displaced by that part. Relative density states that if the specific gravity of an object is less than 1 it will float and if it is greater than 1 it will sink. Hydrostatic pressure is the property of water that places pressure equally on the immersed part.

109. d. Acetic acid is sometimes used in attempts to dissolve a calcium deposit and is driven by the negative pole. Dexamethasone is an antiinflammatory driven by the negative pole. Magnesium sulfate is used to decrease muscle spasms and is driven by the positive pole. Hydrocortisone is also used to treat inflammation and is driven by the positive pole.

110. a. Ultrasound treatments performed on a diabetic patient may cause a reduction in blood sugar. All the other choices are not affected by ultrasound.

111. a. The pulse current improves circulation through the pumping of muscle tissue. The increase in circulation will bring nutrition to the wound and facilitate metabolic waste disposal.

112. c. A PTA can use ultrasound with all of the other choices. Performing an ultrasound over a cemented metal implant is also a contraindication. However, with any ultrasound technique, treatment should be stopped if the patient feels pain.

113. a. Local vasoconstriction is the first response. Nerve conduction velocity decreases after about 5 minutes of ice application.

114. a. This theory supports the use of a transcutaneous electrical nerve stimulation unit for sensory-level pain control. The activation of the larger fibers decreases the amount of sensory information traveling to the brain.

115. d. Tissue with a high collagen content absorbs more ultrasound. Bone absorbs the most ultrasound.

116. c. Correct electrode placement is over the motor points of the involved muscle. On–off cycle time is usually between 1:3 and 1:5. Fused tetany of a muscle usually occurs between 50 and 80 Hz or pps (sources vary).

117. c. Raynaud's phenomenon is a vasospastic disorder of the vessels of the distal parts of the extremities. Patients with Raynaud's phenomenon do not respond well to cold treatment. Choice b is incorrect because it is believed that moist heat may encourage more rapid growth of cancer. Choice d is incorrect because prolonged use of steroids may cause capillaries to lose their integrity, which compromises the body's ability to dissipate heat. Choice a is incorrect because moist heat may encourage hemorrhaging in patients with hemophilia by causing vasodilation.

118. d. The fingers can be bound in paraffin wax as well as in fluidotherapy. When using this technique, the hand remains stationary throughout the heating process, which is necessary for paraffin to be most

effective (when using the standard method of dipping the hand and wrapping with plastic wrap and a towel).

119. c. The electromyogram does not record torque. It assists by showing a linear relationship between the electromyogram and the force produced by the muscle during an isometric contraction.

120. b. This is an example of a bipolar configuration. Another form of bipolar configuration is to have two electrodes of equal size, each from a different lead wire. In a monopolar configuration, one smaller electrode is placed over the intended site, and a larger electrode is placed some distance away. The stimulation is perceived by the patient, in this case, only under the smaller electrode. In a quadripolar configuration, two electrodes coming from two different lead wires are placed over the intended area.

121. c. Choice c is the false statement. Heat decreases spasm by causing the vessels to dilate, which brings more blood (containing oxygen) to the area. Cold decreases spasm by decreasing sensitivity of the muscle spindles.

122. b. Iontophoresis uses direct current to drive medication through the skin by repelling ions. For example, if a medication is positively charged, it can be driven by the anode (the positive electrode); if a medication is negatively charged, it can be driven by the cathode (the negative electrode).

123. d. This is an example of Russian electrical stimulation, which has been shown through limited research to be effective in making gains in muscle forces

124. d. This is the most common placement suggested by sources used in preparation of this book. Spinal level varies, but the overall consensus is that the electrodes are placed higher and on the back initially. Then they are moved lower and to the anterior pubic region as labor progresses.

125. d. This type of stimulation is usually not well tolerated by patients with acute conditions. Acute conditions are usually treated by transcutaneous electrical nerve stimulation with a high frequency, and chronic conditions can be treated with a low frequency (if tolerated by the patient). Treatments providing a noxious stimulus usually have a longer lasting effect.

126. c. Because functional electrical stimulation involves stimulating the paralyzed muscle groups, the same gains that one can expect from the "well" population can be carried over into the spinal cord–injured patient population. There has been no research to prove that osteopenia is reversed with electrical stimulation.

127. a. The lateral knee would cause the most concern because the common peroneal nerve is superficial in this area. The medial elbow near the ulnar nerve would also need extra care during ice application.

128. b. Spinal traction is contraindicated for patients with conditions that may cause spinal instability or fracture such as tumors, acute infections, osteoporosis, and rheumatoid arthritis.

129. c. Positional traction is used to alleviate pressure on an entrapped spinal nerve, which is usually a unilateral occurrence; thus, the side-lying position (nonpainful side) is most commonly used.

130. b. Although all pieces of information are important, the body weight is needed to help determine the maximum intensity for a lumbar traction treatment.

131. b. Pulling the cervical spine into slight flexion is the best way to target your stretch to the posterior cervical musculature. It also reduces tension on the facet joint capsules.

132. c. A force that equals up to 50% of the patient's body weight may be needed to cause distraction of the lumbar vertebra. Much lower forces (about 7%) are needed to distract the cervical vertebrae.

133. d. The pressure setting should never exceed the patient's diastolic blood pressure. Because venous pressure is usually higher in the lower extremities than in the upper extremities, guidelines suggest a range of 30 to 60 mm Hg for the upper extremity and 40 to 80 mm Hg for the lower extremity. Intermittent compression is usually tolerated better, and recommended treatment times are 2 to 3 hours per day, depending on the severity of the condition.

134. a. Congestive heart failure and pulmonary edema are both contraindications for pneumatic compression because the heart and lungs are already overloaded, and compression will just further increase that fluid load. This could result in more breathing difficulties or complete heart failure.

135. b. The active electrode should be the same polarity as the medication. The optimal current dosage (intensity × treatment time) is 40 to 80 mA/min. An amplitude of 8 mA is too high for iontophoresis.

136. b. To move ions continuously into the tissue, a continuous monophasic current (i.e., direct current) is needed.

137. d. Short-wave diathermy produces deep heat and is best absorbed by muscle tissue. Hot packs and infrared radiation are too superficial to

adequately heat the target tissue. Pulsed ultrasound produces little or no thermal effect.

138. c. Diathermy is always contraindicated in patients with pacemakers. Ultrasound is only contraindicated when used to treat a body part in close proximity to the pacemaker. In this case, the patient's thigh is sufficiently distant from the pacemaker.

139. c. Sensory-level TENS is believed to selectively activate the large-diameter A-beta fibers that block (i.e., "close the gait") the slower conduction nociceptive fibers in the dorsal horn of the spinal cord before these neurons can synapse with the second-order neurons in the spinal tracts. Thus, this mechanism is referred to as presynaptic inhibition.

140. a. The application of cold modalities has been shown to reduce nerve conduction velocity.

141. a. Raynaud's disease or phenomenon is induced by exposure to a cold stimulus, so the cold pack should be avoided with this patient.

142. b. Because the soundhead is the active electrode in a combination treatment such as this, you want the dispersive pad to be relatively inactive. Thus, a monopolar technique in which a larger dispersive pad is attached adjacent to the targeted treatment area would be most appropriate.

143. d. Although no evidence has supported prior concerns that ultrasound may damage a growing epiphysis, using ultrasound over these bony sites is still not generally recommended, particularly when other treatment options exist.

144. a. The hydrostatic pressure exerted by the water at deeper depths (near this patient's legs and feet) will help push fluid up and out of the lower extremities and back into the central circulation.

145. a. To increase the extensibility of collagen tissue, you want some thermal effects from the ultrasound treatment; thus, you need to use the continuous mode. To penetrate to the depth of the shoulder joint capsule, you should use the 1-MHz frequency because ultrasound delivered with higher frequencies tends to be absorbed more in the superficial tissues.

146. c. Most heating, compression, and electrical modalities cause some increase in circulation, which can aggravate a metastatic condition. In addition, the presence of an active cancer in local tissue such as bone can weaken the tissue and cause injury, so traction would also be contraindicated. All of the other conditions are either indications or potential precautions for the use of these modalities.

147. b. Electromyography biofeedback requires the patient to consciously attend and respond to a visual or auditory stimulus in order to have a learning effect. An individual with dementia is unlikely to have the attention focus or retention needed to benefit from this type of intervention. All of the other conditions are indicated for either facilitating strength or relaxation of the targeted muscle groups.

148. a. Heat tends to cause local vasodilation, so it is more likely to increase the accumulation of fluid in the interstitial spaces than to decrease it.

149. d. Vapocoolant sprays cause a surface cooling when the liquid spray evaporates.

150. a. Studies have shown an increase in muscle strength following a 5-minute application of a cold modality. Long-term cooling may reduce muscle strength as well as muscle tone. Although cold therapy may reduce the amount of delayed-onset muscle soreness, the modality would need to be applied immediately following the exercise session, not before it.

151. a. Because heat tends to increase circulation, the greatest danger is that heat applied over an infectious lesion will cause the organism to spread to adjacent tissues or get into the central circulation where it can cause a systemic infection.

152. b. Cement and plastic are rapidly heated by ultrasound, so it should be avoided over tissues with these types of implants. Ultrasound can interfere with a cardiac pacemaker when applied over the chest or upper back. The effects of ultrasound on reproductive organs is not known; thus, it should be avoided over these anatomic areas. Metal tends to reflect ultrasound, so metal implants are not a contraindication but rather a precaution.

153. c. Bone has a high attenuation for ultrasound because of both absorption and reflection. Thus, if you are moving the soundhead too slowly or using a unit with a high beam nonuniformity ratio , the heating effect may be more concentrated over the bone tissue and cause discomfort (i.e., deep aching).

154. d. The use of birth control pills does not contraindicate or add precautions to the use of short-wave diathermy, so it is an unnecessary question. All of the other questions may have some relevance to the use of this modality over this particular part of the body.

155. c. Rubbing the skin surface with soap or alcohol will remove any dirt, lotions, or skin oils that may create impedance to the electrical

current and ensure better conductivity using the least amount of intensity.

156. b. Electrotherapy may be used to treat all infected wounds, spasticity, and urinary incontinence (via strengthening of the pelvic floor muscles). However, it is contraindicated in patients with a history of seizures because of the possibility that the stimulus might provoke a seizure.

157. d. This type of current is known as Russian current. The other currents listed have different waveforms and are usually intended for other clinical indications besides muscle strengthening.

158. c. Muscle tetany is usually achieved at a pulse rate between 30 and 50 pulses per second (Hz). Because a smooth contraction is desired for muscle strengthening or range of motion, most neuromuscular electrical stimulation protocols include frequency settings in this range. A muscle contraction can be elicited at lower frequency settings (will present as a twitch response), and higher frequency settings may be used, particularly when the treatment goal is to fatigue a muscle that is in spasm.

159. a. A very weak or partially innervated muscle is easily prone to fatigue, so a lower frequency setting is indicated for these patients.

160. d. When using electrical stimulation to help reduce spasticity, many protocols stimulate the antagonist of the spastic muscle because it is usually in a weakened state. However, if the stimulus is brought on too quickly by using a fast rise/ramp time, it may cause a quick stretch to the spastic muscle, thus exacerbating the problem.

161. d. Because the subluxed humerus is displaced anteriorly and inferiorly, the supraspinatus and posterior deltoid muscles are usually stimulated simultaneously to help reverse the subluxed position.

162. c. When the injury is acute and edema is still forming, stimulation should be kept at the sensory level to avoid further injury to the tissues. Sensory-level stimulation is all that is needed to affect the cell permeability changes that help reduce the edema formation.

163. b. With sensory-level TENS, the body can quickly adapt, or habituate, to the sensation, which diminishes its effects. By modulating the pulse amplitude, frequency, and/or duration, the body does not have the opportunity to get used to the sensation and should continue to respond to it.

164. d. Refractory period is the amount of time it takes for an excitable membrane to be ready for a second stimulus once it returns to its resting state following excitation. In the generation of an action potential, as the membrane potential is increased, both the sodium and potassium ion channels begin to open. This increases both the inward sodium current (which is called depolarization) and the balancing outward potassium current (which is called repolarization). Threshold is the amount of current required for voltage to increase past a critical limit, typically 15 mV higher than the resting value. This results in initiating a process whereby the positive feedback from the sodium current activates even more sodium channels, and this eventually leads to the generation of an action potential.

165. a. Pulse frequency determines the rate of action potential activation. In addition, frequency influences the strength and motor response of a single motor unit. Increasing frequency changes muscle response from twitch to tetany. Tetany is required for most stimulation programs. The frequency range of 25 to 50 pulses per second achieves tetany in most muscles. Anything less will result in twitch muscle responses. Increases in frequency past 50 pps deplete neurotransmitter supply in neuromuscular junction and deplete the muscle's energy supplies (adenosine triphosphate).

166. a. Duty cycle is the percentage of time that stimulation is on or active. Duty cycle = {on time/(on + off time)} × 100%. In this case, 6 seconds on and 18 seconds off = 25% duty cycle (1:3 ratio).

167. c. Electrode placement or electrode configuration is dependent on several factors, including the size of electrodes, orientation of electrodes, distance between electrodes, distance from motor points, polarity of electrodes, and type of waveform used. A monopolar electrode configuration occurs when one electrode is located over the target tissue (active) and a second electrode over a distant site (inactive). A bipolar configuration occurs when both electrodes are over the target area and both electrodes are usually active. Monopolar configurations are often used when current must be kept in a small area. Bipolar is used when current is desired in a larger target area. Asymmetrical or monophase configurations refer to a type of electrical waveform. It is used when current is desired in greater dosages at a specific electrode site. One active electrode is placed close to the motor point, whereas the other electrode is placed at another point to disperse current. Symmetrical or biphasic waveforms are used when both electrodes need to be equally active. This is used in muscles that are larger or require more current. Wrist extensors are a small muscle mass that requires specific current to a small region. The asymmetrical biphasic waveform with monopolar electrode configuration will provide the configuration for this muscle mass.

168. d. Although footdrop can be the result of numerous pathologies (both neurologic and orthopedic), weakness of the tibialis anterior muscle results in an impaired ability to dorsiflex the foot. This deficit is most apparent during the swing phase of gait in which the foot is required to dorsiflex in order to clear the toes as the foot progresses forward in the air.

169. a. The quadriceps are a large muscle group and as a result require a relatively significant amount of current to effectively recruit enough motor units to strengthen the muscle. Studies on the quadriceps indicate that it is difficult to selectively recruit one of the quadriceps muscles individually during functional activities. The focus of treatment is not to improve strength of the muscle but improve the muscle's motor control. Maximal muscle recruitment is not required to improve muscle motor control. Therefore, the clinician could decrease the amount of current (current intensity). This would make the treatment more comfortable for the patient, but the patient should be encouraged to actively recruit the muscle in conjunction with the stimulation. Modifying the pulse rate and pulse duration would affect the ability to recruit muscle fibers and therefore should not be changed. With a muscle group as large as the quadriceps, a biphasic waveform is probably preferable to monophasic; therefore, changing polarity will not affect the comfort of the intervention because a biphasic waveform will have equal current at each electrode.

170. d. Body fluids such as blood and semen are most likely to transmit the HIV virus. Saliva, tears, sweat, or nonbloody urine and feces are not thought to promote HIV transmission.

171. c. Influenza has relatively large particles that do not remain suspended in air but fall within 3 feet of the source. It is spread when the infected individual coughs or sneezes

172. c. The Centers for Disease Control and Prevention have recommended that proper hand hygiene can be met by washing hands with soap and water when the hands are visibly soiled with blood or other body fluid, before and after eating, and after using the restroom. It is advisable to use an alcohol-based rub in the following instances: before and after routine contact with a client, before putting on and after removing gloves for a nonsurgical procedure, and after contact with body fluid or skin that is not intact and before moving to a clean part of the same person.

173. c. Health care workers with localized zoster should not take care of patients until all lesions are dry and crusted.

174. c. The other choices are considerations for cessation of airway clearance techniques. The supervising physical therapist or physician should be consulted if any of these conditions are present.

175. c. Tuberculosis is commonly transmitted by inhalation of infected airborne particles, known as droplet nuclei, which are produced when infected persons sneeze, laugh, speak, sing, or cough.

176. a. The fat globules from the bone marrow or from subcutaneous tissue at the fracture site migrate to the lung and can block pulmonary vessels, decreasing alveolar diffusion of oxygen. The initial symptoms typically occur 1 to 3 days after injury, but this complication can occur a week later. Subtle changes in behavior and orientation occur if there are emboli in the cerebral circulation. There also may be complaints of dyspnea, chest pain, diaphoresis, pallor, or cyanosis.

177. a. The drainage tube should be kept below the level of the chest at all times so that gravity can aid in fluid removal. Upper extremity movement should be monitored so as not to interfere with the tube.

178. b. Any painful stimuli will typically elicit a sympathetic response, resulting in vasoconstriction and hypertension. Following spinal cord injury, sensory nerves below the level of the injury continue to transmit at excitatory impulses, causing this increase in blood pressure and vasoconstriction. In the noninjured individual, the descending sympathetic output compensates for this increase in blood pressure by causing vasodilation to bring blood pressure to a more normal level.

179. a. The vertebral artery test is used to determine whether the extremes of movement of the cervical spine will compromise the vertebral artery. If this test is positive, flow through the cerebral artery could be compromised with high velocity or maintain end-range cervical techniques. Treatment such as cervical spinal traction should be avoided in this patient.

180. d. Choices a, b, and c all involve the lower extremities. The patient is only 3 weeks post fracture and cannot perform any upper extremity activities until cleared by the physician.

181. d. Although all the choices are important, deep vein thrombosis (DVT) is a serious risk for any patient. DVT is most likely to form in the popliteal artery above and below the knee. A DVT could lead to pulmonary embolism and death. Clinicians should be cautious if they suspect DVT in any patient.

182. c. These are classic symptoms of deep vein thrombosis (DVT). This is a medical emergency, and the patient should be immediately referred

to the physician or possibly the emergency department. Further signs of a DVT could be redness along the calf area.

183. a. Superficial skin sensation is often reduced or compromised over the area of surgery after edema has been present for several days, possibly owing to compression of local peripheral superficial nerves. All of the other choices could be infection or deep vein thrombosis. In either of these cases, the physician should be contacted.

184. c. Patients with multiple sclerosis typically present with Uhthoff's phenomenon, which is an adverse reaction to external heat or increased body temperature. This usually occurs with exercise and can be made worse with increased ambient temperatures.

185. b. Patients with Huntington's disease present with chorea movements, making this patient at risk for fractures and bruising of the long bones. Patients cannot control these involuntary movements, which are sometimes forceful. Damage to the long bones is usually not from falls, but from striking the involved extremity on surrounding objects.

186. b. Because this test involves rapidly moving the patient's head from one side to the other then up and down, it should not be performed if there is a possibility of an unstable cervical spine. This test is used to determine cranial nerve function. After the patient's head is moved from side to side, the patient's eyes are watched for movement in the opposite direction to movement of the head, which indicates a positive test or intact reflex.

187. b. Because this patient has a highly communicable disease, a single-use disposable thermometer is the appropriate choice in this scenario. This thermometer is disposed of after use, and there is no danger of transferring the disease to other patients.

188. a. A Borg rating of 12 is within moderate exercise guidelines. Stage 1 on the angina scale is at the onset of angina and is something the patient is familiar with. An increase in heart rate of more than 30 beats/minute over resting is considered a guideline to stopping an exercise test. However, a dyspnea index rating should not exceed 2/4 at any time during rehabilitation.

189. b. Intimate partner violence occurs between current or former partners in both heterosexual and homosexual relationships.

190. c. If the core body temperature is elevated above 104° F, a patient may be experiencing exertional heat stroke. This is a medical emergency.

191. d. Normal intracranial pressure (ICP) ranges from 0 to 15 mm Hg, with a midrange of 8 mm Hg. Sustained ICP above 20 mm Hg requires emergency treatment. A rehab clinician noting a rise in ICP above 15 mm Hg should contact the nurse or physician.

192. b. Status epilepticus is a condition in which seizures are so prolonged or so repeated that recovery does not occur between attacks. These occur when the person has generalized tonic-clonic seizures, and no return to consciousness occurs between seizures. It is a medical emergency.

193. a. You should never restrain someone during a seizure. Attempts to restrain an individual during a seizure could possibly injure the individual. In the event of a seizure, all objects that could possibly harm the person, including chairs, tables, and other movable objects, should be moved away.

194. d. Testicular torsion is an abnormal twisting of the spermatic cord as the testis rotates within the tunic vaginalis. This condition is a medical emergency. Early diagnosis and treatment are imperative to save the testis.

195. d. The risk for postoperative adhesive capsulitis may be decreased with current treatment protocols such as preoperative physical therapy. Postoperative intervention should begin 5 days after the procedure.

196. d. If the blood glucose level is 70 mg/dL or less, a carbohydrate snack should be given and glucose retested in 15 minutes to ensure an appropriate level. Appropriate personnel should be contacted if the glucose level doesn't rise as expected.

197. b. Antihypertensive medication may cause a sharp drop in blood pressure when getting up quickly or leaving a warm pool, which causes vasodilation. This is most evident at the beginning of therapy. Patients must be supervised and warned to get up slowly, to hold onto something firm, and to sit down when leaving the pool.

198. a. Although cooking, canning, and pasteurization can reduce the chances of food-borne infections, handwashing is acknowledged as the single most important measure to prevent spread of infectious diseases. Handwashing with plain soap aids in the mechanical removal of dirt and microbes present on the hands, including potential pathogens, thus preventing the spread of many infectious diseases.

199. d. DVT is a potentially serious condition that requires special studies to properly identify and possible anticoagulant therapy for treatment. Medical referral is indicated as soon as DVT is suspected.

200. b. It is imperative for a rescuer to ensure that the scene is safe to enter before providing emergency rescue. This ensures that the rescuer does not become an additional victim.

201. b. Direct pressure is the first line of defense for external hemorrhage. If it is unsuccessful, then elevation and pressure applied to pulse pressure points are added sequentially. Tourniquets are used as a last resort.

202. c. Pulse, sensation, and motor function are evaluated before splinting to assess the integrity of extremity neurovascular function. They are checked again after splinting to ensure that the splint is not applied too tightly.

203. b. The person should lie down to prevent head injury. Tight clothes are loosened to make sure that nothing is too constricting. Close furniture is moved away for the patient's safety. Nothing should be placed in the patient's mouth because of the danger of obstructing the airway.

204. a. A ground fault interruption circuit protects the patient from a potentially life-threatening situation. The other choices are valid concerns, but choice a is the most important.

205. b. Pressure on the left temporal bone just anterior to the ear helps to occlude blood flow from the temporal artery.

206. d. The therapist does not need to wear a gown, gloves, or mask. These precautions are necessary only if there is a chance that the therapist or his clothing can become contaminated with blood, serum, or feces.

207. b. This maneuver would put undue stress on the upper extremities. Rather, the child should be supported around the shoulders while attempting to sit up.

208. d. Strength training in this group should be closely monitored because of skeletal immaturity. Proper technique should be taught and reinforced.

209. b. With an ongoing tumor in this area, any passive range of motion or mobilization is contraindicated.

210. b. Soreness lasting 24 hours or more is a concern, and care should be taken because of the age of the patient. It is not a contraindication, however. Excessive complaints of pain should be a contraindication. Hemophiliac patients should not be stretched in any joint because of the possibility of effusion.

211. b. Hyperextension is contraindicated because of the anterior approach. This motion would put undue stress on the anterior portion of the hip capsule. Choices a, c, and d are all contraindications for the posterior approach.

212. d. The catheter bag should always be below the level of the waist. This will keep urine in the catheter line from moving back to the patient's urinary tract. Infections can result if urine is allowed to reenter the urinary tract.

213. d. Studies have shown that 15% percent of individuals with Down syndrome have atlantoaxial (C1-2) instability. Instability in that region is a contraindication to cervical traction.

214. d. The uterus moves superiorly in this position. This could cause an air embolism to enter the vagina and uterus. Eventually, the embolism could enter the circulatory system through the placental wound.

215. b. These motions would stretch the tissues that are early in the healing process. Care must be taken not to damage these structures in the anterior capsule.

216. a. Systolic blood pressure should always rise as workload increases. The other values are within normal limits for rest or exercise response.

217. a. DVT usually occurs in sedentary or immobilized people as a result of a decrease in blood flow from inactivity. A serious complication of DVT is pulmonary embolism, which is when a clot travels to the pulmonary system and blocks blood flow. It is a major cause of death in many hospitals.

218. b. The hepatitis vaccine is given in a three-dose series, and anyone born in 1957 or later has been immunized against measles. All adults should have a tetanus booster every 10 years. The flu shot will produce antibodies in the body that will provide protection from the most common strain of influenza viruses found by research that year. Each year, the influenza strains are different, so the immunization is required on an annual basis to prevent recurrent infections.

219. d. Pain that awakens a person from sleep could be due to a malignant tumor. It is important to differentiate this pain from pain that makes it difficult to fall asleep, which is generally not as severe.

220. c. Physiatrists are physicians who specialize in physical medicine and rehabilitation. Physiatrists often oversee the care of patients requiring rehabilitation, referring them to various other physicians and allied health care professionals and following up on the outcome of these referrals.

221. d. According to the Guide, the prognosis should contain "anticipated goals and expected outcomes, predicted level of optimal improvement, specific interventions to be used, and proposed duration and frequency of the interventions that are required to reach the anticipated goals and expected outcomes."

222. a. The PTA provides interventions based on the direction of the physical therapist. PTAs document patient responses to specific interventions and adjust them accordingly.

223. d. The physician does not need to be contacted because this patient is already receiving inpatient medical care. An abnormally high temperature often decreases the patient's tolerance to activity. This patient's session will probably be canceled, but the supervising physical therapist should be consulted first.

224. a. The Guide to Physical Therapist Practice is a pivotal document describing the approach of the physical therapist to patient care.

225. b. An evaluation is conducted to interpret the findings of an examination and is used to establish a diagnosis and prognosis that includes a plan of care.

226. b. Criteria for accreditation stipulate that the degree for a professional-level physical therapy education program must be at the postbaccalaureate level and that the degree for a PTA education program is the associate degree.

227. a. Periodic reassessment ensures program effectiveness and serves as a motivating factor for the client undergoing physical therapy intervention.

228. d. The physical therapist may conduct analysis of ergonomics at the worksite and perform a functional capacity evaluation. After these assessments, the patient may then begin a work-hardening or work-conditioning program.

229. a. The first component of the client management model, examination, is the process of gathering information about the past and current status of the client. It begins with a history to describe the nature of the condition or health status of the client.

230. c. In the final component of the examination, tests and measures, the therapist selects and performs specific procedures to quantify the physical and functional status of the client. The tests and measures than allow the physical therapist to develop the most appropriate plan of care.

231. d. A prognosis is a prediction of the level of improvement and time necessary to reach said level. The therapist designs a plan of care that incorporates the expectation of the client.

232. b. Short-term and long-term goals, outcomes, interventions, and discharge criteria are all part of the plan of care.

233. a. The subjective portion of the SOAP note includes what the client often describes about the current condition. An accurate history should be recorded in this portion of the note.

234. c. The assessment portion of the traditional SOAP note includes clinical judgments based on observations made by the PTA during the treatment; this section can also include goals.

235. d. Procedural intervention is the major therapeutic interaction between the therapist or assistant and the client. A PTA would be involved in a substantial component of the care as delegated by the physical therapist at this point in a patient's rehabilitation.

236. c. Anytime a PTA is unsure of a patient's interventions or response to those interventions, the PTA should immediately consult with the supervising physical therapist.

237. d. The state practice act is the legal statute intended to "protect public health, safety, welfare, and provide for the state administrative control, supervision, licensure, and regulation of the practice of physical therapy." Many state practice acts establish the maximum PT/PTA ratio, type and frequency of communication with the supervising PT, frequency of client reexamination by the PT, and minimum level of supervision.

238. b. Development or modification of a plan of care which is based on the initial examination or reexamination and which includes the physical therapy goals and outcomes is the sole responsibility of the physical therapist.

239. a. The oversight of all documentation for services rendered to each client at each physical therapy session remains the sole responsibility of the physical therapist.

240. a. A supervisory visit by the physical therapist will be made upon the PTA's request for a reexamination, when a change in the plan of care is needed, before any planned discharge, and in response to a change in the client's medical status, at least once a month, or at a higher frequency when established by the physical therapist, in accordance with the needs of the client.

241. d. Choices a, b, and c are all part of the supervisory visit. The referring physician does not need to provide documentation that a supervisory visit is necessary.

242. a. In general supervision, the physical therapist is not required to be onsite for direction and supervision but must be available at least by telecommunication. In choices b and c, telecommunication does not meet the requirement of direct supervision or direct personal supervision.

243. d. Outpatient hospitals, nursing facilities, comprehensive outpatient rehabilitation facilities, and home health agencies require general PTA supervision. PTAs in private practice or in a physician's office require direct supervision.

244. a. Although a PTA can perform all these activities, the only activity listed that can be solely performed by a PTA is ultrasound of a patient's lumbar spine. Physical therapy technicians or aides are authorized to perform the other choices. The client management element of interventions should be represented and reimbursed as physical therapy only when performed by a physical therapist or PTA.

245. c. Selective sharp débridement, which is a component of wound care, and spinal and peripheral joint mobilizations, which are components of manual therapy, are deemed beyond the scope of a PTA's training by the APTA. This, however, remains controversial.

246. c. To remain clinically competent, PTAs must seek ways to improve their clinical skills after graduation. Most jurisdictions require continuing education units to maintain licensure.

247. d. Membership and districts are considered at the local level of the APTA, whereas each state has a chapter. There are several bodies of the APTA at the national level, including sections.

248. c. A prospective physical therapist member must sign a pledge indicating compliance with a Code of Ethics, whereas a perspective PTA member must sign a pledge indicating compliance with the Standards of Ethical Conduct for the Physical Therapist Assistant.

249. b. The Federation of State Boards of Physical Therapy (FSBPT) is particularly helpful for identifying the licensure requirements in each jurisdiction across the nation. Regarding the examinations, the FSBPT develops, maintains, and administers national licensing examination for physical therapists and PTAs.

250. b. The Health Insurance Portability and Accountability Act (HIPAA) requires that among other things, all health care providers who transmit patient information electronically adhere to federal guidelines as to the type of patient information they disclose, to whom they may disclose it, and how they store it in order to protect patient confidentiality.

251. a. Regarding physical therapy practice, the single most important statute is the state physical therapy practice act. The practice act is a legal foundation for the scope and protection of physical therapy practice.

252. b. Among the areas generally provided by a state practice act are the state definition of the physical therapy practice, identification of providers who may legally provide physical therapy services, identification of tasks that may be delegated, and supervisory requirements.

253. d. The consequences of violating state practice acts are often stated in the act itself or accompanying regulations. In some states, such as New York, the unlawful practice of physical therapy is a criminal offense.

254. a. Licensure creates a scope of practice, authorizes the individual of the practice in a given state, and legally protects the use of the professional title. Functionally, certification, without licensure, legally protects the title of the PTA. Unlike licensure, however, it does not create a separate scope of practice by monopoly to provide a particular service. Registration is the least rigorous governmental regulation and requires only that registrants periodically provide the state with updated registrations on their demographic information and pay a registration fee.

255. b. As a general rule, Part A of Medicare covers inpatient services, and Part B provides reimbursement for outpatient services.

256. b. Although the state regulatory board of physical therapy cannot change the practice act adopted by the state legislature, state boards serve many important functions. They may advise the legislature or other government bodies to clarify the scope of practice as well as provide advice to state licensed practitioners seeking guidance on practice issues in the state. They also assist in administering the state licensing procedures and are generally at least consulted by prosecutors in professional misconduct cases.

257. c. The other choices are examples of negligence, which is defined as the failure to act as a reasonably prudent person. Malpractice, or professional negligence, is a failure to act as a member of good

standing of the profession would have acted, resulting in subsequent injury to the patient. It is failure to meet a professional standard of care, a special kind of negligence. An example of malpractice would be when a therapist excessively mobilizes a joint and causes injury.

258. d. Durable medical equipment is medical equipment (such as a wheelchair, hospital bed, or ventilator) that a practitioner may prescribe for a patient's use over an extended period.

259. d. In its simplest form, managed care consists of two components: a predetermined payment schedule established by the insurance company based on utilization data, and a provider network consisting of providers who contract with the insurance company and agree to accept the payment schedule for their services.

260. c. When working with individuals from a culture different from your own, you should avoid stereotyping based on ethnic and cultural expectations. Differences among members of the same ethnic or cultural group may be as great as those among individuals from different ethnic and cultural groups.

261. b. A systems review is included in the O section of the SOAP note. The systems review includes a brief examination of the other systems of the body related to physical therapy and any information about the patient's cognition, communication, and preferred learning style.

262. a. A patient can obtain his or her medical records simply by signing a release form. Charts and records should never be given or faxed to an attorney unless the patient has signed a release.

263. c. The presence of a throw rug could result in a fall, which would be far more hazardous to the health of an elderly client than the other objects in the environment. In elderly people, falls are the major cause of fractures.

264. d. Assessment is the physical therapist's judgment of clients' progress, limitations, and expected benefit from therapy.

265. a. The plan relates to information presented in the O and A sections of the SOAP note and is a description of the interventions, methods, or approaches used to achieve the goals.

266. c. The patient's observations about the right upper extremity are most pertinent to this treatment session because they relate to the entire session. Nursing's comments are important but do not belong in the S section. The S section is usually reserved for the patient's comments.

267. c. The emphasis is on the performance component and the functional application, not the specific media used in the treatment. Many third-party payers also want to see the amount of time per Current Procedural Terminology code charged.

268. b. The behavior was legal because there was no crime and it brought no harm to the patient. It was unethical because the therapist was more concerned about the therapist's needs than the patient's needs. It also violated the principle of veracity.

269. a. Effective communication by supervisors and managers involves communicating expectations, offering constructive criticisms, and expressing interest in an employee's professional growth.

270. d. Informed consent refers to providing and sharing health care information to individuals so that they can make the best decisions about their treatment or health care.

271. c. It is crucial to take the patient's feelings into consideration when you have to let them know that it is unethical to accept gifts. By explaining the situation and acknowledging the gesture, you are more likely to avoid offending the patient.

272. c. The patient's biological father would have the right to access the records whether or not he is on the list, but not the stepfather. Choice b is incorrect because unless he is on the original list, he cannot simply sign a form and receive the records. Choice d is incorrect because you cannot verify that you are speaking to the mother.

273. b. Choice b is the most empathetic response. It also lets the patient know that the therapists will make an effort to prevent the problem from recurring.

274. b. A therapist should never comment on such a serious prognosis before the physician has assessed the lab results and consulted with the patient first.

275. a. The Americans with Disabilities Act allowed structural modifications of federal buildings and protection from discrimination based on disability.

276. d. Choices a, b, and c should all be performed each time a documentation error is made. One should never use erasers or liquid correction.

277. c. All of the above are good advice that needs to be followed, but consent to disrobe is the first and most important choice. Wrinkles

can cause areas of pressure, and patient's clothing could be soiled. Gender situations could obviously cause a concern.

278. c. Examination, evaluation, diagnosis, prognosis is the correct order according to the American Physical Therapy Association.

279. d. Autonomy means self-governance and refers to an individual's right to make his or her own decisions. The term self-determination is synonymous with autonomy. In patient care, this right is protected by a federal statute known as the Patient Self-Determination Act of 1990. This statute codifies the rights of hospitalized patients and long-term care residents to participate in treatment decision making and to control the use of extraordinary treatment measures, including artificial life support.

280. d. Veracity refers to telling the truth. Fidelity refers to faithfulness, justice refers to fairness, and beneficence refers to doing what's best for someone else.

281. b. Beneficence is the ethical principle of acting in a way that reflects the best interests of the patient. In this case, the physical therapist and PTA were attempting to do what they thought was best in terms of protecting the patient from future risk for physical harm resulting from another fall.

282. b. This is an example of ordinary negligence that is incident to health care delivery. Premises liability provides for monetary damages on the part of premise owners for injuries incurred by patrons. The concept of justice refers to fair treatment, or equity. Compensatory justice is one type of justice that compensates individuals fairly for injuries or wrongdoings that they have suffered. The other types of justice listed deal more with fair allocation of health care resources at the societal or individual level.

283. b. Liability for professional negligence occurs when health care professionals fail to care for patients in a manner that complies with legal and professional standards of care. To allege negligence on the part of this therapist, the patient would have to provide evidence that the therapist did not follow standard policies and procedures related to patient safety during transfers and that this action was the direct cause for the injury. Thus, the therapist's best defense is not to place the blame elsewhere, but rather to emphasize that appropriate standard of care was rendered. The Good Samaritan laws do not apply to this case because the situation did not place the patient in eminent or serious peril.

284. c. To protect oneself against allegations of sexual misconduct, health care providers should implement some risk management strategies, including (1) providing same-sex chaperones when conducting

intimate, hands-on procedures or upon patient request; (2) implementing a "knock-and-enter" clinic policy; (3) implementing a general informed consent policy that ensures that patients understand the nature of questions they will be asked and types of therapeutic procedures they may experience; and (4) providing ongoing continuing education to health care professionals and support staff on how to prevent sexual abuse and harassment.

285. c. The ADA legislation applies to public and private businesses employing 25 or more people on July 26, 1992, or those with 15 or more people on July 26, 1994. Title I of the ADA prohibits employment discrimination of "a qualified individual with a disability," which means that the job applicant or employee can perform the essential job functions, with or without reasonable accommodations. The employer determines what the essential job functions are, and the ADA defines what a disability is. The Equal Employment Opportunity Commission (EEOC) provides definitions for "reasonable accommodations."

286. d. According to code, 12 inches of length is necessary for each 1 inch of rise when making an area accessible.

287. a. Giving advice or sending the patient to his doctor to get the decision made is not appropriate therapeutic behavior. The physical therapist or PTA's role is to help the patient review his options and encourage him to make the best decision for himself.

288. d. This answer is correct because patients need a written home program with diagrams and instructions. One-on-one teaching is also necessary to ensure that the patient understands the program. Bringing in another family member is also definitely advisable to assist the patient with the program at home. Although a Social Services consult maybe necessary in the long run, it will not help the patient to perform the exercises over the next several days.

289. b. The supervisor can best handle this situation by discussing the exercise program away from the patient. Correcting the new graduate in front of the patient probably would decrease the confidence of the patient in the treatment and the therapist.

290. c. Posting the inservice date on the bulletin board and sending a memo to the department heads is the most effective way to invite everyone interested. Scheduling during lunch often makes it easier for people to attend.

291. c. This answer is the most appropriate. The therapist cannot guarantee everything will be okay (choice a) or that the physician is the best (choice b). Choice d is too insensitive.

292. b. Attend to nonverbal behaviors and the emotional content of the message. Wernicke's aphasia is a receptive aphasia. Use of a writing board or simpler questions will not be successful because these methods require receptive communication. Frequent correction is not ideal because the patient cannot process receptive feedback.

293. c. Choice c defines experience-based practice. Even though this approach has been used in the past, it does have limitations. Restrictions include the experience of the clinician or the clinician's expertise in providing the intervention.

294. d. Although the latest interventions may be necessary for the best possible outcome, interventions proven by research are more likely to provide expected outcomes.

295. b. A case report is a detailed description of a patient's clinical presentation, the course of treatment, and the changes in clinical presentation that occurred during and generally after that course of treatment. A controlled research study applies an intervention and compares the patient's status with that when the intervention is not applied.

296. c. In vitro subjects are used in studying changes on the cellular level, and animals may not respond as humans. Human subjects with the pathology in question would offer the most accurate response to intervention.

297. c. A study is considered double blind when both the patient and clinician are unaware of whether the treatment is real or placebo. It is difficult to apply this type of study to physical therapy interventions.

298. b. A reliable test gives the same result when applied in the same situation.

299. a. Validity relates a test's usefulness and the degree to which it represents the property it claims to measure.

300. b. A meta-analysis combines and analyzes the numerical data from individual primary randomized clinical trials that meet rigorous predefined standards to determine the efficacy of an intervention. A systematic review is a comprehensive and unbiased integrative descriptive report that provides an overview of the published research on a topic and is considered a qualitative review.

301. d. A narrative report involves articles chosen by the author for review. Often, the methods used to choose studies and interpret data are informal and subjective.

302. b. Sensitivity is also known as the true-positive rate. In contrast, the probability of a negative test result in a person without the pathology is known as specificity, or the true-negative rate.

303. a. Efficacy is the benefit of an intervention in controlled conditions of a research study. Effectiveness takes into account the individual variability of the clinical setting. Effectiveness more closely approximates the "real world."

304. d. During the test and measures portion of the examination (which is in the objective portion of the note), specific numbers or grades may be assigned (quantitative measurement), as is the case with range-of-motion and strength measurements.

305. b. Evidence-based practice includes deciding on an intervention strategy based on research findings, the physical therapist or PTA's own experiences, and family priorities. Basing a decision about how to approach intervention solely on research findings without considering one's own experience and the family's priorities does not allow for consideration of all the unique characteristics and needs of the child and family.

306. b. The mean is the average of the set of numbers. The mode is the number that appears most often in the set of data. The median is the middlemost value.

307. d. Most rating scales represent ordinal levels of measures in that they have scores that are rank-ordered, but do not represent equally spaced measures, as in an interval or ratio-level measurement.

308. c. In addition to being consistent, a measurement must reduce the amount of error in order to be considered reliable. Sources of error may be systematic (e.g., because of poor calibration of an instrument) or random (e.g., changes in subject performance). Statistical tests such as intraclass correlation coefficients take into account these multiple sources of error when estimating the reliability of a measure.

309. d. Scatterplots illustrate the relationship of two variables, one plotted on the x-axis and the other plotted on the y-axis. A line of fit for the data points may also be illustrated. A perfect relationship is illustrated by a diagonal line from one corner of the graph to the opposite corner.

310. b. The outcomes being measured are the dependent variables in a study. The treatment groups would represent the independent variable.

311. a. The Hawthorne effect was named for an experiment conducted at the Hawthorne plant of the Western Electric Company back in the 1920s in which workers' productivity improved no matter what the researchers did to change the work environment. This outcome was attributed to the special attention the workers received from the researchers as opposed to the variables that were introduced into the work setting.

Selected Bibliography and Suggested Readings

Afifi AK, Bergman RA: *Functional neuroanatomy*, ed 2, New York, 2005, McGraw-Hill.

American Association of Cardiovascular and Pulmonary Rehabilitation: *Guidelines for pulmonary rehabilitation programs*, ed 4, Champaign, 2010, Human Kinetics.

American College of Sports Medicine: *ACSM's resources for clinical exercise physiology: musculoskeletal, neuromuscular, neoplastic, immunologic and hematologic conditions*, ed 2, Philadelphia, 2009, Lippincott Williams & Wilkins.

American College of Sports Medicine (editor), Durstine JL, G, Painter P, Roberts S: *ACSMs exercise management for persons with chronic diseases and disabilities*, ed 3, Champaign, 2009, Human Kinetics.

American College of Sports Medicine (editor): *ACSM's health-related physical fitness assessment manual*, ed 3, Philadelphia, 2010, Lippincott Williams & Wilkins.

American College of Sports Medicine: *ACSM's resource manual for guidelines for exercise testing and prescription*, ed 7, Philadelphia, 2013, Lippincott Williams & Wilkins.

American Physical Therapy Association: *Guide to physical therapist practice*, ed 2, (Revised), Alexandria, 2003, American Physical Therapy Association.

Andreoli TE, Griggs RC, Benjamin I, Wing EJ: *Andreoli and Carpenters Cecil essentials of medicine*, ed 8, Philadelphia, 2011, Saunders.

Andrews JR, Harrelson GL, Wilk KE: *Physical rehabilitation of the injured athlete*, ed 4, Philadelphia, 2012, Saunders.

Baldry P: *Acupuncture, trigger points and musculoskeletal pain*, ed 3, St. Louis, 2005, Churchill Livingstone.

Bandy WD, Sanders B: *Therapeutic exercise for physical therapy assistants: techniques for intervention*, ed 3, Philadelphia, 2011, Lippincott Williams & Wilkins.

Baranoski S, Ayello EA: *Wound care essentials: practice principles*, ed 3, Philadelphia, 2011, Lippincott Williams & Wilkins.

Barrett KE, Barman SM, Boitano S, Heddwen B: *Ganongs review of medical physiology*, ed 24, New York, 2012, McGraw-Hill Medical.

Baxter RE: *Pocket guide to musculoskeletal assessment*, ed 2, St. Louis, 2003, Saunders.

Bear MF, Connors BW, Paradiso MA: *Neuroscience: exploring the brain*, ed 3, Philadelphia, 2006, Lippincott Williams & Wilkins.

Belanger AY: *Therapeutic electrophysical agents: evidence behind practice*, ed 2, Philadelphia, 2009, Lippincott Williams & Wilkins.

Beam W, Adams G: *Exercise physiology laboratory manual*, ed 7, New York, 2013, McGraw-Hill.

Benjamin PJ: *Tappans handbook of healing massage techniques*, ed 5, Stamford, 2010, Prentice Hall/Pearson.

Berg KE, Latin RW: *Essentials of research methods in health, physical education, exercise science, and recreation*, ed 3, Philadelphia, 2007, Lippincott Williams & Wilkins.

Berk LE: *Development through the lifespan*, ed 5, Boston, 2009, Pearson.

Berman J: *Color atlas of basic histology*, ed 3, New York, 2003, McGraw-Hill.

Bickley LS: *Bates' guide to physical examination and history taking*, ed 11, Philadelphia, 2012, Lippincott Williams & Wilkins.

Bogduk N: *Clinical and radiological anatomy of the lumbar spine*, ed 5, St. Louis, 2012, Churchill Livingstone.

Boissonnault WG: *Primary care for the physical therapist: examination and triage*, ed 2, St. Louis, 2011, Saunders.

Brotzman SB, Manske RC: *Clinical orthopaedic rehabilitation: an evidence-based approach*, ed 3, St. Louis, 2011, Mosby.

Brukner P, Khan K: *Brukner and Khans clinical sports medicine*, ed 4, New York, 2011, McGraw-Hill.

Bryant DP, Bryant BR: *Assistive technology for people with disabilities*, ed 2, Boston, 2012, Pearson.

Bryant R, Nix D: *Acute and chronic wounds: current management concepts*, ed 4, St. Louis, 2012, Mosby.

Cameron MH: *Physical agents in rehabilitation: from research to practice*, ed 4, St. Louis, 2013, Saunders.

Cameron MH, Monroe L: *Physical rehabilitation for the physical therapist assistant*, St. Louis, 2011, Saunders.

Campbell SK, Palisano RJ, Orlin MN: *Physical therapy for children*, ed 4, St. Louis, 2012, Saunders.

Cantu RI, Grodin AJ: *Myofascial manipulation: theory and clinical application*, ed 3, Austin, 2011, Pro-ED.

Carr JH, Shepherd CJ: *Movement science: foundations for physical therapy in rehabilitation*, ed 2, Dallas, 2000, Pro-Ed.

Carr JH, Shepherd RB: *Stroke rehabilitation: guidelines for exercise and training to optimize motor skill*, Philadelphia, 2003, Butterworth-Heinemann.

Carr JH, Shepherd RB: *Neurological rehabilitation: optimizing motor performance*, ed 2, Philadelphia, 2010, Churchill Livingstone.

Case-Smith J: *Occupational therapy for children*, ed 6, St. Louis, 2010, Mosby.

Cech DJ, Martin S: *Functional movement development across the life span*, ed 3, St. Louis, 2012, Saunders.

Ciccone CD: *Pharmacology in rehabilitation*, ed 4, Philadelphia, 2007, FA Davis.

Cleland J, Koppenhauers S: *Netters Orthopaedic clinical examination: an evidence-based approach*, ed 2, Philadelphia, 2011, Saunders.

Cole MB: *Group dynamics in occupational therapy*, ed 4, Thorofare, 2011, Slack.

Cook AM, Polgar JM: *Cook and Husseys assistive technologies: principles and practice*, ed 3, St. Louis, 2008, Mosby.

Cottrell RR, Girvan JT, McKenzie JF: *Principles and foundations of health promotion and education*, ed 5, San Francisco, 2011, Benjamin Cummings.

Crossman AR, Neary D: *Neuroanatomy: an illustrated colour text*, Philadelphia, 2010, Churchill Livingstone.

Cuppett M, Walsh K: *General medical conditions in the athlete*, ed 2, St. Louis, 2012, Mosby.

Dandy DJ, Edwards DJ: *Essential orthopaedics and trauma*, ed 5, Philadelphia, 2009, Churchill Livingstone.

DeDomenico G: *Beard's massage: principles and practice of soft tissue manipulation*, ed 5, St. Louis, 2008, Saunders.

DePoy E, Gitlin LN: *Introduction to research: understanding and applying multiple strategies*, ed 4, St. Louis, 2011, Mosby.

Domholdt E: *Rehabilitation research: principles and applications*, ed 4, St. Louis, 2011, Saunders.

Donatelli RA: *Physical therapy of the shoulder*, ed 5, St. Louis, 2012, Churchill Livingstone.

Donatelli RA, Wooden MJ: *Orthopaedic physical therapy*, ed 4, St. Louis, 2011, Churchill Livingstone.

Dorland (editor): *Dorland's illustrated medical dictionary*, ed 32, Philadelphia, 2011, Saunders.

Drake RL, Vogl W, Mitchell AWM: *Gray's anatomy for students*, ed 2, New York, 2010, Churchill Livingstone.

Drench ME, Noonan A, Sharby N, Ventura S: *Psychosocial aspects of healthcare*, ed 3, Stamford, 2011, Prentice Hall.

Dutton M: *Duttons orthopaedic examination, evaluation, and intervention*, ed 3, New York, 2012, McGraw-Hill.

Echternach J: *Introduction to electromyography and nerve conduction testing*, ed 2, Thorofare, 2002, Slack.

Edelman CL, Mandle CL, Kudzma EC: *Health promotion throughout the lifespan*, ed 8, St. Louis, 2009, Mosby.

Edmond SL: *Joint mobilization manipulation: extremity and spinal techniques*, ed 2, St. Louis, 2006, Mosby.

Edmunds MW, Mayhew MS: *Pharmacology for the primary care provider*, ed 4, St. Louis, 2014, Mosby.

Effgen SK: *Meeting the physical therapy needs of children*, ed 2, Philadelphia, 2013, FA Davis.

Esterson SH: *Starting and managing your own physical therapy practice*, Jones and Bartlett Learning, 2004.

Felton DL: *Netter's neuroscience flash cards*, ed 2, Philadelphia, 2010, Saunders.

Field D, Owen-Hutchinson J: *Fields anatomy, palpation and surface markings*, ed 5, Philadelphia, 2012, Churchill Livingstone.

Fritz S: *Mosby's fundamentals of therapeutic massage*, ed 5, St. Louis, 2013, Mosby.

Frontera WR, Slovik DM: *Exercise in rehabilitation medicine*, ed 2, Champaign, 2006, Human Kinetics.

Frownfelter D, Dean E: *Cardiovascular and pulmonary physical therapy: evidence to practice*, ed 5, St. Louis, 2013, Mosby.

Gateley C, Borcherding S: *Documentation manual for occupational therapy: writing SOAP notes*, ed 3, Thorofare, 2011, Slack.

Gelb D: *Introduction to clinical neurology*, ed 3, Philadelphia, 2005, Butterworth Heinemann.

Gillen: *Stroke rehabilitation: a function-based approach*, ed 3, St. Louis, 2011, Mosby.

Gladson B: *Pharmacology for rehabilitation professionals*, ed 2, St. Louis, 2011, Saunders.

Goodman CC, Fuller KS: *Pathology for the physical therapist assistant*, St. Louis, 2011, Saunders.

Goodman CC, Snyder TEK: *Differential diagnosis for physical therapists: screening for referral*, ed 5, St. Louis, 2013, Saunders.

Greene D, Roberts SL: *Kinesiology: movement in the context of activity*, ed 2, St. Louis, 2005, Mosby.

Greenspan A, Chapman MW: *Orthopedic imaging: a practical approach*, ed 5, Philadelphia, 2010, Lippincott Williams & Wilkins.

Guccione AA, Wong R, Avers D: *Geriatric physical therapy*, ed 3, St. Louis, 2012, Mosby.

Gulick D: *Ortho notes clinical examination pocket guide*, ed 3, Philadelphia, 2013, FA Davis.

Gutman SA: *Quick reference neuroscience for rehabilitation professionals*, ed 2, Thorofare, 2007, Slack.

Haines DE: *Neuroanatomy: an atlas of structures, sections, and systems*, ed 8, Philadelphia, 2011, Lippincott Williams & Wilkins.

Haines DE: *Fundamental neuroscience for basic and clinical applications*, ed 4, Philadelphia, 2013, Saunders.

Hall JE: *Guyton and Hall textbook of medical physiology*, ed 12, Philadelphia, 2011, Saunders.

Hall JE: *Pocket companion to Guyton and Hall textbook of medical physiology*, ed 12, Philadelphia, 2012, Saunders.

Hall SJ: *Basic biomechanics*, ed 5, Boston, 2006, McGraw-Hill.

Hamill J, Knutzen KM: *Biomechanical basis of human movement*, ed 3, Philadelphia, 2008, Lippincott Williams & Wilkins.

Hansen JT: *Essential anatomy dissector: following Grant's method*, ed 2, Philadelphia, 2002, Lippincott Williams & Wilkins.

Hay WW, Levin MJ, Deterding RR, Abzug M: *Current diagnosis and treatment pediatrics*, ed 21, New York, 2012, McGraw-Hill Medical.

Henderson G, Bryan WV: *Psychosocial aspects of disability*, ed 4, Springfield, 2011, Charles C. Thomas Publisher.

Hertling D: *Management of common musculoskeletal disorders: physical therapy principles and methods*, ed 4, Philadelphia, 2005, Lippincott Williams & Wilkins.

Heuer A: *Wilkins clinical assessment in respiratory care*, ed 7, St. Louis, 2014, Mosby.

Hicks CM, Hicks C: *Research methods for clinical therapists: applied project design and analysis*, ed 5, New York, 2010, Churchill Livingstone.

Hillegrass EA: *Essentials of cardiopulmonary physical therapy*, ed 3, St. Louis, 2011, Saunders.

Hillman SK: *Interactive functional anatomy*, ed 2, Champaign, 2006, Primal Pictures.

Hislop HJ, Montgomery J: *Daniels and Worthingham's muscle testing: techniques of manual examination*, ed 9, St. Louis, 2013, Saunders.

Houglum PA, Bertoti DB: *Brunnstroms clinical kinesiology*, ed 6, Philadelphia, 2012, FA Davis.

Huber FE, Wells CL: *Therapeutic exercise: treatment planning for progression*, Philadelphia, 2006, Saunders.

Irion G: *Comprehensive wound management*, ed 2, Thorofare, 2009, Slack.

Jacobs MA, Austin NM: *Splinting the hand and upper extremity: principles and process*, Philadelphia, 2002, Lippincott Williams & Wilkins.

Jenkins DB, Hollinshead WH: *Hollinshead's functional anatomy of the limbs and back*, ed 9, St. Louis, 2009, Saunders.

Jensen GM, Mostrom E: *Handbook of teaching and learning for physical therapists*, ed 3, St. Louis, 2013, Saunders.

Jones MA, Rivett DA: *Clinical reasoning for manual therapists*, Philadelphia, 2004, Butterworth-Heinemann.

Kandel ER, Schwartz JH, Jessell TM, Siegelbaum S, Hudspeth AJ: *Principles of neural science*, ed 5, New York, 2002, McGraw-Hill Medical.

Katzung BG, Masters S, Trevor A: *Basic and clinical pharmacology*, ed 12, Boston, 2012, McGraw-Hill Medical.

Kauffman TL, Barr JO, Moran ML: *Geriatric rehabilitation manual*, ed 2, St. Louis, 2007, Churchill Livingstone.

Kendall FP, McCreary EK, Provance PG, Rodgers M, Romani W: *Muscles: testing and function, with posture and pain*, ed 5, Philadelphia, 2005, Lippincott Williams & Wilkins.

Kisner C, Colby LA: *Therapeutic exercise: foundations and techniques*, ed 6, Philadelphia, 2013, FA Davis.

Konin JG, Wiksten D, Isear J, Brader H: *Special tests for orthopedic examination*, ed 3, Thorofare, 2006, Slack.

Kumar V, Abbas AK, Fausto N, Aster J: *Robbins and Cotran pathologic basis of disease*, ed 8, Philadelphia, 2010, Saunders.

Leonard PC: *Building a medical vocabulary: with Spanish translations*, ed 8, St. Louis, 2012, Saunders.

Levangie PK, Norkin CC: *Joint structure and function: a comprehensive analysis*, ed 5, Philadelphia, 2011, FA Davis.

Levine D, Richards J, Whittle MW: *Whittles gait analysis*, ed 5, Philadelphia, 2012, Churchill Livingstone.

Lewis CB: *Aging: the health care challenge*, ed 4, Philadelphia, 2002, FA Davis.

Lewis CB, Bottomley JM: *Geriatric rehabilitation: a clinical approach*, ed 3, Stamford, 2008, Prentice Hall/Pearson.

Lippert LS: *Clinical kinesiology and anatomy*, ed 5, Philadelphia, 2011, FA Davis.

Long T, Toscano K: *Handbook of pediatric physical therapy*, ed 2, Philadelphia, 2001, Lippincott Williams & Wilkins.

Los Amigos Research and Education Center: *Observational gait analysis*, Downey, 2001, Los Amigos Research and Education.

Lowe WW: *Orthopedic massage*, ed 2, St. Louis, 2009, Churchill Livingstone.

Lundy-Ekman L: *Neuroscience: fundamentals for rehabilitation*, ed 4, St. Louis, 2013, Saunders.

Magee DJ: *Orthopedic physical assessment*, ed 5, Philadelphia, 2008, Saunders.

Magee DJ, Zachazewski JE, Quillen WS: *Scientific foundations and principles of practice of musculoskeletal rehabilitation*, St. Louis, 2007, Saunders.

Magill RA: *Motor learning and control: concepts and applications*, ed 9, New York, 2010, McGraw-Hill.

Maitland GD, Hengeveld E, Banks K, English K: *Maitland's vertebral manipulation*, ed 7, Philadelphia, 2006, Butterworth-Heinemann.

Mansfield PJ, Neumann DA: *Essentials of kinesiology for the physical therapist assistant*, ed 2, St. Louis, 2014, Mosby.

Martin S, Kessler M: *Neurologic intervention for physical therapy*, ed 2, Philadelphia, 2007, Saunders.

Maxey L, Magnusson J: *Rehabilitation for the postsurgical orthopedic patient*, ed 3, St. Louis, 2013, Mosby.

McArdle WD, Katch FI, Katch VL: *Essentials of exercise physiology*, ed 4, Philadelphia, 2010, Lippincott Williams & Wilkins.

McCance KL, Huether SE: *Pathophysiology: the biologic basis for diseases in adults and children*, ed 6, St. Louis, 2010, Mosby.

McGill S: *Low back disorders*, ed 2, Champaign, 2007, Human Kinetics.

McKinnis LN: *Fundamentals of musculoskeletal imaging*, ed 4, Philadelphia, 2013, FA Davis.

McPhee SJ, Papadakis MA, Rabow MW: *Current medical diagnosis and treatment 2013*, ed 52, New York, 2012, McGraw-Hill Medical.

Mettler FA: *Essentials of radiology*, ed 3, Philadelphia, 2014, Saunders.

Moore KL, Dalley AF, Agur AMR, Dalley AF: *Clinically oriented anatomy*, ed 7, Philadelphia, 2013, Lippincott Williams & Wilkins.

Moore KL, Persaud TVN, Torchia MG: *Before we are born: essentials of embryology and birth defects*, ed 8, Philadelphia, 2013, Saunders.

Mosby (editor): *Mosby's dictionary of medical, nursing and health professions*, ed 9, St. Louis, 2013, Mosby.

Myers BA: *Wound management: principles and practice*, ed 3, Stamford, 2012, Prentice Hall/ Pearson.

Netter FH: *Atlas of human anatomy*, ed 5, Philadelphia, 2010, Saunders.

Neumann DA: *Kinesiology of the musculoskeletal system: foundations for rehabilitation*, St. Louis, 2010, Mosby.

Nieman DS: *Exercise testing and prescription*, ed 7, New York, 2010, McGraw-Hill.

Nolte: *The human brain: an introduction to its functional anatomy*, ed 6, St. Louis, 2009, Mosby.

Nordin M, Frankel VH: *Basic biomechanics of the musculoskeletal system*, ed 4, Philadelphia, 2012, Lippincott Williams & Wilkins.

Norkin CC, White DJ: *Measurement of joint motion: a guide to goniometry*, ed 4, Philadelphia, 2009, FA Davis.

Nosse LJ: *Managerial and supervisory principles for physical therapists*, ed 3, Philadelphia, 2009, Lippincott Williams & Wilkins.

Nowak TJ, Handford AG: *Pathophysiology: concepts and applications for health care professionals*, ed 3, New York, 2004, McGraw-Hill.

Oatis CA: *Kinesiology: the mechanics and pathomechanics of human movement*, ed 2, Philadelphia, 2008, Lippincott Williams & Wilkins.

Oschman JL: *Energy medicine in therapeutics and human performance*, Philadelphia, 2003, Butterworth-Heinemann.

OShea RK: *Pediatrics for the Physical therapist assistant*, St. Louis, 2009, Saunders.

O'Sullivan SB, Schmitz TJ, Fulk G: *Physical rehabilitation*, ed 6, Philadelphia, 2013, FA Davis.

Pagana KD, Pagana TJ: *Mosby's diagnostic and laboratory test reference*, ed 11, St. Louis, 2013, Mosby.

Pagliarulo MA: *Introduction to physical therapy*, ed 4, St. Louis, 2012, Mosby.

Palastanga N, Soames R, Field D: *Anatomy and human movement: structure and function*, ed 6, Philadelphia, 2012, Churchill Livingstone.

Palisano RJ: *Movement sciences: transfer of knowledge into pediatric therapy practice*, London, 2004, Routledge.

Payne VG, Isaacs LD: *Human motor development: a lifespan approach*, ed 8, New York, 2011, McGraw-Hill.

Paz JC, West MP: *Acute care handbook for physical therapists*, ed 4, St. Louis, 2014, Saunders.

Peckenpaugh NJ, Poleman CM: *Nutrition essentials and diet therapy*, ed 11, St. Louis, 2010, Saunders.

Pierson FM, Fairchild SL: *Pierson and Fairchilds principles and techniques of patient care*, ed 5, St. Louis, 2013, Saunders.

Portney LG, Watkins MP: *Foundations of clinical research: applications to practice*, ed 3, Stamford, 2008, Prentice Hall/Pearson.

Powers SK, Howley ET: *Exercise physiology: theory and application to fitness and performance*, ed 8, New York, 2011, McGraw-Hill.

Purnell LD, Lattanzi JB: *Developing cultural competence in physical therapy practice*, Philadelphia, 2006, FA Davis.

Purtilo RB, Doherty R: *Ethical dimensions in the health professions*, ed 5, St. Louis, 2011, Saunders.

Purtilo RB, Haddad AM, Doherty R: *Health professional and patient interaction*, ed 8, Philadelphia, 2014, Saunders.

Quinn L, Gordon J: *Documentation for rehabilitation: a guide to clinical decision making*, ed 2, St. Louis, 2010, Saunders.

Reese NB: *Muscle and sensory testing*, ed 3, St. Louis, 2012, Saunders.

Reese NB, Bandy WD: *Joint range of motion and muscle length testing*, ed 2, Philadelphia, 2010, Saunders.

Reynolds F: *Communication and clinical effectiveness in rehabilitation*, Philadelphia, 2005, Butterworth-Heinemann.

Richmond T, Powers D: *Business fundamentals for the rehabilitation professional*, ed 2, Thorofare, 2009, Slack.

Royeen M, Crabtree JL: *Culture in rehabilitation: from competency to proficiency*, Stamford, 2006, Prentice Hall/Pearson.

Sahrmann S: *Diagnosis and treatment of movement impairment syndromes*, St. Louis, 2002, Mosby.

Schmidt RA, Lee TD: *Motor control and learning: a behavioral emphasis*, ed 5, Champaign, 2011, Human Kinetics.

Scott RW: *Promoting legal and ethical awareness: a primer for health professionals and patients*, St. Louis, 2009, Mosby.

Scott RW: *Legal, ethical, and practical aspects of patient care documentation: a guide for rehabilitation professionals*, ed 4, Sudbury, 2013, Jones & Bartlett.

Scott RW, Petrosino CL: *Physical therapy management*, St. Louis, 2008, Mosby.

Shamus E, Stern DF: *Effective documentation for physical therapy professionals*, ed 2, New York, 2011, McGraw-Hill.

Shankman GA, Manske RC: *Fundamental orthopedic management for the physical therapist assistant*, ed 3, St. Louis, 2011, Mosby.

Shiland BJ: *Mastering healthcare terminology*, ed 4, St. Louis, 2013, Mosby.

Shumway-Cook A, Woollacott MH: *Motor control: translating research into clinical practice*, ed 4, Philadelphia, 2011, Lippincott Williams & Wilkins.

Sine R, Liss SE, Roush RE: *Basic rehabilitation techniques: a self-instructional guide*, ed 4, Gaithersburg, 2000, Aspen Publishers.

Sisto SA, Durin E, Sliwinski MM: *Spinal cord injuries: management and rehabilitation*, St. Louis, 2009, Mosby.

Skinner HB: *Current diagnosis and treatment in orthopedics*, ed 5, New York, 2013, McGraw-Hill.

Skinner JS: *Exercise testing and exercise prescription for special cases: theoretical basis and clinical application*, ed 3, Philadelphia, 2005, Lippincott Williams & Wilkins.

Snell RS: *Essential clinical anatomy*, ed 4, Philadelphia, 2010, Lippincott Williams & Wilkins.

Somers MF: *Spinal cord injury: functional rehabilitation*, ed 3, Stamford, 2009, Prentice Hall/Pearson.

Springhouse (editor): *Clinical pharmacology made incredibly easy*, ed 3, Philadelphia, 2008, Lippincott Williams & Wilkins.

Staheli LT: *Fundamentals of pediatric orthopedics*, ed 4, Philadelphia, 2007, Lippincott Williams & Wilkins.

Standring S: *Gray's anatomy: the anatomical basis of clinical practice*, ed 40, New York, 2009, Churchill Livingstone.

Stone RJ, Stone JA: *Atlas of skeletal muscles*, ed 6, Boston, 2008, McGraw-Hill.

Straus SE, Glasziou P, Richardson WS, Haynes RB: *Evidence-based medicine*, ed 4, New York, 2011, Churchill Livingstone.

Swisher LL, Page CG: *Professionalism in physical therapy: history, practice, and development*, Philadelphia, 2005, Saunders.

Tortora GJ, Derrickson BH: *Principles of anatomy and physiology*, ed 13, New York, 2012, Wiley.

Trevor AJ, Katzung BG, Masters SB, Knuidering-Hall M: *Katzung and Trevor's pharmacology examination and board review*, ed 10, New York, 2012, McGraw-Hill.

Umphred DA, Lazaro RT, Roller M, Burton G: *Neurological rehabilitation*, ed 6, St. Louis, 2013, Mosby.

Voight ML, Hoogenboom B, Prentice WE: *Musculoskeletal intervention: techniques for therapeutic exercise*, Philadelphia, 2006, McGraw-Hill.

Watchie J: *Cardiovascular and pulmonary physical therapy: a clinical manual*, ed 2, St. Louis, 2010, Saunders.

Watson T: *Electrotherapy: evidence-based practice*, ed 12, New York, 2008, Churchill Livingstone.

Weir J, Abrahams PH: *Imaging atlas of human anatomy*, ed 4, S.t Louis, 2011, Mosby.

West JB: *Respiratory physiology: the essentials*, ed 9, Philadelphia, 2011, Lippincott Williams & Wilkins.

White AA: *Clinical biomechanics of the spine*, ed 3, Philadelphia, 20130, Williams & Wilkins.

Whitmore I, et al: *Human anatomy: color atlas and textbook*, ed 5, St. Louis, 2009, Mosby.

Index